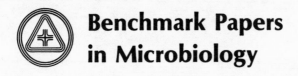

Benchmark Papers
in Microbiology

Series Editor: Wayne W. Umbreit
Rutgers—The State University

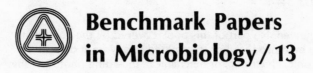

**Benchmark Papers
in Microbiology / 13**

A BENCHMARK® Books Series

MICROBIAL
RESPIRATION

Edited by
WALTER P. HEMPFLING
University of Rochester

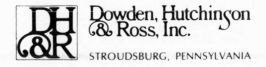

Dowden, Hutchinson & Ross, Inc.
STROUDSBURG, PENNSYLVANIA

Copyright © 1979 by **Dowden, Hutchinson & Ross, Inc.**
Benchmark Papers in Microbiology, Volume 13
Library of Congress Catalog Card Number: 78–22097
ISBN: 0–87933–344–8

81 80 79 1 2 3 4 5
Manufactured in the United States of America.

LIBRARY OF CONGRESS CATALOGING IN PUBLICATION DATA
Main entry under title:
Microbial respiration.
   (Benchmark papers in microbiology ; 13)
   Includes bibliographical references and indexes.
   1. Microbial respiration—Addresses, essays, lectures. I. Hempfling, Walter P.
QR89.M5   576'.11'2   78–22097
ISBN 0–87933–344–8

Distributed world wide by Academic Press,
a subsidiary of Harcourt Brace Jovanovich,
Publishers.

SERIES EDITOR'S FOREWORD

Knowledge of the respiration of procaryotes is not as extensive as the knowledge of mitochondrial respiration. As Dr. Hempfling points out, this is partly because the procaryotic cell had potentially wide respiratory capability compared to the eucaryotic mitochondria, and that the mitochondrion, since it could be isolated in a functional condition, was an experimentally simpler system. It is, therefore, important to assemble what we do know about the respiration of procaryotes lest it be assumed, as it so often is, that the mitochondrial system is *the* respiratory system of all living cells. True, there are many similarities between the procaryotes and mitochondria, but there are distinctive and important differences which should not be neglected. If, indeed, the mitochondria are the result of the establishment of an endosymbiotic relationship between a procaryote (specifically suggested to be *Micrococcus denitrificans*) and a eucaryote at a time when eucaryotes had not yet achieved a respiratory capability, it would seem surprising that the establishment of this relationship should have occurred only once. It would seem worthwhile to examine the possibility that not all mitochondria follow the same pattern, and perhaps one may trace their origin by the presence of procaryotic respiratory processes.

The general lack of really good oxidative phosphorylation among the procaryotes makes rather a shambles of energy calculations based upon the assumption of three energy rich phosphates per mole of 2H. Presumably, the endosymbiotic relationship permitted an increase in the phosphorylating ability.

Dr. Hempfling is an excellent guide to the field of microbial respiration and his selection of papers gives one a sampling of the major contributions to the field. It is a pleasure to have these scattered contributions available in one handy volume. And I feel certain that this volume will prove to be useful as well as a starting point for a new look at microbial respiration.

WAYNE W. UMBREIT

v

PREFACE

What are the mechanics of the electron transport-dependent esterification of inorganic phosphate? This is the greatest question facing fundamental biochemistry today. The unique properties of the procaryotes have been insufficiently employed in answering this question. These convictions prompted me to accept the invitation of Professor Wayne W. Umbreit to compile a Benchmark volume on *Microbial Respiration*, selecting the contributions that, in my view, formed the corpus of accomplishment in this vital area of bioenergetics. With this volume, I hoped to facilitate the future use of non-mitochondrial respiratory systems by the judicious selection of outstanding experimentation and exemplary exposition.

In assembling the articles for this volume I have naturally favored my own tastes in content and style of investigation and in manner of presentation, limited only by the reasonable constraints of space. Those inclinations were acquired largely during the years, too few in number, of my association with the general microbiologist Wolf V. Vishniac.

I acknowledge with pleasure the organizational talent of Rita Nielsen Rasmussen, without whose participation this volume would not have been completed. Sue Hall Hoke Hempfling, my wife, typed the final manuscript and provided liberal allotments of her immense reserves of patience. George Hoch and Craig Rice offered much-needed criticism and encouragement.

WALTER P. HEMPFLING

CONTENTS

Contents

Contents

PART IV: ADAPTIVE RESPONSES

CONTENTS BY AUTHOR

INTRODUCTION

Life demands energy, and exists on this planet because of the ability of living organisms to couple the energy-requiring reactions of biosynthesis and maintenance to energy-liberating chemical transformations. The linkage between endergonic and exergonic reactions is achieved principally by the use of phosphate anhydride bonds. Reaction pathways that yield biologically conservable energy usually involve electron transfer. We define fermentation as an energy-yielding sequence of reactions in which the final electron acceptor arises from the initial substrate, and respiration as a series of reactions in which the final electron acceptor is exogenously supplied and is not itself an intermediate product of metabolism. The processes of respiration in procaryotes and the phenomena associated with trapping and converting energy liberated thereby to biologically useful forms concern us here.

Hypotheses have been offered which rationalize the mitochondrial localization of the eucaryotic respiratory apparatus as a result of establishment of an endosymbiotic relationship between a respiring procaryote and a nascent eucaryote.[1] Similarities between the respiratory systems of procaryotes and eucaryotes are extensive, and have prompted such notions, but important overt differences between the two kinds of respiration exist. While eucaryotes are restricted to oxygen-dependent respiration, many bacteria may employ oxygen or nitrate ion; for still other procaryotes, sulfate ion or carbon dioxide may serve as terminal oxidant. The nonphotosynthetic eucaryotes are limited to the use of organic reductants to supply respiration, but the chemoautotrophic bacteria make use of inorganic electron donors. The capability of adaptive response of procaryotes to changing edaphic conditions exceeds that of eucaryotes respiring with mitochondrial systems, in part due to the many choices of respiratory reductant and oxidant. *Escherichia coli*, for example, reacts to changes of dissolved oxygen concentration by adjusting the concentrations of multiple terminal oxidases (Paper 29), reacts to the absence of oxygen by carrying out fermentation of suitable substrates or by respiring with nitrate[2] and responds to changes of the identity of the growth substrate by modifying the net amount of conserved energy available for biomass formation (Paper 31).

Although these manifold capabilities would seen to make the procaryotes ideal experimental subjects for the study of respiration and associated mechanisms of energy conservation, investigations of isolated mitochondria have furnished most of the information extant about such processes, and work with microbial respiration has been largely imitative. A comparison of the contributions of studies of procaryotic systems to bioenergetics and to the elucidation of the mechanism of heredity provides a sharp contrast. The simplicity of growth requirements, short generation times, and convenience of manipulation of bacteria made their patterns of inheritance indispensable as models of the heredity of evolutionarily higher creatures. A surrogate mitochondrion was unnecessary, however, since the organelle could be isolated in a functional state and in good yield from multicellular organisms at about the same time that suitable techniques were developed to exploit its availability. Above all, the ability of nucleotide-permeable mitochondrial preparations to carry out oxidative phosphorylation was markedly superior to that of extracts of bacteria. It has only recently become feasible to study oxidative phosphorylation in intact bacteria, the proper analogs of intact mitochondria.

To some extent the inability to measure phosphorylation efficiency during coupled procaryotic respiration has been circumvented by studies of respiration-driven membrane transport processes. It thereby has become practicable to examine the mechanisms by which respiration is linked to energy-requiring phenomena other than oxidative phosphorylation. Models have been provided in which the maintenance of transmembrane solute disequilibria and oxidative phosphorylation share a common intermediate derived from respiration. A portion of this work has already been summarized in the Benchmark Series,[3] and the coupling to respiration of membrane transport processes will not be treated further here.

We will consider the present state of understanding of microbial respiration as the outcome of results obtained during three periods of investigation, each of which may be identified by their guiding hypotheses and by the techniques devised to test them. The first is the era of establishment of the role of intermediate electron-transferring compounds in respiratory processes, specifically the demonstration of the participation and characterization of the pyridine nucleotides,[4] flavoproteins,[5] and "oxygen-transferring iron" by Otto Warburg (Papers 1 and 2) and the rediscovery of "cytochrome" by D. Keilin.[6] Keilin has also prepared an account of this period entitled *The History of Cell Respiration and Cytochrome*,[7] which includes a thoughtful and sympathetic appreciation of the contributions of C. A. MacMunn.[8] Paper 3 is a contribution by A. Bertho and H. Glück, associates of Heinrich Wieland, one of Warburg's scientific adversaries.

During the third and fourth decades of this century the overt events of microbial respiration were described. Compounds serving as reductants and oxidants were identified, as described in the inimitable text, *Bacterial Metabolism*,[9] by Marjory Stephenson, who, along with Keilin, J. H. Quastel, and their associates at Cambridge, obtained much of the information presented. Even though M. W. Beijerinck had pointed out as early as 1903 the importance of understanding biological energy conservation as a means of rationalizing microbial growth,[10] it was not until the demonstration of oxidative phosphorylation (that is, esterification of inorganic phosphate obligatorily linked to respiration by V. A. Belitser and E. T. Tsybakova[11] in 1939 that experimental approaches to the mechanisms of respiratory energy conservation became possible. This and related contributions have been collected by H. Kalckar as *Biological Phosphorylations. Development of Concepts.*[12]

A major issue examined in the succeeding years was that of the mechanism of oxidative phosphorylation; and we identify the second era as that dominated by a view of oxidative phosphorylation modelled after substrate-level phosphorylation, or the "chemical intermediate" hypothesis as articulated by E. C. Slater (Paper 16).

As embodied in Lemberg's and Legge's *Haematin Compounds and Bile Pigments*,[13] development of techniques in porphyrin chemistry had progressed far enough to facilitate the chemical characterization of the cytochromes of bacteria. Excellent examples of such work are found in Papers 4 and 10. Yet such procedures did not allow the investigator to probe the dynamic interactions *in situ* of the components of the respiratory sequence. Keilin, Warburg, and others had approached this task, but it was Britton Chance who developed an array of powerful techniques allowing the rapid sensing of the state of reduction of electron transport components in highly optically scattering suspensions of mitochondria and bacteria (Papers 7 and 9). These and related tools, as well as the procedures of microbial genetics as successfully applied by Butlin, Cox, Gibson, and their associates (Paper 27), are employed in the third and current period of investigation in which the "chemiosmotic" model of P. Mitchell dominates as the regnant hypothesis to explain the coupling of respiration to energy-requiring functions (Papers 20, 21, and 22).

Although the chemiosmotic hypothesis could reasonably account for the coupling of respiration to active transport processes by means of electrical and proton transmembrane gradients, the intimate chemical details of the phosphorylation of adenosine diphosphate catalyzed by the membrane adenosine triphosphatase were not equally well provided. Papers 23 through 26 represent the most recent trend toward amplification of the role of the membrane ATPase in the mechanistic account of oxidative phosphorylation. This approach has produced a significant modification of the chemiosmotic mechanism in the view of some investigators, and the vitality and excitement attending the resultant controversy is depicted nicely in Paper 23, a communication in the series of exchanges between P. D. Boyer and P. Mitchell, in which the major features of Boyer's "conformational" hypothesis are outlined.

The final group of selections (Papers 29–31) illustrates the plasticity of respiratory mechanisms and their associated energy-conserving systems in bacteria. Greater usage should be made of the unique properties of procaryotic bioenergetic phenomena in working toward solutions of the problems of respiratory energy conservation.

REFERENCES

1. Broda, E. *The Evolution of the Bioenergetic Processes.* Pergamon Press, New York, pp. 123–125, 1975.
2. Taniguchi, S. *Z. Allg. Mikrobiol.,* **1**, 341–375, 1961.
3. Reeves, J. P., ed. *Microbial Permeability* (Benchmark Papers in Microbiology). Dowden, Hutchinson & Ross, Inc. Stroudsburg, Pa., 1973.
4. Warburg, O., W. Christian, and A. Griese. *Biochem. Z.,* **282**, 157–164, 1935 (Paper 16 in reference 14).
5. Warburg, O., and W. Christian. *Biochem. Z.,* **254**, 444–454, 1932 (Paper 15 in reference 14).
6. Keilin, D. *Proc. Roy. Soc. London,* ser. B, **98**, 312–339, 1925 (pp. 178–191 in reference 12).
7. Keilin, D. *The History of Cell Respiration and Cytochrome* (J. Keilin, ed.), Cambridge Univ. Press, Cambridge, 1966.
8. MacMunn, C. A. *Phil. Trans. Roy. Soc. London,* **177**, 267–298, 1886.
9. Stephenson, M. *Bacterial Metabolism,* 3rd ed. Longmans, Green and Co., Ltd., London, 1949.
10. Beijerinck, M. W., *Handelingen van het G. Nederlandsch. Natuuren Geneeskundig. Congres,* 195, 1903. See also *Maly Jahresbericht* **33**, 1014, 1904.

11. Belitser, V. A., and E. T. Tsybakova. *Biokhymiya,* **4**, 516–534, 1939 (pp. 211–227 in reference 12).
12. Kalckar, H. M. *Biological Phosphorylations. Development of Concepts.* Prentice-Hall, Englewood Cliffs, N. J., 1969.
13. Lemberg, R., and J. W. Legge. *Haematin Compounds and Bile Pigments.* Interscience, New York, 1949. (See also Lemberg, R., and J. Barrett. *Cytochromes.* Academic Press, New York, 1973.)
14. Doelle, H. W., ed. *Microbial Metabolism* (Benchmark Papers in Microbiology). Dowden, Hutchinson & Ross, Inc. Stroudsburg, Pa. 1974.

Part I

HISTORICAL BACKGROUND

Editor's Comments
on Papers 1, 2, and 3

1   WARBURG
Iron, the Oxygen Transporting Constituent of the Respiration Enzyme

2   WARBURG
Cytochrome

3   BERTHO and GLÜCK
The Formation of Hydrogen Peroxide by Lactic Acid Bacteria

Otto Warburg dominated the field of respiration during most of the period prior to the discovery of oxidative phosphorylation. Even before David Keilin's epochal rediscovery of MacMunn's "histohaematins" and "myohaematins," Warburg had established the function of pyridine nucleotides and flavoprotein enzymes in oxidative metabolism, posited and obtained evidence for the participation of iron-containing compounds in respiration, and contended for a decade with Heinrich Wieland concerning the chemical nature of oxygen reduction in respiration.

Warburg's views of the development of the concepts of the functions of "oxygen-transporting" iron and of cytochrome at the end of World War II are presented in Papers 1 and 2. They are two chapters from his book *Schwermetalle als Wirkungsgruppe von Fermenten*. The Kaiser-Wilhelm-Institut für Zellphysiologie in Berlin-Dahlem, wherein much of Warburg's work was carried out, was destroyed by an Allied bombing attack in 1943.

The dispute with Wieland need never have arisen. As now accepted, either hydrogen peroxide (as predicted by Wieland) or water may arise as the terminal product of oxygen reduction depending upon the nature of the respiratory system employed. In the words of Warburg:

> Oxygen transporting iron and oxidation by dehydrogenation are not incompatible. On the contrary, "oxidation by dehydrogenation" can almost be regarded as a consequence of oxygen transporting iron, for when molecular oxygen has oxidized the ferro-iron to the ferri-state, it has played its part in respiration. All further oxidations must proceed anaerobically and

these oxidations can only be brought about through loss of electrons or loss of hydrogen.[1]

Alfred Bertho and Hans Glück, Wieland's associates, nevertheless continued to support the "dehydrogenation" theory of their senior. In the course of their experiments they established the nearly stoichiometric production of hydrogen peroxide from molecular oxygen by lactic acid bacteria. The hemeless homo- and heterolactic eubacteria are now known to be capable of respiration through routes involving flavoprotein oxidases catalyzing the formation of hydrogen peroxide and oxygen-inducible flavoprotein peroxidases.[2] Although procedures used in cultivation of the bacteria employed by Bertho and Glück were not described, it is apparent that the organisms were not oxygen-adapted, or peroxide probably would not have been produced in significant amounts.[3]

REFERENCES

1. Warburg, O. *Heavy Metal Prosthetic Groups and Enzyme Action,* translated by Alexander Lawson, Oxford Univ. Press. London, 1949, p. 6.
2. Dolin, M. I. Cytochrome-independent electron transport enzymes of bacteria. In I. C. Gunsalus and R. Y. Stanier, eds. *The Bacteria, II, Metabolism.* Academic Press, New York, 1961, pp. 425–460.
3. Seeley, H. W., and P. J. VanDemark. *J. Bact.,* **61**, 27–35, 1951.

Reprinted from pp. 46–52 of *Heavy Metal Prosthetic Groups and Enzyme Action*,
A. Lawson, trans., Oxford University Press, Oxford, 1949, 230 pp.

IRON, THE OXYGEN TRANSPORTING CONSTITUENT OF THE RESPIRATION ENZYME

Otto Warburg

1. Historical

IN Liebig's *Tierchemie* published in 1843 there is a chapter entitled 'Theorie der Respiration' in which combustion in the animal body is connected with the presence of iron. Liebig's iron, however, is not the iron of the tissue cells, but the haemoglobin iron of the red blood cells. Liebig believed that the combustion took place in blood, where the haemoglobin iron oxidized the biological substrates. 'Die Blutkörperchen enthalten eine Eisenverbindung, kein anderer Bestandteil der lebendigen Körperteile enthält Eisen.' If Liebig were right, the combustion would be of no value to the tissue cells since the energy of combustion can only be changed into work at the point where it is liberated. Liebig soon realized this and omitted the theory of respiration from the next edition of his *Tierchemie*. But the confusion surrounding oxygen transport has continued, and has not even to-day disappeared from chemical literature. Leaving aside all this confusion between oxygen transport and combustion, and between haemoglobin and catalytically active cell iron, there remains one historical work of note, that of Spitzer† in 1897. In this work the opinion was expressed that oxygen transfer was associated with iron in the cells, and an attempt made to prove this experimentally. Spitzer minced up tissue, precipitated it with acetic acid, and found that the precipitate promoted oxidations when in contact with air. For example, the oxidation of salicylaldehyde to salicylic acid, and that of the Nadi mixture to indophenol blue were brought about. Spitzer also found that the precipitate contained iron, and he expressed the view that the iron content and the oxidizing action were related.

Experimentally, the work of Spitzer was unsatisfactory, since the main bulk of the precipitate was inactive cell substance,

† W. Spitzer, *Pflügers Archiv*, **67**, 615 (1897).

and any decision as to whether the iron was associated with the inactive or the catalytically active part was impossible to make. Actually this iron was really haemoglobin iron. Nevertheless, Spitzer was right, because his precipitate did contain some oxygen transporting iron protein and cytochrome, i.e. the iron system of aerobic cells.

On account of the imperfect experimental proof, Spitzer's views attracted little attention. It happened that Röhmann,† under whose direction Spitzer's work had arisen, recalled in the year 1912 all the essentials of it. The year 1912 saw the birth of the Wieland theory and Röhmann's recapitulation was really published as a result of this. From then on, however, cell respiration was regarded as a direct autoxidation of biological substrates, oxygen transport by metals being super-fluous.

A publication‡ on the part played by iron in the respiration of sea urchin's eggs which appeared in 1914 did nothing at first to alter the state of affairs at the time. Then the researches on iron catalysis at surfaces and in solutions, which have been dealt with in the previous chapter, caused some doubt as to whether science had followed the right road. This was roughly the position when, in 1924, I put forward a theory which was perhaps premature, but which future work has proved to be correct.

2. The theory§

Molecular oxygen which is used up by the respiration of aerobic cells never reacts directly with the biological substrates, but always and exclusively with divalent iron combined in a complex. Iron of a higher valency is thereby formed, and this is reduced back again to the divalent state by organic substances. Thus, in so far as the iron is concerned, the original state is regained. We therefore have a valency change in a complex iron compound by which the oxygen for the cell respiration is

† F. Röhmann and T. Shmamine, *Bioch. Zeitschr.* **42**, 235 (1912).
‡ O. Warburg, *Zeitschr. f. physiologische Chem.* **92**, 231 (1914).
§ O. Warburg, *Bioch. Zeitschr.* **152**, 479 (1924); *Chemische Berichte*, **58**, 1001 (1925).

transported, and in this sense iron is the oxygen transporting
part† of the respiration enzyme.

In order to avoid any misunderstanding as to what is meant
by the expression oxygen transport, I have graphically illus-

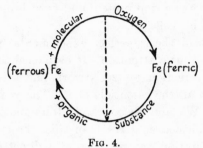

FIG. 4.

trated the theory, the valency changes of the iron being made
clear by a cycle.

The arrow in the diagram connects the molecular oxygen with
the organic substance. It is shown as a dotted line in order to
indicate that reactions in the direction of the arrow do not take
place in cell respiration.

3. Range of application of the theory

It has been said that the greater the value of a theory, the
more specialized it is, and the more general is its application.
The theory of oxygen transport by the valency change of an
iron complex compound was very specialized. Its application
was, as the future has shown, very general, since the reaction of
divalent iron is really that reaction by which molecular oxygen
most often reacts in biochemistry. An exception to this, which
the theory of 1924 admitted, was the substitution of other
heavy metals for the iron. 'Es mag Ausnahmen geben — man
denke an das Kupfer der Oktopoden oder an Henzes Ent-
deckung des Vanadiums im Blut der Aszidien — aber derartige
Fälle gehören nicht in eine allgemeine Theorie der Atmung.'

Thirteen years later we discovered that, in the respiration of

† 'Iron, the oxygen transporting part', could be more correctly written as
'iron, the autoxidizable part of the respiration enzyme'. [Compare
Chapter XVI.]

the potato and of several fungi, the oxygen is transported, not by iron, but by copper.

The yellow enzymes which could have been used to attack the theory have, as was shown soon after their discovery, detracted nothing from the truth and applicability of the iron theory. The yellow enzymes transport oxygen in cell extracts and in such anaerobic cells as have a degenerating oxygen transporting system. In the aerobic cells, however, the yellow enzymes are intermediate members of the enzyme chain at the head of which stands oxygen transporting iron.

4. The iron compound

There are three types of substances mentioned in the theory, molecular oxygen, the iron compound and the organic substance.

As regards the iron compound, it was only stated in the theory that this was a complex. There are several reasons for this assumption. The ferrous ion is not autoxidizable, and cannot therefore transport oxygen. Ferrous hydroxide is, however, autoxidizable, but it combines so firmly with cyanide that the cyanide inhibition of respiration could not be reversible if this compound were involved.

In spite of our experiments with the blood charcoal no mention was made of haematin in the theory of 1924. Meyerhof and D. C. Harrison, however, believed our experiments sufficiently conclusive for their assertion that the oxygen transporting complex was a haematin derivative.

'We may imagine the structural surfaces of the cell to be like the charcoal surface, a mosaic of fields with and without iron, iron in definite combination similar to haematin.'†

'It is probable that oxidations in the tissue may be catalysed by organic compounds allied to haematin.'‡

If this were right then all aerobic cells would contain haematins. Actually the haematin of yeast was discovered by Hans Fischer and Hilger§ in 1924.

---

† O. Meyerhof, *Chemical Dynamics of Life Phenomena*, p. 22 (Philadelphia, 1924).   ‡ D. C. Harrison, *Biochem. Journ.* **18**, 1009 (1924).
§ H. Fischer and J. Hilger, *Z. f. physiologische Chem.* **138**, 288 (1924).

5. The organic substance

In the graphic representation of the theory the 'organic substance' follows after the higher valency iron. The intention was to leave the relationship between these two as indefinite as possible since the course of the reaction of the ferric iron was really more problematical than was the oxidation of the ferrous iron. If the question were asked to-day, which substance reduces the iron of the oxygen transporting enzyme, the answer would be ferrous cytochrome. If, however, one includes the cytochrome iron with the oxygen transporting iron, then the course of the reduction of the iron is still a problem not completely solved. According to the work of A. v. Szent-Györgyi,† it is succinic acid in muscle which reduces the iron.

The organic substance mentioned in our theory of 1924 was immediately changed by others into 'activated substrate', so that the iron theory and that of Wieland could be combined. Thus the original iron theory was falsified, and the incorrect theory of Wieland was not made any less incorrect. The substrates, whether activated or unactivated, do not reduce the iron, but reduce the alloxazine—or the nicotinamide—conjugated proteins, about which nothing was known in 1924.

The indefinite expression 'organic substance' was therefore appropriate in 1924. Anyone taking exception to this demanded too much of the theory. The limiting of the theory to 'iron, the oxygen transporting part of the respiratory enzyme' was no defect in 1924, but rather an asset.

6. Hydrogen cyanide

The fact that cyanide combines with the oxygen transporting iron to give an inactive complex was no consequence of the theory, quite the reverse. From a knowledge of the chemical properties of the anticatalyst, the chemical nature of the catalyst was recognized.

As a result of the theory of 1924, the question was often asked whether the cyanide combined with the divalent or the trivalent iron, or both. This question was answered in 1927 by deter-

† A. v. Szent-Györgyi et al., Z. f. physiologische Chem. 236, 1 (1935).

mining the cyanide inhibition at different oxygen tensions.†
The cyanide combines with the trivalent iron. We found that
the cyanide inhibition of the respiration is independent of the
oxygen pressure.

If the cyanide had reacted with the divalent iron, the molecular oxygen and the cyanide would have competed for the
iron, and the inhibition of the respiration would have become
smaller with increasing oxygen pressure.

7. Inhibition by narcotics

Oxygen transport by iron has in the theory been designated
'catalysis at surfaces', because narcotics inhibit cell respiration
according to the same law as applies to the respiration of charcoal.

Kurt H. Meyer‡ opposed this on the grounds that it was mere
analogy, and that decisive biological proof was not available.
He was quite right. On the other hand he was unable to suggest
a single model experiment or analogy for his own view that
narcotic inhibition of biochemical reactions is brought about by
solution of the narcotics in the fatty constituents of the cells.
By this I mean that he could not put forward any chemical
reactions which were inhibited by narcotics in accordance with
his theory. On the contrary, Kurt Meyer's view has become less
probable as our knowledge of the chemistry of enzymes has
developed. How could the chemical reactions of conjugated
proteins be inhibited by the solution of chemically indifferent
substances like narcotics in the fatty constituents of the cell?
If we take the opposite view that chemical reactions which are
inhibited by narcotics according to the homologous series rule
are invariably surface reactions, then the question might still
be asked to-day, why should it be the first reaction of the enzyme chain that is affected by narcotics when they inhibit
respiration? The answer is that possibly all the stages of the
enzyme chain of reactions are surface reactions, but that the

† O. Warburg, *Bioch. Zeitschr.* **189**, 354 (1927) [p. 372].
‡ Kurt H. Meyer and H. Hopff, *Z. f. physiologische Chem.* **126**, 281 (1923);
Kurt H. Meyer and H. Hemmi, *Bioch. Zeitschr.* **277**, 39 (1935).

iron system has a special position of its own because it is insoluble in water, whilst the other enzymes in the chain are all soluble. Enzymes dissolved in water are not inhibited by narcotics except when the concentration of the latter is increased to that causing coagulation.

It must, however, be emphasized with regret that the problem of narcotic inhibition has not been as sufficiently studied quantitatively as befits its importance. The chemical problem of respiration has pushed the physical problem, the inhibiting action of narcotics, into the background. In a more complete theory of cell respiration which would deal with the energy changes taking place, the study of narcotic inhibition would take an outstanding place.

2

Reprinted from pp. 62–72 of *Heavy Metal Prosthetic Groups and Enzyme Action*, A. Lawson, trans., Oxford University Press, Oxford, 1949, 230pp.

CYTOCHROME

Otto Warburg

1. The experiments of MacMunn††‡

MACMUNN in 1885 discovered by spectroscopic examination that all animal cells 'from echinoderms to man throughout the animal kingdom' contain hæm compounds. These are present in two forms according to whether the cell is saturated with, or is cut off from, oxygen. 'They are joined proteids.' 'They are capable of oxidation and reduction and are therefore respiratory.'

Whilst the oxidized hæm compounds give no characteristic spectrum with visible light, in the reduced condition they show a four-banded spectrum. MacMunn found that the positions of the bands were about the same in all cells, the mean values being:

605 mμ	567 mμ	550 mμ	522 mμ
yellow-red strong	green strong	green very strong	blue-green weak

In accordance with their presence in muscle or in other tissues, MacMunn called the hæm compounds 'myohaematins' or 'histohaematins'. He found the greatest concentration in the wing muscles of rapidly flying insects. MacMunn was able to extract a part of the hæms from the cells, and he was surprised that after the extraction they lost their ability to be oxidized by atmospheric oxygen. He observed:

In studying the chromatology of many invertebrates, I have been struck by the fact that while some of their colouring matters can be reduced by such agents as sulphide of ammonium, yet by shaking with air or by passing a stream of oxygen into them, they cannot be reoxidised; in this point they afford a parallel to the histohaematins. Krukenberg has noticed the same thing, and he has justly concluded that the respiratory process of many of these animals is not as simple a matter as it is supposed to be.

† C. A. MacMunn, *Phil. Trans. Royal Soc. London*, **177**, 267 (1885).
‡ Id., *Journ. Physiology*, **8**, 51 (1887).

Thus there arose at a remarkably early date a problem which has only been solved in recent years, namely, that there are cell pigments which appear to react inside the cell with molecular oxygen and yet are not autoxidizable. To this class many yellow enzymes also belong. The solution to this problem was the enzyme chain. The first link in the chain is always an autoxidizable enzyme, though it may not be recognizable spectroscopically, whilst the oxidation of the later links in the enzyme chain is brought about by those preceding them.

2. Hoppe-Seyler's objections

The views of MacMunn were challenged in 1889 by Hoppe-Seyler's co-worker Levy[†] who took the view that the myohaematins and histohaematins were substances of no physiological function, but decomposition products of haemoglobin. MacMunn[‡] replied quite rightly that the histohaematins were also to be found in animals having no haemoglobin and that their concentration was greatest in the muscles of insects without haemoglobin. But Hoppe-Seyler[§] thought MacMunn's reply invalid. The conditions in the lower forms of animal life might not apply to the higher animals.

I have reported this discussion because it shows how dangerous it is when people allow themselves to be influenced by false objections. MacMunn remained silent, and the result was that nothing more was heard of histohaematins during the next 33 years.

3. Experiments of Hans Fischer

MacMunn's discovery that not only the red blood cells, but that all cells contained haems was verified analytically in the years 1923 and 1924 by Hans Fischer.[||] 'I am convinced of the correctness of MacMunn's results.' Fischer's starting point was porphyria, a disease of man in which large amounts of porphyrin

† L. Levy, *Z. f. physiologische Chem.* **13**, 309 (1889).
‡ C. A. MacMunn, ibid. **13**, 497 (1889); **14**, 328 (1890).
§ F. Hoppe-Seyler, ibid. **14**, 106 (1890).
|| Hans Fischer, *Strahlentherapie*, **18**, 185 (1924).

are excreted in the urine and faeces. In 1916 Fischer† isolated a porphyrin which he called coproporphyrin I. He proved that the substance was different from the porphyrin of the blood haem, protoporphyrin. Coproporphyrin I is tetramethyl-porphin-tetrapropionic acid; protoporphyrin is dimethyl-divinyl-porphin-dipropionic acid. The arrangement of the methyl or vinyl groups and the propionic side chains in the two porphyrins indicated that the one could not have been formed from the other. Hans Fischer therefore concluded that there are either red blood pigments the haems of which are different, or there must occur naturally haem compounds which are not blood pigments. The connexion with the work of MacMunn was thus established.

The question as to how coproporphyrin I arises remains still unanswered to-day, but the discovery of two naturally occurring porphyrins started Fischer‡ looking for haems everywhere in living nature. He thus discovered that yeast contains haems, and moreover, to such an extent that if a pyridine extract is made of a little fresh baker's yeast, it appears quite red. Fischer also found haems in plant cells and he isolated the corresponding porphyrins.

4. Cytochrome§

Keilin's work in 1925 confirmed the results of the spectro-scopic studies of MacMunn, and he attempted, moreover, to show‖ the connexion between MacMunn's work and the oxygen transporting iron of 1924, embodying ideas of Meyerhof and Harrison on the haem nature of the enzyme.

Although Keilin in his work of 1925 erroneously identified MacMunn's histohaematin with the oxygen transporting en-zyme, this work was nevertheless of great importance in the solution of the respiration problem. Keilin then gave MacMunn

† Hans Fischer, *Münchener Med. Wochenschr.* 1916, p. 377 and 1923, p. 1143.
‡ Hans Fischer *et al., Z. f. physiologische Chem.* **135**, 253; **138**, 288; **140**, 57 (1924); **144**, 101 (1925).
§ D. Keilin, *Proc. Royal Soc. London,* B **98**, 312 (1925); **100**, 129 (1926); **104**, 206 (1929); **106**, 418 (1930).
‖ Cf. chap. VI, section 4.

his rightful place. He showed, however, that haems are more widely distributed in nature than MacMunn had believed. He confirmed the existence of Fischer's yeast haem using the spectroscopic method, and by applying the 'inhibition technique' to histohaematin, he paved the way to the recognition of these haem compounds as being links in the chain of respiration enzymes. It was, however, unnecessary to change the name of MacMunn's histohaematin into cytochrome. Keilin replaced a name which correctly expressed the chemical constitution by a name which did not differentiate the histohaematin from other cell pigments. We shall, however, use the name cytochrome in accordance with Keilin's wishes.

Keilin attributed three of the MacMunn bands to three different haem compounds which he called cytochrome a, cytochrome b, and cytochrome c.

The fourth MacMunn band (522 mμ) ought to be common to all three cytochromes. Actually the band at 522 on closer examination appears to consist of two or three separate bands as MacMunn had previously observed. Nevertheless it is probable that the 522 band belongs to cytochrome c and that the corresponding bands for cytochrome a and b cannot be seen on spectroscopic examination of cells owing to their low concentration.

All four MacMunn bands are so-called secondary bands. The main bands which are situated in the blue region were discovered by us in 1931 using blue light.† We found in the blue region bands at 417 mμ, 433 mμ, and 449 mμ. Of these, however, the last, as Keilin and Hartree‡ showed in 1939, belongs probably in part to the oxygen transporting enzyme.

To summarize: Cytochrome consists of three haem compounds which in the reduced or ferrous condition show the following bands:

	Cytochrome a	Cytochrome b	Cytochrome c
1. Secondary bands	605 mμ	567 mμ	550 mμ
2. Secondary bands	?	?	522 mμ
3. Main bands	449 mμ	433 mμ	417 mμ

† O. Warburg and E. Negelein, *Bioch. Zeitschr.* **233**, 486 (1931); **238**, 135 (1931).
‡ D. Keilin and E. F. Hartree, *Proc. Royal Soc.* B **127**, 167 (1939).

5. The experiments of Anson and Mirsky†

Anson and Mirsky in 1925 showed that the haemochromogens are dissociating compounds of ferrohaem (ferroporphyrin) with nitrogen-containing bases, such as ammonia, pyridine, and protein:

$$\text{ferrohaem} + \text{base} \rightleftharpoons \text{haemochromogen}.$$

Whilst the ferrohaems have no characteristic spectra, the haemochromogens are distinguished by sharp band spectra, the positions of the bands being determined by both components, the haem and the base. The same haem forms different haemochromogens according as it is coupled with ammonia, with pyridine, or with a protein. Different proteins coupled with the same haem give different haemochromogens distinguishable by the position of the bands.

Since the haemochromogens are dissociating compounds, any haemochromogen can be converted into another by reaction with a nitrogenous base. If the affinity and the concentration of the added base are adequate a new haemochromogen is formed by displacement.

On account of its great affinity for haem, pyridine is a particularly active substance in this respect. If a haemochromogen is dissolved in concentrated aqueous pyridine, the whole of the haem is converted into pyridine haemochromogen. Anson and Mirsky applied this to the cytochrome problem. They came to the conclusion that the haems of cytochrome b and c were identical and, moreover, that it was protohaem. The bands of cytochrome b and c are different, therefore, not on account of the haem, but on account of the protein component. Further, cytochrome a differs from cytochrome c in respect of both the haem and the protein. All that has been discovered since then is in agreement with this conclusion.

6. Oxidation and reduction of cytochrome

A stoppered glass vessel with plane parallel sides and of about 200 c.c. capacity and 2 cm. internal width is two-thirds filled with a 20 per cent. suspension of baker's yeast which has been

† M. L. Anson and A. E. Mirsky, *Journ. Physiology*, **60**, 50, 161, 221 (1925).

previously washed with sodium chloride solution. On the near side of the vessel the filament of a powerful metal-filament lamp is arranged, and on the other side a spectroscope is fitted up. If nitrogen is passed through this yeast suspension, or if the suspension is allowed to stand undisturbed, the bands of reduced cytochrome can be seen. If, however, oxygen is passed through the suspension, the bands disappear because saturation of the cells with oxygen converts the cytochrome into the oxidized form. In this way it can be seen how cytochrome in respiring cells is oxidized and reduced. As MacMunn said, 'They are capable of oxidation and reduction and are, therefore, respiratory.'

7. Inhibition of cytochrome action by cyanide

Keilin studied the oxidation and reduction of cytochrome using the same methods which we had employed for cell respiration. He found that the two processes were completely analogous. We found that cyanide and hydrogen sulphide inhibit yeast respiration: Keilin found that the action of yeast cytochrome was likewise inhibited by the same concentrations. We found that hydrogen cyanide ethyl ester and pyrophosphate, in spite of their being complex-forming substances, do not inhibit yeast respiration; Keilin found that these compounds did not inhibit the action of yeast cytochrome. We found that indifferent narcotics inhibit yeast respiration by a different mechanism from that of cyanide; Keilin found that this was also the case for the action of yeast cytochrome.

In view of this, anyone would have drawn the conclusion that cytochrome is the oxygen transporting enzyme. However, certain points of disagreement arose when the inhibition of the cytochrome action was more closely investigated, for example with cyanide.

If oxygen is passed through a yeast suspension till the absorption bands of cytochrome disappear and cyanide in sufficient quantity (N/10,000) to inhibit the respiration is added, the bands of the reduced cytochrome reappear in spite of the oxygen, and, moreover, these bands are exactly the same as those to be seen in the absence of cyanide and oxygen. Cyanide, therefore, appeared to inhibit the oxidation of cytochrome without reacting with it—a contradiction in terms.

8. Keilin's theory†

Keilin did not consider this anomaly, but on the grounds of the concordant behaviour of cell respiration and cytochrome function towards inhibiting agents, he put forward the theory that cytochrome was the oxygen transporting enzyme. He replaced the iron in our scheme of 1924 by cytochrome iron.

$$O_2 \rightarrow \text{ferro-cytochrome} \rightarrow \text{ferri-cytochrome} \rightarrow \text{substrate.}$$

'Cytochrome is oxidized by the air and reduced by the tissue itself.' 'The oxygen is constantly taken up by this pigment and given up to the cells.'

The cytochrome, according to this theory, was therefore autoxidizable and, moreover, sufficiently so to transfer oxygen in respiration.

9. Inhibition by carbon monoxide‡

In 1926 we examined the action of carbon monoxide on yeast cytochrome and found that it inhibited the oxidation of cytochrome iron at concentrations which were the same as those inhibiting respiration.

In this case, too, as with the cyanide in Keilin's experiments, the carbon monoxide did not affect the cytochrome bands. This substance, therefore, also appeared to inhibit the oxidation of cytochrome without reacting with it.

10. The Warburg theory

If it were assumed that in respiring cells the oxygen transporting enzyme oxidized the cytochrome, all difficulties would be eliminated.

$$O_2 \rightarrow \text{oxygen transporting enzyme} \rightarrow \text{cytochrome} \rightarrow \text{substrate.}$$

Cytochrome, although not autoxidizable, would be immediately oxidized when oxygen was present in the respiring cell, but only

† D. Keilin, *Proc. Royal Soc.* B **98**, 312 (1925).
‡ O. Warburg, *Bioch. Z.* **177**, 471 (1926), and A. Reid, ibid. **242**, 159 (1931).

through the agency of the oxygen transporting enzyme. More-over, cyanide and carbon monoxide, although they did not react with the cytochrome, would inhibit its oxidation by their reaction with the oxygen transporting enzyme.

This theory was put forward by me at the Royal Society[†] in London on 12 May 1927, and by Keilin[‡] in Paris on 27 May 1927. It was generally accepted. The discussion which then arose with Keilin and which is dealt with in Chapter XVI con-cerned the further question: What is the oxygen transporting enzyme? Is it an iron compound or a haem compound or neither?

11. The sequence of the components[§]

If the three cytochrome components in the respiring cell are arranged in an oxidation-reduction chain, the question arises as to the sequence of the components. Eric G. Ball in 1938 attempted to answer the question by the following experiment:

A suspension of washed heart muscle was treated with enough hydrosulphite to allow the bands of the three ferrocytochromes to appear in full strength. By preventing access of oxygen, the oxygen transporting iron and also the reoxidation of the ferro-cytochrome were excluded. Then, oxidation-reduction systems of different potentials were added and their effect on the ferro-cytochrome bands observed. Large differences in the effect on the three cytochromes were seen. For example, the methylene blue system caused disappearance of only cytochrome b bands. With systems of considerably higher oxidation potentials only were the bands of cytochrome a and c made to disappear.

In this way Ball determined the oxidation potential E_0 (potential at which [ox.] = [red.]) of the three cytochromes and found:

	Cytochrome a	Cytochrome b	Cytochrome c
$E_0 =$	$+0.29$ volt	-0.04 volt	$+0.27$ volt

Ball concluded, therefore, that in the respiring cell, cytochrome

† O. Warburg, *Die Naturwissenschaften*, **15**, 546 (1927).
‡ D. Keilin, *Soc. de Biologie Paris, Réunion Plénière*, 27 and 28 May 1927.
§ Eric G. Ball, *Bioch. Zeitschr.* **295**, 262 (1938).

a oxidized cytochrome *c*, which in its turn oxidized cytochrome *b*, so that the sequence of the iron atoms in the chain would be

$O_2 \rightarrow$ Oxygen transporting $Fe \rightarrow Fe_{\text{cytochrome } a} \rightarrow Fe_{\text{cytochrome } c} \rightarrow Fe_{\text{cytochrome } b}.$

If in the stationary state of respiration cytochromes *a* and *c* were present almost completely in the reduced state, whilst cytochrome *b* was almost completely in the oxidized state, then the E_0 values would not determine the sequence of the cytochromes since

$$E = E_0 + RT \ln\frac{[\text{ox.}]}{[\text{red.}]}.$$

The sequence could therefore be different from that postulated by Ball. But under such conditions in the resting state of the respiration the ferro bands of cytochrome *a* and *c* would have to be fully developed, whilst that of cytochrome *b* need be hardly visible. Actually the situation appears to be just the reverse. The theory of Ball is, therefore, probably correct.

12. Rate of cytochrome reduction†

If a yeast suspension takes up *A* moles of oxygen per minute, and *v* mole of cytochrome component are reduced per minute, then if the whole respiration proceeds over the cytochrome,

$$A = \tfrac{1}{4}v,$$

since $\tfrac{1}{4}$ mole oxygen is necessary to reoxidize 1 mole cytochrome.

Using 1 c.c. bakers' yeast at 0° we found

$A \equiv 0.34$ c.mm. oxygen per minute,

$v \equiv 4 \times 0.32$ c.mm. cytochrome per minute.‡

Thus the expected relationship between the oxygen requirement and the cytochrome reduction was realized.

It was shown by this experiment that the route over cytochrome is not just one of alternative routes, but that it is the main route by which the oxidation equivalent of the respired oxygen is carried forward.

Note. The rather cumbersome arrangement of the experiment which we described in 1934 can be simplified in the following way:

† E. Haas, *Die Naturwissenschaften*, **22**, 207 (1934).
‡ 1 millimole Fe $\equiv$ 22,400 c.mm.

The spectra of two similar yeast suspensions through which oxygen is continuously passed are projected one over the other. To suspension I, which serves as a control, a small measured amount of ferrocytochrome c is added. This, in spite of the oxygen, remains reduced as it does not penetrate into the cells and is not autoxidizable in solution. To suspension II there is added at a time t_0 enough hydrogen cyanide to inhibit completely the respiration. The band at 550 mμ then appears in II also, and the intensity increases until at a time t it has reached that in suspension I. If n mole ferrocytochrome had been added to I, then the cells in suspension II must have reduced n mole ferricytochrome to ferrocytochrome in a time $t-t_0$.

The experiment must be arranged so that the amount of cytochrome added to I is not greater than one-third of the amount present in the yeast cells. Only then does the initial rate of cytochrome reduction correspond to that of the respiration in the resting state.

13. Cytochrome c†

Of the three cytochromes, the components a and b are so firmly combined with the insoluble cell constituent that it was not possible in the past to dissolve them out. Contradictory statements are to be ascribed to the fact that the insoluble material, particularly in alkaline media, forms suspensions which are difficult to centrifuge and which appear to be solutions.

Cytochrome c which is soluble in water was isolated by Hugo Theorell. It is a conjugated protein of molecular weight 13,000 and contains 1 molecule of protohaem which corresponds to the determined iron content of 0·43 per cent.

In contrast to haemoglobin, cytochrome cannot be reversibly broken down into the haem and protein. This is because the haem and the protein are joined together by two strong bonds, which one can visualize as being formed by the union of two

† Hugo Theorell, *Bioch. Zeitschr.* **279**, 463 (1935); **285**, 207 (1936). Hugo Theorell and Akeson, *Journ. Amer. Chem. Soc.* **63**, 1804 (1941). Hugo Theorell, *Ergebnisse der Enzymforschung*, **9**, 231 (1943).

cysteine residues in the protein to the vinyl groups in the haem, thus giving two thioether linkages. On mild acid hydrolysis the di-cysteine compound of the protoporphyrin is split off, but on strong acid hydrolysis, haematoporphyrin is obtained, as was shown in 1933 by Zeile and Reuter.

The colour changes of cytochrome which Theorell observed in the titration of the acid groups and which he determined colorimetrically are explained by the reversible action between the iron of the cytochrome and the imidazole groups of the protein, since the colour of the cytochrome during the titration changes just at those pH ranges at which the titratable acidity could only correspond to imidazole residues.

3

THE FORMATION OF HYDROGEN PEROXIDE BY LACTIC ACID BACTERIA

Alfred Bertho and Hans Glück

This translation was prepared expressly for this Benchmark volume by Walter P. Hempfling from "Die Bildung von Wasserstoffperoxyd durch Milchsäurebakterien," in Naturwissenschaften 19:88 (1931)

The facultatively anaerobic, catalase-free lactic acid formers *B. Delbrücki, B. iugurt,* and *B. acidophilus* produce hydrogen peroxide during oxidative metabolism. Oxygen uptake was followed using Barcroft manometers with living bacteria in the presence of glucose as the donor substance. M/2000 HCN has no effect on the process. The hydrogen peroxide thus formed is determined qualitatively with titanosulfuric acid or quantitatively by trapping as cerium peroxide [I, II, V, VI, IX, X—see Wieland and Rosenfeld, *Liebigs. Ann.* **477,** 69 (1930)], sometimes by direct titration (III, IV). The amount of oxygen uptake (I–VI, IX, X) and the observed amounts of peroxide correspond within experimental error to the equation $2H + O_2 = H_2O_2$. The addition of catalase, in spite of the presence of the cerium salt, diminishes the oxygen uptake practically by half according to expectation. If the hydrogen peroxide is not trapped, increasing damage to the cells occurs along with its increasing formation. The amount of peroxide that is trapped is less than expected for this reason (I–VI). These results demonstrated for the first time with *living** cells such an *exact** relation between oxygen consumption and peroxide formation as to require the dehydrogenation theory. Hydrogen peroxide has repeatedly been observed in pneumococcus cultures (McLeod and Gordon, Avery and Niell). Acetone preparations do not show these phenomena. Blank titrations were always parallel and the test with catalase was negative.

B. Delbrücki. I, II: 3 ml bacterial suspension containing 10.4 mg dry weight, 3 ml M/10 glucose solution, 3 ml M/5 borate buffer pH 9.0, 1 ml M/500 cerous sulfate, starting pH 8.2–8.3. III, IV: as above, except without the cerium salt and with 3 ml M/5 borate buffer pH 8.2.

---

*Author's italic—ed.

Editor's note: The reference given is to H. Wieland and B. Rosenfeld, Über den mechanismus der Oxydationsvorgänge. XXI. Uber die dehydrierenden Enzyme der Milch. *Liebigs Ann.*, **477**, 32–77, 1930.

Min.	I ml O_2	II ml O_2	III ml O_2	IV ml O_2
60	20.5	26	15	15.5
120	31.5	29	25.5	24.5
180	27	30	4.5	6
240	23	23	3.5	4
Total after 240 min.	102	108	48.5	50
Titrated	86	90	51.5	56

B. acidophilus. V, VI: contents corresponding to I, II, except 3 ml bacterial suspension containing 13.2 mg dry weight and 2 ml M/500 cerous sulfate. VII, VIII: as above, except with about 2 mg of a preparation of liver catalase.

Min.	V ml O_2	VI ml O_2	VII ml O_2	VIII ml O_2
60	92	88	12.5	10.5
180	45	52	37.5	31
240	45	46	34	21
300	33	38	16	26.5
Total after 300 min.	215	224	100	89
Titrated	193	210	—	—

B. iugurt. IX, X: contents corresponding to I, II, except 3 ml bacterial suspension containing 4.9 mg dry weight.

Min.	IX ml O_2	X ml O_2
120	23.5	27.5
300	21	28
Total after 300 min.	44.5	55.5
Titrated	42.5	51.5

In the facultatively anaerobic, catalase-free lactic acid producer *Streptococcus casei*, "respiration" is likewise not inhibited by M/2000 HCN, but hydrogen peroxide has not as yet been found by the same method. Further research will show whether the "incomplete respiration system" described principally requires two mechanisms.

We have chosen these primitive oxidative metabolic processes of the simplest intact cellular material for consideration since a positive result has actually been obtained with regard to the demonstration of hydrogen peroxide. The way is thereby also smoothed to attempt the demonstration of peroxide in bacteria containing weak catalase activity (certain lactic acid producers, propionic acid bacteria) and in bacteria containing strong catalase activity (acetic acid bacteria).

Part II

THE APPARATUS OF TERMINAL ELECTRON TRANSPORT

Editor's Comments
on Papers 4, 5, and 6

DISTRIBUTION OF CYTOCHROMES

Cytochromes, originally obseved in aerobically grown organ-isms,[1,2] are also found in anaerobic procaryotes. This is reasonable, since the function of cytochromes other than terminal oxidases is electron transfer rather than oxygen reduction, without concomit-ant hydrogen transfer, and no observation better confirms War-burg's contention quoted in our comments about Papers 1, 2, and 3. It is therefore logical to expect that certain cytochromes might be oxidized by electron acceptors other than oxygen. The following selections illustrate the wide distribution of cytochromes among procaryotes, and include a sulfate reducer, a facultative photo-heterotroph, and an obligately anaerobic rumen bacterium.

John Postgate provides in Paper 4 an account of the proper-ties and function of cytochrome c_3 from *Desulfovibrio*, an electron transfer component active in sulfate respiration linked to oxida-tive phosphorylation (see also Paper 19). This work is part of Post-gate's comprehensive investigation of such bacteria.[3] Considered with the information available about dissimilatory nitrate reduc-tion,[4] it is apparent that oxygen-independent respiratory systems deserve greater attention than they have so far received. It is of further interest that desulfoviridin, only briefly described in Paper 4, has since been characterized as a sirohydrochlorin active in sul-fite reduction.[5]

Following the initial description of the carbon monoxide-bind-ing "*Rhodospirillum* heme protein" (RHP) by Vernon and Kamen,[6] considerable interest was aroused by the possibility that RHP might prove to be a novel terminal oxidase active when facultative photoheterotrophs were grown aerobically in the dark. RHP was, accordingly, extensively investigated. Paper 5 describes the preparation of RHP and characterizes it. Further investigation has disclosed that RHP (currently "cytochrome *c'*, *cc'''*", see Editor's Comments on Papers 9, 10, and 11) is without oxidase function, but may participate in photosynthetic electron transport.

Involvement of a cytochrome in electron transport associated with a true fermentation by an obligate anaerobe is strongly suggested by White, Bryant, and Caldwell in Paper 6. Reddy and Peck have recently reported that small amounts of uncoupler-sensitive phosphate esterification accompany fumarate reduction in extracts of the obligately anaerobic rumen bacterium *Vibrio succinogenes*.[7]

REFERENCES

1. Yaoi, H., and H. Tamiya. *Proc. Imp. Acad. Tokyo*, **4**, 435–439, 1929.
2. Smith, L. Cytochrome systems in aerobic electron transport. In I. C. Gunsalus and R. Y. Stanier, eds. *The Bacteria, II, Metabolism*. Academic Press, New York, 1961, pp. 365–396.
3. Postgate, J. R. *J. Gen. Microbiol.*, **5**, 725–738, 1959. Paper 31 in Doelle.
4. Taniguchi, S. *Z. Allg. Mikrobiol.*, **1**, 341–375, 1961.
5. Murphy, M. J., and L. M. Siegel. *J. Biol. Chem.*, **248**, 6911–6919, 1973. (We are grateful to Professor Postgate for bringing this work to our attention).
6. Vernon, L. D., and M. D. Kamen. *J. Biol. Chem.*, **211**, 643–662, 1954.
7. Reddy, C. A., and H. D., Peck, Jr. *J. Bact.*, **134**, 982–991, 1978.

4

Reprinted from *J. Gen. Microbiol.* **14**:545–572 (1956)

Cytochrome c_3 and Desulphoviridin; Pigments of the Anaerobe *Desulphovibrio desulphuricans*

By J. R. POSTGATE

Chemical Research Laboratory, Teddington

SUMMARY: Suspensions of various mesophilic strains of *Desulphovibrio desulphuricans* show absorption bands attributable to a cytochrome and a green protein; there are small differences in the position of absorption maxima depending on the strain and culture medium. Both pigments have been extracted, together with flavins rich in flavinadenine dinucleotide; an electrophoretically and chromatographically pure preparation of the cytochrome has been obtained and is designated c_3. The green protein has been termed 'desulphoviridin'.

Cytochrome c_3 is a soluble autoxidizible thermostable haemoprotein (reduced bands at 553, 525 and 419 mμ.) of low redox potential (-205 mV.), high iso-electric point (pH > 10) and containing 0·9 % Fe. Degradation studies indicate that it is a bifunctional haemato-haematin with the thio-ether haem-apoprotein links also found in cytochromes c and f; its M.W. is approx. 13,000 ($S_{20,\,w} = 1·93 \times 10^{-13}$). Spectroscopic data for various derivatives including haemin c_3 and a porphyrin derivative are recorded. Material purified to at least 94 % by cellulose and ion-exchange chromatography acts as carrier in the reduction in hydrogen of sulphite, thiosulphate, tetrathionate or dithionite by detergent-treated bacterial preparations; a similar role has been demonstrated with cell-free systems which reduce sulphite, thiosulphate and tetrathionate. Benzylviologen would replace cytochrome c_3. No preparation has been obtained showing c_3-linked sulphate reduction; the evidence for this depends on difference spectra and competition by known sulphate antagonists.

Oxidation of H_2 or organic compounds with O_2 has been demonstrated with these bacteria; the H_2/O_2 reaction takes place fastest in an atmosphere containing 4 % O_2, when oxygen is frequently reduced faster than sulphate. The reaction requires the mediation of cytochrome c_3 and is probably a consequence of the autoxidizibility of c_3.

Desulphoviridin is a thermolabile, soluble, acidic porphyroprotein absorbing at 630, 585 and 411 mμ.; no metabolic function has been detected. It is stable over a limited pH range and decomposes readily, yielding a chromophoric group which fluoresces red in ultraviolet light, absorbs at 595 mμ. in neutral and alkaline solution (solution red) and at 612 mμ. in acid solution (solution blue-green). This material can be purified by chromatography on 'Florisil' or paper. It is very photo-sensitive and water-soluble. Its character is obscure; it may be a highly carboxylated chlorin. Spectroscopic data are recorded.

The cytochromes have for long been regarded as pigments characteristic only of aerobic or facultatively anaerobic bacteria. For many years they were believed to be absent from obligate anaerobes (see Keilin, 1933; Keilin & Slater, 1953), a view which was supported by a recent examination of seven anaerobes, which allowed for the possibility of adaptive cytochrome formation in air (Schaeffer & Nisman, 1952). However, a cytochrome has now been observed in the sulphate-reducing bacterium *Desulphovibrio desulphuricans* (Butlin & Postgate, 1953; Ishimoto, Koyama & Nagai, 1954*a, b*; Postgate,

1954*a*, *b*), though this bacterium is an exacting anaerobe (Grossman & Postgate 1953*a*, *b*); cytochromes have also been demonstrated in species of the obligately anaerobic photo-autotrophs *Chromatium* and *Chlorobium* (Kamen & Vernon, 1954*a*, *b*; Vernon & Kamen, 1954; Gibson & Larsen, 1955). The present paper describes the spectroscopic properties of a strain of sulphate-reducing bacteria, the extraction of the components responsible for the spectroscopic absorption bands, the purification of the cytochrome component, and some of its chemical and biological properties.

METHODS

Spectroscopy. The behaviour of suspensions of bacteria was observed in a Hartridge reversion spectroscope modified for use with relatively opaque material and calibrated with the emission lines of neon; quoted readings were taken at limiting dilution as recommended by Lemberg & Legge (1949). Spectrophotometric measurements were made in the Hilger 'Uvispek' instrument. Measurements on intact organisms were made by the procedure of Barer (1955), in which scattering was reduced to a minimum by suspending the organisms in a medium of refractive index similar to that of themselves. The refractive index of the bacteria used in this work was shown by phase-contrast microscopy to be $1·383 \pm 0·001$; therefore a solution of bovine serum albumin (Armour Laboratories, Fraction V) of *c.* 34 % (w/w; refractive index, measured in the hand refractometer, equivalent to 31·5 % sucrose) was the most suitable suspending medium.

Manometry. Conventional Warburg manometers were used for experiments involving gas exchanges; details of procedure were given by Grossman & Postgate (1955).

Organisms used and their cultivation. Desulphovibrio desulphuricans strain Hildenborough (National Collection of Industrial Bacteria NCIB 8303), purified according to Postgate (1953) was used, except where otherwise mentioned; its origin, maintenance and methods of subculture were described by Postgate (1951*a*). Large quantities of organisms for fractionation were obtained from continuous culture experiments being conducted elsewhere in this laboratory (Report, 1953); the conditions of culture changed in detail from time to time, but normally the bacteria were grown in a medium containing Na_2SO_4 equivalent to 0·4 % (w/v) S, yeast extract (Difco) 0·4 % (w/v) and small amounts of NH_4^+, K^+ and Mg^{++} (Report, 1954, p. 53). Effluent containing 0·4–0·8 mg. air-dry wt. organisms/ml. was harvested during several days, centrifuged in 100 l. lots in a Sharples centrifuge, the organisms washed with distilled water and dried by addition to 10 vol. cold acetone (4°), followed by washing with acetone and then ether. Yield: 30–35 g. dried material/100 l. culture medium. Organisms freshly harvested during the logarithmic phase of growth were used for metabolic experiments; a few experiments were done with bacteria from batch cultures.

Chromatography. Cellulose columns were packed with Whatman cellulose powder (standard grade) and washed with 4 vol. of distilled water. Ammonium

'Amberlite' columns were prepared as follows: a finely divided form of Amberlite IRC 50 (XE 97, Chas. Lennig and Co. Ltd.) was obtained and the fraction which sedimented between 3 and 20 min. in water was collected. This was converted to the ammonium form by adding excess 2 N-NH_4OH, packed and washed with distilled water (c. 8 vol.) until the effluent contained less than 0·0025 N-HN_4OH (pH 9·5 to 10). Mean flow rate: 75 ml./hr. The resin XE 97 was also used for chromatography with sodium phosphate buffers (0·34 g.-ion Na^+/l.) following the procedure described by Boardman & Partridge (1955). It was washed successively with 2 N-NaOH, 2 N-HCl, then water and buffer; the columns (12 × 0·9 cm. diam.) were then packed and run at room temperature; mean flow rate 0·8–1·1 ml./hr. Florisil (30/60 mesh; Floridin Co., Florida, U.S.A.) was packed in water and washed with 20 vol. of 0·1 N-HCl followed by 20 vol. distilled water. Cross-linked polymin P columns were prepared following the advice of Mr D. K. Hale of this Laboratory. Polymin P (Badische Anilin und Soda Fabrik, Germany; a soluble polyethylenimine; 40 g.) was mixed with 40 ml. methanol, 4 ml. epichlorhydrin and 36 g. powdered cellulose (above) in that order; this mixture was allowed to polymerize at 60° for 3 days, and the product broken up in 2 N-HCl and washed successively with water, 2 N-NaOH, water, 2 N-acetic acid and 0·02 N-sodium acetate buffer (pH 5·0). The column, after packing, was washed with distilled water. Paper chromatography was conducted at room temperature on Whatman no. 1 filter-paper sheets, using the ascending method.

Electrophoresis. Electrophoresis on strips of Whatman no. 1 paper was carried out in the EEL instrument (Evans Electroselenium Ltd., Harlow, Great Britain).

Potentiometry. The Cambridge pH meter was used for fine pH measurements with a glass electrode, and for potentiometric titrations with a bright Pt electrode and a calomel reference electrode. Redox potentials were studied by titrating the test material in KH_2PO_4 (1 %, w/v, adjusted to pH 7 ± 0·02 with 2 N-NaOH) against $Na_2S_2O_4$ (30 mg./ml. buffer) in a current of O_2-free N_2 in a thermostat at 30 ± 0·05°.

Units of cytochrome. The millimolar extinction coefficient of the cytochrome studied here is not known. Evidence is presented in this paper that the cytochrome has a similar molecular weight to cytochrome c but two haemin groups per molecule. Hence ϵ_{mM} should theoretically be 54 (compare 27 for cytochrome c); the units used in this paper are derived from spectrophotometric measurements at the α-peak in the reduced form: 1 mUnit (mU.) = 1 mMole if $\epsilon_{mM} = 54$.

Abbreviations. The following abbreviations are used in this paper: CTAB for cetyltrimethylammonium bromide, FAD for flavin adenine dinucleotide, FMN for flavin mononucleotide, DPN for diphosphopyridine nucleotide, TPN for triphosphopyridine nucleotide, ATP for adenosine triphosphate, TCA for trichloracetic acid.

RESULTS

Observations with whole bacteria

Suspensions of the Hildenborough strain heavier than 10 mg. dry wt./ml. KH_2PO_4 (0·5 %, w/v; pH 6·9) showed strong adsorption bands at 553 and at 630 mμ. when viewed through a depth of 0·5 cm. A weaker band at 525 mμ. was seen, and old suspensions showed a shading about 595 mμ. This last band was later shown to be due to a chromophore liberated by partial decomposition of the 630 mμ.-component. The bands at 525 and 553 mμ. disappeared on

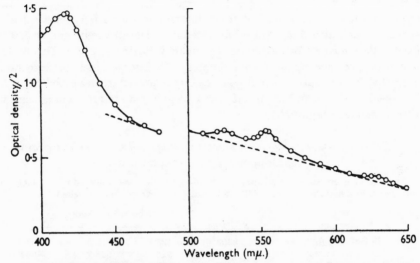

Fig. 1. Absorption spectra of *Desulphovibrio desulphuricans* (Hildenborough). Organisms were suspended in strong bovine plasma albumin and examined spectrophotometrically through a depth of 0·5 cm. after addition of $Na_2S_2O_4$. Visible range: 65 mg. dry wt./ml.; Soret range: 20 mg./ml. Dotted lines represent hypothetical scatter curve of a suspension of bacteria devoid of pigments.

shaking in air and returned on (*a*) standing, (*b*) passing in H_2, (*c*) adding $Na_2S_2O_4$. The band at 630 mμ., and the 595 mμ. band when present, were not affected by these procedures, nor by addition of H_2O_2, $K_3Fe(CN)_6$, or on passing in pure O_2. The bands at 525, 553 and 630 mμ. intensified and shifted to shorter wavelengths on freezing and de-vitrifying a suspension in 50% glycerol with liquid N_2, but remained single; hence they represented single compounds (Keilin & Hartree, 1955). Inspection of the suspension through a blue filter (dilute methylene blue) showed that the limit of visibility in the violet shifted from about 420 mμ. to about 410 mμ. with aerated suspensions. The absorption bands were recorded spectrophotometrically by Barer's procedure (Fig. 1).

This sulphate-reducing organism thus contained a reversibly oxidizible pigment resembling the cytochrome *c* of muscle, responsible for absorption peaks at 553 and 525 mμ. as well as at about 420 mμ. in the reduced condition. The absorption peak at 630 mμ., though similar in position to cytochrome a_2, had none of the properties of a conventional cytochrome. The cytochrome probably represented the sole intracellular haematin, because treatment of a suspension of bacteria with $Na_2S_2O_4$ in the presence of alkali and pyridine led to a shift of the cytochrome band to about 550 mμ., but no increase in its intensity; hence no additional haemochromogens were formed.

The presence of cytochrome and the 630 mμ.-component was confirmed with five other mesophilic strains of *Desulphovibrio desulphuricans* examined in washed suspension at 8–12 mg. dry wt. organisms/ml. (Table 1). Small differences in the position of the bands occurred between strains, wider variation occurred with bacteria derived from different media: El Agheila Z had its strongest band at 555 mμ. when harvested from lactate media and at 559 mμ. from malate media (for media see Grossman & Postgate, 1955). This was not due to the presence of another or a different cytochrome, since: (*a*) cytochrome extracted from malate-grown organisms by the procedure described below had its α-peak at the usual 553 mμ.; (*b*) the α-band in malate-grown organisms was homogeneous in liquid N_2.

Table 1. *Visible absorption spectra of suspensions of various strains*
of Desulphovibrio desulphuricans

Bacteria were harvested from lactate media except in the case indicated when El Agheila Z was grown in a malate medium. All strains halophilic except those marked *.

Strain	NCIB no.	Absorption peaks (mμ.)		
Hildenborough*	8303	525	553·8	630·0
California 43:63	8364	525	555·2	630·0
El Agheila Z	8380	525	555·2	630·8
El Agheila Z (malate)	—	525	559·8	629·0
Canet 41	8393	525	553·6	630·0
Wandle*	8305	525	555·7	630·0
Venice 2	8323	525	554·0	628·5

Oxidation by sulphate

It was possible that the cytochrome was concerned as a carrier in the reduction of sulphate and other reducible anions (see Postgate, 1951*b*), but addition of sulphate or sulphite to washed suspensions in anaerobic conditions led to no obvious change in the visible absorption bands. This was not surprising, however, since the end product of reduction of these compounds—sulphide—is a powerful reducing agent and might well mask any oxidation. To avoid this difficulty, suspensions of bacteria were incubated *in vacuo* in Thunberg tubes containing $CdCl_2$ (10 %, w/v) in the side arm to remove sulphide continuously, and, after 30 min. at room temperature at pH 7·0, the visible cytochrome bands were clearly less intense, by some 40 %, in the presence of excess sodium sulphate, sulphite, thiosulphate or tetrathionate, than in a control suspension without these. The peak at 630 mμ. did not alter in these conditions, except that, after prolonged exposure to sulphite, evaporation of SO_2 produced conditions sufficiently alkaline to cause decomposition, as a result of which a band appeared at 595 mμ. and the suspension fluoresced red in ultraviolet light. Ishimoto, Koyama & Nagai (1954*b*) reported observation of cytochrome oxidation by certain sulphur-containing anions without taking these precautions; the discrepancy between our results may be attributable either to the use of different strains or to difference in the amount of sulphide present at the moment of adding the oxidizing agent.

The oxidation of cytochrome by sulphate was recorded by difference spectra (Fig. 2). Since the modified spectrophotometric apparatus recommended by Chance (1954) was not available, Fig. 2 was obtained with suspensions of organisms rendered translucent by Barer's procedure. The introduction of sulphate caused a slight change in the refractive index of the suspending medium as compared with the control; in consequence the difference spectrum in Fig. 2 did·not lie exactly about the abscissa.

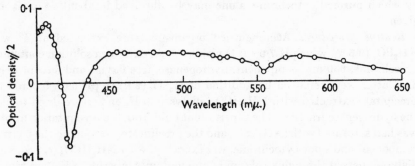

Fig. 2. Difference spectrum of *Desulphovibrio desulphuricans* (Hildenborough). The absorption of a bacterial suspension (7·2 mg. dry wt./ml. plasma albumin) containing excess sulphate was measured with a reference cell containing a similar suspension without sulphate.

Effect of inhibitors

Selenate or monofluorophosphate, which are competitive inhibitors of sulphate reduction (Postgate, 1949, 1952), inhibited the oxidation of the cytochrome by sulphate for several hours, though they did not affect oxidation by sulphite. The absorption bands were unaffected by passing in pure CO, adding KCN (10^{-2} M), Na_2S (5×10^{-3} M), or NH_2NH_2 (10^{-2} M); their reaction with air took place normally in the presence of these compounds. CTAB (recrystallized from acetone; 100 μg./mg. dry wt. organisms) inhibited the reduction of the oxidized cytochrome on standing, but did not prevent its reduction in H_2.

Mode of action of CTAB

Salton (1951) showed that CTAB rendered Gram-positive aerobes permeable to substances of low molecular weight. Suspensions of *Desulphovibrio desulphuricans* treated with CTAB (100 μg./mg. dry wt.) were killed: the viable count by the method of Grossman & Postgate (1953*b*) decreased from $1·7 \times 10^9$/ml. to $2·4 \times 10^3$/ml. Material absorbing at 265 mμ. was demonstrated in the supernatant liquid after centrifugation together with free cytochrome, though hydrogenase and the 630 mμ.-component were absent. Thus CTAB rendered the organisms permeable to the cytochrome; this conclusion was supported later by the observation that untreated bacteria reduced added purified cytochrome only slowly in H_2, though CTAB-treated organisms reduced it practically instantaneously. CTAB-treated organisms did not reduce sulphate in H_2, though they reduced methylene blue at a normal rate; they also did not reduce methylene blue with lactate or pyruvate.

Extraction of the pigments and purification of the cytochrome

The routine procedure given below for extraction of the cell pigments was devised to give maximum yields, as well as preparations of hydrogenase and of denatured cytochrome; it is therefore more complicated than if cytochrome only had been required and if yield had been unimportant. A rapid procedure by which purified cytochrome alone may be obtained in about 24 hr. is also given.

Routine procedure. Acetone-dried organisms were extracted at 4° with KH_2PO_4 (0·5 %, w/v; pH 7·0 $\pm$ 0·1) yielding a green-brown solution containing cytochrome, 630 mμ.-component, hydrogenase, free flavins and flavoproteins. The latter were removed by addition of H_2SO_4 (2 N) to pH 5·0 $\pm$ 0·2 and the precipitate extracted with NH_4HCO_3, dialysed in H_2 and freeze-dried to yield the hydrogenase fraction. The supernatant fluid from the precipitation at pH 5 was half saturated with $(NH_4)_2SO_4$ and the precipitate, containing the 630 mμ.-component and some cytochrome, was extracted with NH_4HCO_3 (c. 1 %, w/v), dialysed, passed through a column of ammonium Amberlite-XE 97 to remove as much cytochrome as possible, dialysed and freeze-dried as the 630 mμ.-component. Some purified cytochrome was eluted from the Amberlite column with NH_4OH (0·25 N) and added to the major fraction obtained later. The supernatant from the $(NH_4)_2SO_4$ precipitation was brought to pH 2·6 $\pm$ 0·2 with 2 N-H_2SO_4 and the precipitate, whose cytochrome content increased the longer it was left in contact with the supernatant, was dissolved in $NaHCO_3$ solution and dialysed. The supernatant fluid was passed through a column of Whatman 'standard grade' cellulose powder, the effluent (containing flavins) discarded and the adsorbed cytochrome eluted, together with some flavin, with NH_4OH (0·25 N) and dialysed. The combined dialysed products from the last two steps were adsorbed on to a column of ammonium Amberlite-XE 97 and washed with water. The coloured effluent contained denatured cytochrome which was collected and freeze-dried; it had no enzymic activity and reacted with CO. The native protein was eluted with NH_4OH (0·25 N), dialysed and freeze-dried. Fig. 3 records the steps in a typical preparation. Sulphuric acid was used in preference to TCA for pH adjustment because some earlier fractionations with TCA had yielded wholly denatured products—consistent with Lewis's (1954) observation that TCA has a more drastic effect than H_2SO_4 on haemoproteins. Verhoeven & Takeda (1956) encountered similar difficulties during the extraction of bacterial cytochrome *c* from nitrate-reducing bacteria, and finally chose citric acid for their fractionation procedure. Filtrations were avoided at all stages since the cytochrome was readily absorbed on cellulose; Keilin & Hartree (1945) reported that salt-free solutions of cytochrome *c* behaved similarly. Ishimoto & Koyama (1955) used an essentially similar procedure based on acetone precipitation in place of acid fractionation.

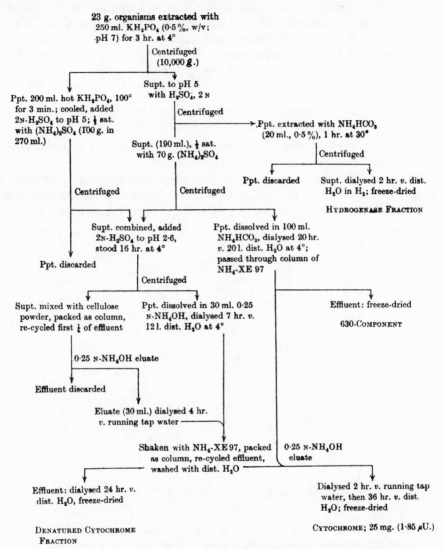

Fig. 3. Fractionation of acetone-dried *Desulphovibrio desulphuricans* (Hildenborough). The bacteria contained *c.* $0.22 \mu U.$ cytochrome c_3/g. air-dry mass; assuming their acetone-dried mass was similar, the yield was *c.* 28 % of theory.

Rapid procedure. Rapid procedures based on the release of cytochrome by CTAB or by heat were sometimes used; a record of a typical preparation follows: wet centrifuged bacteria (28 g. dry wt./100 ml. distilled water) were added slowly to 1 l. boiling and stirred KH_2PO_4 solution (0.5 %, w/v;

pH 7·0 ± 0·05), boiled 3 min. and allowed to cool at 4°. After 4 hr. the mixture was centrifuged, the supernatant fluid dialysed for 16 hr. against 12 vol. distilled water and shaken with 50 ml. ammonium Amberlite XE 97, packed as a column, and the first portion of effluent re-cycled to ensure complete absorption of cytochrome. As in the earlier procedure, a portion of 'denatured' material, able to react with CO, was not held by the resin. The pink column was washed with distilled water, the cytochrome eluted with 0·25 N-NH₄OH, and the product dialysed against 100 vol. distilled water and freeze-dried. The yield was 16·6 mg. purified powder (*c.* 19 % theory).

THE PROPERTIES OF THE CYTOCHROME OF
DESULPHOVIBRIO DESULPHURICANS

A preliminary account of the chemical and physical properties of the bacterial cytochrome has appeared elsewhere (Postgate, 1955*b*).

Spectrum. The cytochrome prepared by the procedure above had typical haematin spectra (Fig. 4). The analogy of the ferricytochrome spectrum at pH 7·0 to that of ferricytochrome *c* type III (Theorell & Akesson, 1941) is

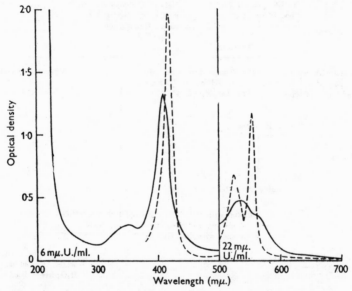

Fig. 4. Spectrum of purified cytochrome *c₃* from *Desulphovibrio desulphuricans* (Hildenborough). Readings were taken at 1 mμ. intervals at absorption peaks, 5 mμ. intervals elsewhere; pH 7·00 ± 0·02; *t* = 20°; 22 mμU. cytochrome/ml. in visible range, 6 mμU./ml. in ultraviolet; - - - -, reduced form; ———, oxidized form.

marked, even to the inflexion about 565 mμ., but the band at 280 mμ. was missing and no evidence for a band about 685 mμ. (Theorell, 1948) was found. The ferrocytochrome spectrum was not examined in the ultraviolet region since it was not stable in the absence of dithionite, which absorbs in this region, but the visible and Soret peaks again resembled those of cytochrome *c* except that they were shifted a few mμ. towards the red. The visible peaks were measured with greater precision in the optical spectroscope and were $\alpha = 553 \cdot 2$ mμ. and $\beta = 525 \cdot 2$ mμ. at pH $7 \cdot 00 \pm 0 \cdot 02$ and $19°$. Some ratios of the intensities of various peaks are given in Table 2.

Table 2. *Ratios of heights of absorption peaks in cytochrome* c$_3$

$\alpha = 553$ mμ., $\beta = 525$ mμ., $\gamma = 419$ mμ., $\delta = 350$ mμ.

Peaks	Ratio
$\gamma : \alpha$ (reduced)	5·75
$\gamma : \alpha$ (oxidized)	12·6
γ (reduced) : (oxidized)	1·51
$\gamma : \delta$ (oxidized)	6·6
$\alpha : \beta$ (reduced)	1·52

The specific extinction coefficient was obtained by dissolving known amounts of well-dialysed, freshly chromatographed cytochrome in buffer; at $20°$ and pH $7 \cdot 0$ $\epsilon_{sp.} = 4 \cdot 20 \pm 0 \cdot 06$ in the reduced condition at 553 mμ., and $1 \cdot 60$ in the oxidized condition at 535 mμ.

Purity. Electrophoresis on paper in KH_2PO_4 ($0 \cdot 5 \%$, w/v, pH $7 \cdot 0$) showed only the single cytochrome zone even after staining with bromothymol blue. Chromatography in buffer on a cation exchange resin (Boardman & Partridge, 1955) indicated small amounts of a colourless impurity which absorbed light at 280 mμ.; the pH value of the buffer used was less than pH $7 \cdot 0$ recommended by Boardman & Partridge for cytochrome c, since at the latter pH value the band due to the bacterial cytochrome spread badly. A typical experiment showing the presence of impurity absorbing at 280 mμ. is recorded in Fig. 5; the R_f value of the impurity was $0 \cdot 9$–$1 \cdot 0$ (that of the cytochrome was $0 \cdot 38$), and a rough integration indicated that it amounted to less than 6% of the total protein. Since purification by chromatography in buffer was laborious and conveniently applicable only to small amounts of material, the work reported in this paper was done with material containing this impurity.

Reactions in solution. The freeze-dried powder had a deep red colour. It dissolved completely in phosphate buffer or $0 \cdot 25$ N-NH_4OH to give a clear solution; it also dissolved in distilled water but much more slowly, and salt-free solutions were best prepared by dialysis of salt-containing solutions. Pre-parations stored for over 1 month at $-12°$ sometimes contained insoluble brown material, but the supernatant fluid was enzymically active. Exposure of solutions to preparations of organisms caused some denaturation, since cyto-chrome recovered from metabolic experiments (below) always contained a por-tion of material which was not retained by ammonium Amberlite XE 97, and which reacted with CO.

No spectroscopic change occurred in any of the following conditions: heating at pH $7 \cdot 0$ to $100°$ for 5 min.; passing in pure CO; adding KCN up to 10^{-2} M; adding excess ascorbic acid, $NaBH_4$, $K_4Fe(CN)_6$ or $FeSO_4$. With cysteine the reduced form of the cytochrome appeared slowly and incompletely, with Na_2S it appeared slowly but completely, and with $Na_2S_2O_4$ it appeared at once. Sodium nitrite and diluted acetic acid gave a nitroso-derivative of the oxidized form (visible bands of equal intensity at 532·5 and 563·5 mμ.; compare 531·1 and 563·4 mμ. for muscle cytochrome c); treatment with 2 N-NaOH denatured the preparation, since it then reacted with CO (absorption peaks: 415, 530, 565 mμ.; compare 415, 531·5, 564·5 mμ. for muscle cytochrome c) or with pyridine+dithionite (absorption peaks of 'pyridine haemochromogen':

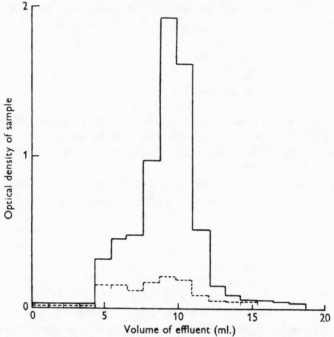

Fig. 5. Chromatography of purified cytochrome from *Desulphovibrio desulphuricans* (Hildenborough). 2 mg. cytochrome c_3 was chromatographed in phosphate buffer (pH 6·40 ± 0·02) on Amberlite XE 97 (see text), flow rate 1·1 ml./hr.; room temperature; retention volume of column 3·8 ml. Absorptions of 1·1 ml. samples at 410 and 280 mμ. (dotted lines) were plotted; R_f of cytochrome c_3 (410) = 0·38.

413, 521·5, 551·8 mμ.; compare 415, 521·8, 550·6 mμ. for muscle cytochrome c). The denatured form had no enzyme activity, and its reduced absorption spectrum at pH 7·0 had bands at 418, 552·6 and 524·9 mμ. which were indistinguishable from the native protein without special care.

Autoxidizibility. The cytochrome was apparently autoxidizible, but it was desirable to prove that this was a property of the native protein since apparent autoxidizibility might also be due to denaturation or contamination with an oxidase. The following evidence is in favour of the view that the native protein is autoxidizible: (i) enzymically active preparations were fully autoxidizible but did not react with CO; (ii) the oxidation was not affected by KCN (10^{-2} M), a powerful inhibitor of cytochrome c oxidase; (iii) no sign of a cytochrome c oxidase was detected at any stage in the purification of the cytochrome; (iv) the standard redox potential (below) was such that, on physico-chemical grounds, the reduced form was unlikely to be stable in air.

Iso-electric point. The fact that the cytochrome could be purified by ion-exchange with an ammonium Amberlite XE 97 suggested a basic iso-electric point; this was confirmed by paper electrophoresis in KH_2PO_4 buffers (0·5 %, w/v) adjusted to various pH values with 20 % (w/v) NaOH, on paper strips of 5 cm. width with the instrument setting at 2 mA./strip (potential between buffer compartments about 380 V.). At pH 6·99, 8·10, 9·23 (borate buffer) and 10·15 the protein migrated towards the cathode rather more slowly than chromatographically purified cytochrome *c* on the same strips. At pH values in the region of ten paper strips took up CO_2 with a decrease in pH value, so that a precise determination of the iso-electric point was not attempted. However, during a 2 hr. run starting at pH 10·66 (the iso-electric point of cytochrome *c*) and ending at pH 10·30 the protein migrated slowly towards the cathode together with a control spot of cytochrome *c*. Hence the iso-electric point probably lies between these values.

Redox potential. Careful reduction with $Na_2S_2O_4$ in the presence of redox dyes indicated a standard potential between that of sodium indigo disulphonate ($E'_0 = -125$ mV.) and benzylviologen ($E'_0 = -395$ mV.) and lying in the range of Janus green ($E'_0 = -225$ mV.); Ishimoto *et al.* (1954*b*) obtained a similar value with their preparation. This strongly reducing potential accounted for the failure of ascorbic acid, $K_4Fe(CN)_6$, etc., to reduce the protein, and also made impracticable the measurement of the standard redox potential by spectrophotometric procedures (e.g. Davenport & Hill, 1952) since there is no stable redox system in this range. The potential was therefore determined by potentiometric titration in O_2-free nitrogen with excess anthraquinone-2-sulphonic acid ($E'_0 = -250$ mV.), which did not absorb significantly in visible light and which poised in the appropriate potential range. Three titrations of 0·15 μU. cytochrome + 1·5 mg. anthraquinone-2-sulphonic acid in 29 ml. sodium phosphate buffer (0·34 g. ion Na^+/l.; pH 7·0 ± 0·02) at 30 ± 0·3° against $Na_2S_2O_4$ indicated a standard potential of $E'_0 = -205 ± 4$ mV.

Molecular weight. The sedimentation coefficient of a preparation of the cytochrome was determined by Dr A. G. Ogston at the Department of Biochemistry, University of Oxford. A solution of *c.* 0·5 % cytochrome in NH_4OH (0·25 M), dialysed overnight against 1000 vol. of a solution containing NaCl (0·1 M) + Na_2HPO_4 (0·0627 M) + KH_2PO_4 (0·0133 M) had a sedimentation coefficient $S_{20, w} = 1·93 \times 10^{-13} ± 2$ % (compare $1·83 \times 10^{-13}$ quoted for cytochrome *c* of 0·43 % Fe content; Paul, 1952). The sedimenting boundary seemed symmetrical, no obvious sign of heterogeneity was observed, and all the light-absorbing material appeared to be associated with the sedimenting material. This sedimentation coefficient implies a minimum possible value of 10,200 for the molecular weight, on the assumption that $f/f_0 = 1$, the particles being spherical, unhydrated and with a hydrodynamic specific volume equal to the partial specific volume taken as 0·71, the value given by Theorell (1936) for cytochrome *c*. Since most globular proteins have values of f/f_0 considerably greater than 1, the sedimentation coefficient above would be consistent with a molecular weight in the region of 13,000 (see Discussion).

Iron content. Analysis of some residues recovered from metabolic experiments indicated a high iron content (0·75 %), and a single analysis of 8·1 mg freshly chromatographed, well-dialysed cytochrome, by the o-phenenthroline procedure (Sandell, 1944) indicated an iron content of 0·92 %.

Linkage of prosthetic groups. The haemin of cytochrome c is linked to the apoprotein by thio-ether links to the porphyrin ring, as well as by co-ordination to the iron atom; as a result the molecule shows considerable thermo-stability and resistance to cleavage of its prosthetic group from the apoprotein by acids. Moreover, the molecule readily yields, with mineral acids, an ether-insoluble porphyrin in which the sulphur-containing amino acid groups remain attached to the porphyrin residue.

The bacterial cytochrome showed similar thermal and acid stability. Porphyrin was released from the oxidized form only by concentrated H_2SO_4 (bands at 404, 550·8, 593 mμ. in 2 N-HCl; HCl number, 0·05 ± 0·01 %); the reduced form was less stable and 3·3 N-HCl in the presence of $Na_2S_2O_4$, released mainly a porphyrin which was insoluble in ether + glacial acetic acid (15 %, v/v), and which had its main band at 554 mμ. (compare 553 mμ. quoted by Keilin (1933) for 'porphyrin c').

Ice-cold acetone containing 10 % (v/v) glacial acetic acid, which removes the haemin from haemoglobin, catalase, etc. (see Lewis, 1954), precipitated the bacterial cytochrome unchanged. Ice-cold acetone containing 1 ml. 5 N-H_2SO_4/50 ml. acetone did not yield an ether-soluble haemin, although the protein was converted to a brown water-soluble material from which ether-soluble haemin could be obtained by Paul's (1950) procedure. These properties all suggest that thio-ether links participate in the binding of prosthetic groups and protein in the bacterial cytochrome.

Nature of prosthetic groups. A haemin was released from the cytochrome by Paul's (1950) procedure. A typical experiment was as follows: 1 ml. chromatographed cytochrome solution (0·7 μU/ml.) was treated with 0·2 ml. glacial acetic acid and 1 ml. $AgSO_4$ (8 mg./ml.) for 30 min. at 75–80°, cooled and the haemin extracted three times into ether containing 25 % (v/v) acetic acid, dried, dissolved in KH_2PO_4 (0·5 % w/v, pH 7·0) and examined spectrophotometrically. The product had a Soret band at 390 mμ. as compared with 391 mμ. found in a control preparation of haematohaemin from cytochrome c. Pyridine haemochromes prepared from these haemins were spectroscopically closely similar: pyridine haematohaemochrome had peaks at 409, 518·5 and 546·0 mμ.; the pyridine haemochrome found from the isolated haemin of the bacterial cytochrome absorbed at 408, 517·2 and 546·0 mμ. It is interesting that, as with cytochrome c, the spectrum of the 'pyridine haemochromogen' formed directly from the protein (quoted earlier, p. 555) differed from that obtained from the separated haemin.

These observations suggested that the prosthetic groups of cytochrome c and the bacterial cytochrome were closely similar, and further evidence for this was obtained by reductive fission of the protein to porphyrin. Davenport (1952) obtained mesoporphyrin and a chlorin from cytochrome c by reduction *in vacuo* with sodium amalgam; degradation of the bacterial cytochrome in this manner gave a porphyrin spectroscopically resembling mesoporphyrin as well as a chlorin (α-band at 648 mμ. in ether, identical with a control preparation from cytochrome *c*). The wavelengths in mμ. of the absorption peaks of the porphyrin, freed of chlorin, in dioxane and in 2 N-HCl are given below:

In dioxane	Mesoporphyrin from cytochrome *c*	402, 496·5, 529·8, 566·8, 621·5
	Porphyrin from bacterial cytochrome	402, 497, 530·2, 566·5 621·5
In 2 N-HCl	Mesoporphyrin from cytochrome *c*	402, 547·5, 570·5, 590·5
	Porphyrin from bacterial cytochrome	402, 549·2, 571, 591

These observations permit the tentative conclusion that the prosthetic groups of the bacterial cytochrome are OH-substituted haematohaemins linked to the protein by thio-ether bridges as in cytochrome *c*, a view further supported by the close spectroscopic similarities of the pyridine, carboxy- and nitroso-derivatives of the two proteins (p. 555).

Metabolic function of the bacterial cytochrome

The probability that the cytochrome acted as electron carrier during the biological reduction of sulphate and related ions was investigated further by studying preparations of bacteria able to oxidize the cytochrome anaerobically with these substrates and by measuring the effect of the cytochrome on the rates of substrate reduction in hydrogen by these preparations. Owing to shortage of cytochrome the quantitative aspects of its effect on these reactions could not be studied thoroughly, but some qualitative impressions of its relative activity are recorded. A preliminary account of this work was given elsewhere (Postgate, 1955*a*).

Anaerobic cytochrome oxidation

Bacteria treated with CTAB (50 μg./mg. dry wt.) oxidized the cytochrome anaerobically with Na_2SO_3, $Na_2S_2O_3$ or $Na_2S_4O_6$, but not with Na_2SO_4, provided precautions were taken to remove sulphide continuously as in the earlier experiments with living organisms (above). In a typical experiment a suspension of 0·2 mg. CTAB-treated cells/ml. at pH 7·0 was placed in a double side-arm Thunberg tube under H_2 until all added cytochrome (5 mμU./ml.) was reduced. One side arm contained $CdCl_2$ (10 %, w/v) on filter-paper to absorb sulphide, the other contained substrate. The hydrogen was then pumped out, the substrates added *in vacuo* and the suspension examined spectroscopically. The intensities of the cytochrome bands, compared with controls without substrate or with Na_2SO_4, diminished markedly during 5 min., though the bands did not disappear entirely even after several hours.

While this work was in progress, Millet (1955) obtained a cell-free sulphite reductase from another strain of *Desulphovibrio desulphuricans*, and kindly provided instructions on how to prepare active extracts. Such preparations, made from the Hildenborough strain, contained, in addition to a sulphite reductase and hydrogenase, thiosulphate and tetrathionate reductases. Being

transparent they permitted quantitative measurement of the extent of cytochrome oxidation by sulphite, thiosulphate and tetrathionate (Table 3).
A constant percentage oxidation was reached much more slowly with Na_2SO_3
than with $Na_2S_2O_3$ or $Na_2S_4O_6$; quoted values in Table 3 are corrected for a slow
oxidation which occurred in the control tubes without substrate.

Table 3. *Anaerobic oxidation of cytochrome* c_3 *by cell-free extracts*
of Desulphovibrio desulphuricans (*Hildenborough*)

Vacuum-dried organisms were shaken with distilled water (25 mg./ml.) for 1 hr. at 37°
under N_2 and the debris removed at 15,000 *g* (15 min.). The supernatant fluids were diluted
1/3 with KH_2PO_4 (0·5 %, w/v; pH 7·0 ± 0·05) containing 25 mμU. cytochrome/ml., added
to double side-arm Thunberg tubes containing substrate in one arm and $CdCl_2$(10 %, w/v) on
filter-paper in the other. After reducing the cytochrome in H_2 the substrates were added *in
vacuo* and the optical density at 554 mμ. was measured at intervals until a constant percentage
oxidation was reached.

		Percentage oxidation of cytochrome	
Substrate	expt:	1	2
Na_2SO_3		19	14
$Na_2S_2O_3$		70·5	76
$Na_2S_4O_6$		82	84

Substrate reduction in hydrogen

CTAB released cytochrome from the bacteria. Consequently, cytochrome-
linked reactions would be expected to be inhibited by CTAB owing to dilution
of the co-factor, and the inhibition should be overcome by adding large
amounts of purified cytochrome. This approach was used to investigate the
effect of cytochrome on the reduction of substrates in hydrogen.

Thiosulphate reduction. CTAB (50 μg./mg. dry wt. organisms) prevented the
reduction of sulphate in H_2 by bacterial suspensions, but permitted slow
reduction of sodium thiosulphate. Addition of the cytochrome augmented the
reaction rate (Fig. 6), thus indicating a carrier action. FAD, DPN, TPN and
ATP had no carrier action.

Tetrathionate reduction. Similar experiments, using sodium tetrathionate
in place of thiosulphate, showed that the cytochrome acted as a carrier for
the tetrathionate reductase system (Fig. 6).

Sulphite reduction. Similar experiments, with sulphite in place of thiosulphate, showed that the cytochrome acted as a carrier in this system, but its
effect was much less marked than with thiosulphate and tetrathionate (Fig. 6).
This may be due to: (*a*) a greater requirement for cytochrome in this system;
(*b*) need for additional co-factors; (*c*) greater damage to the sulphite reductase
caused by CTAB. The latter explanation was favoured by the further observations that doubling the CTAB concentration totally inhibited the sulphite
reductase, though the thiosulphate reductase remained active. A mixture of
FAD, DPN, TPN and ATP did not augment the effect of the cytochrome.

Dithionite reduction. Sodium dithionite hydrolyses in anaerobic solution
to a mixture of thiosulphate and metabisulphite, hence the ability of the

cytochrome to act as carrier in its reduction by CTAB-treated bacteria (Fig. 6) was not unexpected. The experiment is of interest however, since it demonstrated that cytochrome augmented the reaction rate in an environment having, at least initially, a redox potential of about -350 mV. (that of a weak dithionite solution), some 150 mV. more reducing than the standard potential of the cytochrome itself.

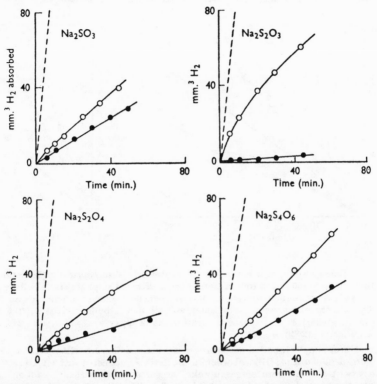

Fig. 6. Cytochrome-linked reductases in CTAB-treated *Desulphovibrio desulphuricans* (Hildenborough). Organisms (1·5 mg./vessel) were treated CTAB (50 μg./mg. dry wt. bacteria) and their ability to reduce substrates in H_2 with and without cytochrome c_3 was measured manometrically. Cytochrome: 50 mμU./ml.; vessels preincubated 1 hr. before adding c. 1 mg. substrate (dithionite added as solid); centre well: $CdCl_2$ (0·25 ml., 10 %, w/v); reaction fluid 1·25 ml. final; pH 6·9 $\pm$ 0·05; 37°, H_2 gas phase; dotted lines indicate average rates of substrate reduction without CTAB, $\bigcirc$; cytochrome; $\bullet$, without added cytochrome.

Sulphate reduction. The cytochrome did not influence the rate of reduction of sulphate in H_2 by intact bacteria. None of the following preparations reduced sulphate in hydrogen: organisms treated with CTAB, acetone-dried or vacuum-dried bacteria and soluble extracts therefrom; extracts of cells ground with Al_2O_3; hence experiments analogous to those recorded above were not undertaken. The failure of acetone-dried bacteria to reduce sulphate conflicts with a report by Sadana & Jagannathan (1954), who stated that sulphate acted as hydrogen acceptor for crude preparations of acetone-dried organisms. Indirect evidence pointing to a function in sulphate reduction is summarized later (see 'Discussion').

Oxygen reduction. The fact that the cytochrome is autoxidizible gave theoretical reasons for suspecting that the sulphate-reducing bacteria could reduce oxygen in spite of their anaerobic habit; synthesis of water from H_2/O_2 mixtures was detected and reported earlier (Postgate, 1954 *b*). The reaction took place at a maximum rate with H_2/air mixtures containing 4 % (v/v) O_2

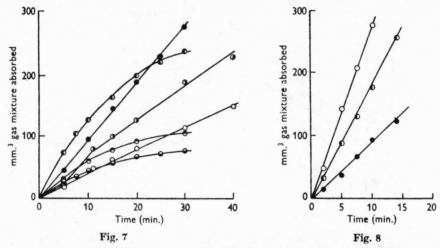

Fig. 7

Fig. 8

Fig. 7. Hydrogen-oxygen reaction in *Desulphovibrio desulphuricans* (Hildenborough). Bacteria were harvested from a lactate yeast extract + sulphate static culture and the rates of gas uptake in hydrogen-air mixtures were determined manometrically. 9·25 mg. dry wt. organisms/vessel; total fluid volume 3 ml.; buffer: KH_2PO_4 (0·5 %, w/v; pH 6·3±0·05); 37°, gas phase concentrations of O_2 (v/v): ○, 1 %; ◑, 2 % ●, 4 %; ◐, 8 %; ◓, 12 %; ◒, 16 %.

Fig. 8. Effect of cytochrome c_3 on hydrogen-oxygen reaction by CTAB treated *Desulphovibrio desulphuricans* (Hildenborough). Bacteria were treated with CTAB (100 μg./mg. dry wt.) and the rate of gas uptake measured manometrically. 4·3 mg. dry wt. organisms/vessel; fluid volume 1·5 ml.; buffer: KH_2PO_4 (0·5 %, w/v; pH 6·9±0·05). ○, without CTAB; ●, with CTAB; ◐, with CTAB + cytochrome c_3 (250 mμU./ml.).

(Fig. 7); at lower pO_2 values availability of oxygen presumably limited the reaction velocity, and at higher pO_2 values oxidation of hydrogenase inhibited the reaction. This situation is familiar in the biological aerobic oxidation of hydrogen, but the system in *Desulphovibrio desulphuricans* appears to be more sensitive to oxygen inhibition than most (compare optimal pO_2 values of 8 % for *Hydrogenomonas flavus*, Kluyver & Manten, 1942; 4–10 % for *Azotobacter vinelandii*, Wilson, Lee & Wilson, 1942; about 9 % for *Escherichia coli*, Lascelles & Still, 1946; 5–15 % for an unspecified *Hydrogenomonas* sp., Schlegel, 1953).

A remarkable feature of the H_2/O_2 reaction was that, in the optimum atmosphere of 4 % (v/v) O_2, oxygen was frequently reduced faster than sulphate. The Q_{O_2} of the control curve in Fig. 8 is −129 mm.³/mg. dry wt. organisms/hr., corresponding to an oxygen reduction rate of 5·8 μmole/mg./hr.

The mean Q_{H_2} value in several experiments with sulphate as hydrogen acceptor was -440 mm.^{3}/mg./hr., corresponding to a sulphate reduction rate of 4.9 μmole/mg./hr.

CTAB (100 μg./mg. dry wt. organisms) decreased the reaction velocity to a low value, and addition of cytochrome increased the reaction rate again (Fig. 8). Oxidation of lactate, pyruvate, fumarate and malate with O_2 as terminal H-acceptor ($N_2 + 4$ % (v/v) O_2) was demonstrated with strain Hildenborough (Postgate, 1954*b*) and strain El Agheila Z (Grossman & Postgate, 1955), but was not studied further.

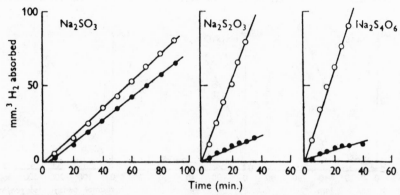

Fig. 9. Influence of cytochrome c_3 on hydrogen uptake by cell-free reductase preparations from *Desulphovibrio desulphuricans* (Hildenborough). Vacuum-dried bacteria were extracted under N_2 at $37°$ with distilled water (1 ml./25 mg.; 1 ml./50 mg. for sulphite reductase) and the supernatant fluids (0.5 ml.) used in the manometers. Fluid volume 1.5 ml.; buffer: KH_2PO_4 (0.5 %, w/v; pH 6.3 ± 0.05); centre well: $CdCl_2$ (0.25 ml., 10 %, w/v); substrates: 5 μmole; H_2 gas phase; $37°$. $\bigcirc$, with cytochrome c_3 (560 mμU./ml.; 680 mμU./ml. with sulphite reductase); $\bullet$, control without cytochrome.

Reduction by cell-free preparations. The demonstration of cytochrome-linked reductases by the use of CTAB was open to the criticism that the cytochrome may act, not as an electron carrier, but merely by reversing chemically an inhibitory effect of CTAB. It was thus desirable to demonstrate carrier action by a technique not involving CTAB.

Extracts of vacuum-dried bacteria prepared following Millet's advice reduced thiosulphate, tetrathionate or sulphite in hydrogen, unlike extracts of acetone-dried cells, which reduced only thiosulphate in these conditions. The reduction rate was augmented by addition of the bacterial cytochrome (Fig. 9). As in the experiments with CTAB-treated organisms, the effect of the cytochrome on $Na_2S_2O_3$ and $Na_2S_4O_6$ reduction was much more marked than on Na_2SO_3 reduction. The reason for this seemed most likely to be that the total sulphite-reductase content of the extracts was low since benzylviologen, which also has a cytochrome-like effect on the sulphite reductase system, did not much augment the activity of these preparations.

Cytochrome-like effect of benzylviologen. Ishimoto, Koyama & Nagai (1955) extracted a soluble thiosulphate-reductase system from their strain of *Desulphovibrio desulphuricans* which conducted the reaction: $S_2O_3'' + H_2 = SO_3'' + H_2S$, and whose reaction rate was augmented by benzyl- or methyl-viologen. Later Ishimoto & Koyama (1955) showed that their bacterial cytochrome had a similar effect on these preparations. It was of interest to see whether benzyl-viologen had a cytochrome-like effect on the major systems examined in the present work. Suspensions of CTAB-treated bacteria reduced benzylviologen with $Na_2S_2O_3$, $Na_2S_4O_6$ or Na_2SO_3, but not with Na_2SO_4. In a typical experiment a suspension of 0·33 mg. CTAB-treated bacteria/ml. at pH 7 was treated as in the comparable experiments with the bacterial cytochrome except that benzyl viologen (2 μmole/ml.) replaced the added cytochrome. The time taken to decolorize the reduced benzylviologen at 37° was noted. In contrast to

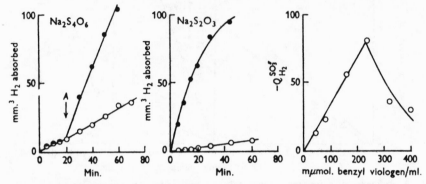

Fig. 10. Cytochrome-like effect of benzyl viologen. Organisms of *Desulphovibrio desulphuricans* (Hildenborough) were treated with CTAB (50 μg./mg. dry wt.) and the rates of hydrogen uptake in the presence of reducible substrate measured manometrically. Cell contents as for Fig. 6 except that benzylviologen replaced cytochrome c_3. With sulphite as substrate a curve illustrating the effect of benzylviologen concentration on substrate reduction rate is given; with tetrathionate the benzylviologen was tipped in after the start of the experiment (A). ●, with 200 mμmol benzylviologen/ml.; ○, control.

their behaviour with cytochrome, the suspensions re-oxidized reduced benzyl viologen completely with the substrates mentioned; re-oxidation with Na_2SO_3 was markedly slower (70 min.) than with thiosulphate (15 min.) or tetrathionate (8 min.); without substrate or with Na_2SO_4 the dye remained reduced for more than 170 min. Jebb (1949) used a somewhat similar technique to show that the 'tetrathionase' of a coliform organism re-oxidized reduced Nile blue. Benzylviologen augmented the rate of reduction of thiosulphate, tetrathionate or sulphite in hydrogen by CTAB-treated bacteria and by cell-free reductase preparations. A selection of curves illustrating this is given in Fig. 10; the findings confirm and extend those of the Japanese workers.

THE COMPOUND ABSORBING AT 630 mμ.

Concentrates of the material prepared as described always contained variable amounts of cytochrome and material insoluble in water. The material was purified further by extracting into distilled water and passing the solution through a column of cellulose coated with an aliphatic polyimine resin in the acetate form (see 'Methods'). The effluent contained cytochrome and flavo-protein, and the 630 mμ.-component remained on the column as an emerald green zone. It was eluted with sodium acetate + acetic acid buffer (5 M, pH 5·0) and dialysed against distilled water.

Properties. After prolonged dialysis, preparations of the 630 mμ.-component precipitated in the dialysis sac, but the precipitate re-dissolved, on adding traces of phosphate buffer or $NaHCO_3$, to give an emerald-green solution. This solution had the spectrum shown in Fig. 11; the Soret peak at 411 mμ. did not change in height or position on adding dithionite, indicating that the material was free from cytochrome; there was an inflexion at c. 390 mμ., a minor peak at 585 mμ. and a strong peak at 632·5 ± 0·2 mμ. Paper electro-

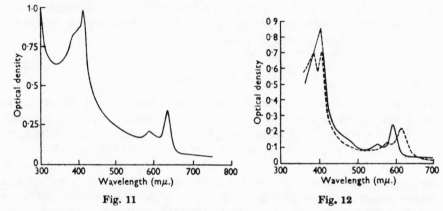

Fig. 11   Fig. 12

Fig. 11. Spectrum of chromatographed '630 mμ.-component'. Readings taken at 1 mμ. intervals at the Soret peak, 2·5 mμ. at α-peak, 5 mμ. at β-peak, 10 mμ. elsewhere. Protein in KH_2PO_4 (0·5 %, w/v; pH 7·0 ± 0·05); 20°.

Fig. 12. Spectra of chromophore from '630 mμ.-component'. Spectra obtained after chromatography on 'Florisil' (see text). ——, in acetic acid (0·1 N); - - - -, in HCl (N). Readings every 1 mμ. at Soret peaks, 2·5 mμ. at visible peaks, 10 mμ. elsewhere.

phoresis showed an iso-electric point on the acid side of pH 7·0. On heating above 70° or treatment with acid to pH < 4 or alkali to pH > 9 the 630 mμ.-band shifted towards the green and the solution fluoresced red in ultraviolet light (365 mμ.). No evidence for formation of a pyridine haemochrome was obtained; the main visible band moved to 595 mμ. with alkali with or without pyridine and/or dithionite.

Chromophoric group. The red fluorescent material was readily photo-oxidized with loss of fluorescence, and had to be handled in the dark, where it survived 3 min. in contact with warm conc. H_2SO_4. It was slightly soluble in ether containing 15 % (v/v) glacial acetic acid, but was not extracted quantitatively from aqueous solution with this mixture; it returned to the aqueous phase on shaking with distilled water. It was chromatographed in the dark on paper in 5 % (w/v) Na_2HPO_4, running as a single spot of $R_f = 0·74$ (20°). The chromophore was also adsorbed as a blue-green band from acid solution by 'Florisil' and was eluted with aqueous pyridine (1 % v/v) as a pink-brown solution with an intense red fluorescence; with dilute mineral acids the colour changed to blue-green and the fluorescence became more purple. The spectra of preparations obtained in this fashion depended on the pH value of the solution (Fig. 12). Both acid and neutral forms showed their major visible absorption peak in the red, unlike a simple aetioporphyrin; the absorption peaks lay at 404, 594·5 and 551·0 mμ. (alkaline or neutral) and 385, 404, 575·0 and 613·5 (N-HCl). The position and height of the double Soret peak of the acid form were unchanged in 2 N-HCl. A neutral spectrum of this material was not successfully obtained owing to its insolubility in organic solvents.

The chromophore was also observed by its fluorescence in old cultures that had become alkaline owing to loss of H$_2$S from the medium. Red fluorescence in u.v. light after adding NaOH to a culture was a sensitive test for the presence of the 630 mμ.-component in various strains. The chromophore was undoubtedly responsible for the shading at 595 mμ. sometimes observed in the spectrum of washed bacterial suspensions.

OTHER PIGMENTS

The spectrum of crude extracts of acetone-dried organisms showed a hump at about 450 mμ. which disappeared on adding dithionite or on passing in hydrogen; simultaneously the extracts ceased to fluoresce yellow in ultraviolet light, a change characteristic of flavins. Protein was removed from such extracts with TCA (4 %, w/v), the TCA was removed by extraction of the tri-n-octylamine salt into chloroform (Hughes & Williamson, 1951), and the extracts concentrated and chromatographed in the dark on paper in n-butanol/acetic acid/water (4 : 1 : 5) or aqueous Na$_2$HPO$_4$ (5 %, w/v). The chromatograms indicated the presence of FAD, FMN and traces of riboflavin. An examination of freshly harvested *Desulphovibrio desulphuricans* was undertaken by Dr J. L. Peel, who showed that the Hildenborough strain has a low flavin content compared with most other anaerobes he has examined, but an unusually high ratio of FAD to FMN; the riboflavin observed was probably an artefact of the acetone-drying procedure; Dr Peel's results are reported elsewhere (Peel, 1955). As would be expected, these flavins exist in the normal cell as conjugates, since CTAB at concentrations able to release cytochrome into the medium released no flavin. No evidence was obtained for association of flavin with the cytochrome, unlike the cytochrome b_2-lactic dehydrogenase system of Appleby & Morton (1954).

DISCUSSION

The cytochrome. Table 4 lists the properties of a number of cytochromes which have an α-peak within 1 mμ. of that of the cytochrome described here, and shows that it is not identical with any of them. It may be identical with a degradation product of heart muscle cytochrome b (Hübscher, Kiese & Nicolas, 1954), but insufficient published data are available to judge. Hence the systematic name 'Desulphovibrio desulphuricans cytochrome 553' should be applied to the material studied here (see Scarisbrick, 1947), but since this name is cumbersome and does not bring out its relation to muscle cytochrome c, the trivial name of cytochrome c_3 has been adopted.

The relationship to cytochrome c may be summarized: c_3 is thermostable, soluble, has firm chemical linkings between the haemin and apoprotein and is strongly basic. It differs mainly in (a) its low redox potential and consequent autoxidizibility; (b) its different metabolic function; (c) details of its spectrum.

Table 4. *Some properties which distinguish various cytochromes from that present in* Desulphovibrio desulphuricans ('*cytochrome c_3*')

Pigment	Reference	Source	Major distinctive properties
Cytochrome c_1 (e)	1	Heart muscle	Thermolabile, not autoxidizible
Cytochrome f	2	Green leaves	Not autoxidizible, positive E_0'
Cytochrome b_4	3	Halotolerant bacterium	Not autoxidizible, acid iso-electric point
'*Chlorobium limicola* cytochrome 553'	4, 5	*C. limicola*	Not autoxidizible, positive E_0'
'*Acetobacter suboxydans* cytochrome 554'	6	*A. suboxydans*	Insoluble, not autoxidizible
'Hemoprotein 554'	7	Heart muscle	Positive redox potential
'*Chromatium*' cytochrome	8	*Chromatium* 'D'	High m.w., limited pH stability
Cytochrome c_3	—	*D. desulphuricans*	Thermostable, low m.w., soluble, autoxidizible, negative E_0', basic iso-electric point

References: 1, Keilin & Hartree (1955); 2, Davenport & Hill (1952); 3, Egami *et al.* (1953); 4, Kamen & Vernon (1954a); 5, Gibson & Larsen (1955); 6, Smith (1954), also personal communication; 7, Widmer *et al.* (1954); 8, Newton & Kamen (1955).

A further difference from cytochrome c may be noted. The specific extinction coefficient of ferrocytochrome c at 550 mμ. is about 2·1, whereas $\epsilon_{sp.}$ for cytochrome c_3 at 553 is about double this (4·2). Since the molecular weights of cytochromes c and c_3 are of a similar order, it follows that c_3 has two haemin groups/molecule. This view is confirmed by the high iron content (0·92 %) of c_3, more than twice that of the purest c recorded (see Paul, 1952).

Though c_3 can act as carrier in reactions in which oxygen is terminal hydrogen acceptor, the strictly anaerobic character of these bacteria emphasized by Grossman & Postgate (1953a) leaves little doubt that these reactions are of limited metabolic significance and merely reflect the low redox potential of c_3. Such reactions might, however, provide a mechanism by which the organism could remove traces of O_2 from its environment since O_2, while not lethal, prevents growth and sulphate reduction. The absence of inhibition by KCN, CO, etc. indicates that no ordinary cytochrome c oxidase is present, and the presence of a cytochrome c oxidase insensitive to cyanide like that of *Myrothecium verrucaria* (Darby & Goddard, 1950) is excluded since neither suspensions nor preparations of the strain studied here oxidized reduced cytochrome c. However, though no preparation has been obtained in which a linkage between cytochrome c_3 and sulphate reduction could be demonstrated directly, difference spectra, the effect of sulphate antagonists, and the demonstration of a role in the reduction of sulphite (the one established intermediate; Millet, 1955) makes such a function plausible. The sulphite-, thiosulphate-, and tetrathionate-reductases of *Desulphovibrio desulphuricans* perform a metabolic function analogous to the cytochrome c oxidase of aerobes; it seems probable, but is not proven, that the sulphate-reductase acts similarly. A cytochrome of the b group may perform a similar function in nitrate reduction by *Escherichia coli* (Sato & Egami, 1949) and *Pseudomonas stutzeri* (Allen & van Niel, 1952); a cytochrome of the c group is involved in the oxidation of nitrite by *Nitrobacter* spp. (Lees & Simpson, 1955) and in the reduction of nitrate by various denitrifying bacteria (Verhoeven & Takeda, 1956) and *Thiobacillus denitrificans* (Baalsrud & Baalsrud, 1954; Dr S. Elsden, personal communication). Cytochrome c is concerned in the oxidation of sulphite to sulphate by plant mitochondria (Tager & Rautanen, 1956). The failure to obtain preparations of sulphate-reducing bacteria able to reduce sulphate in hydrogen may be due to (*a*) need for a second co-factor in the sulphate→sulphite step, (*b*) chemical instability on the part of the sulphate reductase or (*c*) need for coupled reactions, perhaps yielding energy, in the primary attack on sulphate which are sensitive to CTAB.

The E'_0 of cytochrome c_3 of -205 mV. is related to the free energy of its oxidation at pH 7·0. This may be written

$$\underset{\text{M}}{Fe_2^{+++++}} + \underset{10^{-7}\,\text{M}}{2H^+} = \underset{\text{M}}{Fe_2^{++++++}} + \underset{\text{atm.}}{H_2}; \quad \Delta G'_1 = -9{,}500 \text{ cal.} \tag{1}$$

The free energy of reduction of sulphate by these bacteria may be calculated from standard free energy data (Rossini, Wagman, Evans, Levine & Jaffe, 1952)

$$\underset{\text{M}}{SO_4''} + \underset{\text{atm.}}{4H_2} = \underset{\text{M}}{S''} + \underset{\text{liq.}}{4H_2O}; \quad \Delta G'_2 = -29{,}660 \text{ cal.} \tag{2}$$

but at pH 7·0 the sulphide ion is largely hydrolysed to $HS' + H_2S$. Using the two dissociation constants of H_2S (Hodgman, 1949) one can evaluate a correction for this:

$$\underset{\text{M}}{S''} + \underset{10^{-7}\,\text{M}}{H^+} = \underset{}{S''} + \underset{\underbrace{HS' + H_2S}_{\text{M}}}{}; \quad \Delta G'_3 = -11{,}500 \text{ cal.} \tag{3}$$

The oxidation of reduced cytochrome c_3 by sulphate at pH 7 can be written

$$SO_4'' + 4\,Fe_2^{+++++} + 8H^+ \rightarrow (S'' + HS' + H_2S) + 4\,Fe_2^{++++++} + 4H_2O, \tag{4}$$

and free energy change in this reaction (ΔG_4) is given by

$$\Delta G'_4 = \Delta G'_2 + \Delta G'_3 - 4\,\Delta G'_1 = -3{,}460 \text{ cal./mole } SO_4'' \text{ or } -865 \text{ cal./mol } c_3.$$

Thus the oxidation of cytochrome c_3 with sulphate would provide a net energy yield. The point can be expressed differently by calculating the redox potential corresponding to the reduction of sulphate in H_2 at pH 7·0 from the free energies of reactions (2) and (3), and observing that the value, $E'_0 = -188$ mV., is less negative than E'_0 of c_3 (-205 mV.).

The failure to observe complete oxidation of c_3 by sulphate and other ions, in contrast to benzy viologen, could be because sulphide was incompletely removed from solution in the test conditions, with the result that sufficient remained in solution to hold some cytochrome reduced. This explanation is unlikely, however, since the percentage oxidations quoted in Table 3 should then be independent of the substrate, which they are not. The phenomenon might be accounted for if the E_0' values of the reductions of sulphite, thiosulphate, etc., were of an order similar to that of c_3; the ions would then come to redox equilibrium with c_3 rather than oxidize it completely. If $\Delta G'$ values at pH 7 are calculated for the reductions of sulphite, thiosulphate and tetrathionate (ΔG° for S_2O_3'' obtained from Mel, 1954), in the manner used above for sulphate, and the values are converted to potentials, the quantities below are obtained:

$$SO_3'' + 3H_2 = S'' + 3H_2O; \qquad \Delta G' = -43{,}700 \text{ cal.}; \qquad E_0' = -96 \text{ mV., (5)}$$

$$S_2O_3'' + 4H_2 = S'' + H_2S + 3H_2O; \qquad \Delta G' = -46{,}340 \text{ cal.}; \qquad E_0' = -162 \text{ mV., (6)}$$

$$S_4O_6'' + 9H_2 = S'' + 3H_2S + 6H_2O; \qquad \Delta G' = -107{,}600 \text{ cal.}; \qquad E_0' = -152 \text{ mV. (7)}$$

These potentials do not lie in the order necessary to account for the results in Table 3; hence no simple thermodynamic formulation of the reactions involved will account for the phenomenon.

The low E_0' values of cytochrome c_3 and of the reduction of sulphate, sulphite, etc., are consistent with the strictly anaerobic habit of these bacteria. Starkey & Wight (1945) showed that the initiation of growth of sulphate-reducing bacteria was accompanied by a decrease in redox potential of the environment to below -200 mV.; ZoBell & Rittenberg (1948) quoted an E value of -100 to -300 mV. as being most favourable to growth of marine strains; Stárka (1951) showed that the ripening of medicinal muds, attributed to thermophilic strains of *Desulphovibrio*, was associated with a decline of E_0' value to between -200 and -300 mV.; Grossman & Postgate (1953a, b) showed that small inocula did not multiply unless the medium was supplemented with Na_2S or cysteine, which would bring the redox potential into this range. Clearly, then, one can regard *D. desulphuricans* as an organism which conducts oxidative reactions at the strongly reducing potential of about -200 mV.

The presence of c_3 in *Desulphovibrio desulphuricans* accounts, at least partly, for the iron requirement first demonstrated by Butlin, Adams & Thomas (1949). The fact that cytochrome c_3 is present in relatively large amounts (a typical content of 0.22 μU. cytochrome c_3/g. dry wt. organisms, observed spectroscopically by Barer's procedure, corresponds to a c_3 content of about 3 mg./g.; i.e. 0.3% of the air-dry bacterial mass) and is very easily extracted and purified, makes it surprising that c_3 was not observed earlier. The explanation must lie in (*a*) the convention of growing *D. desulphuricans* in the presence of excess ferrous salts, thus producing a spectroscopically impenetrable black mass of bacteria and FeS; (*b*) the relative difficulty of obtaining and maintaining pure cultures of these bacteria; (*c*) the low yields obtained in even the best batch cultures; (*d*) the belief, supported by earlier studies among the clostridia, that looking for cytochromes in obligate anaerobes was a waste of time.

The 630 *mμ.-component.* This pigment, though a protein, is clearly not a cytochrome in the conventional sense of the word, and the spectroscopic resemblance to cytochrome a_2 is misleading. The present work provides no clue to its metabolic function. Oxidation and reduction lead to no spectroscopic change; there is no obvious reaction with CO, KCN or NaN$_3$ and no compound that can be definitely classed as a haemochrome was observed, in contrast to the report of Ishimoto *et al.* (1954*b*). The name 'desulphoviridin' is proposed for this pigment. It appears to be a simple porphyro-protein since heat, acid or alkali treatment all yield the same product: the fluorescent photo-oxidizible chromophoric group. Verhoeven & Takeda (1956) obtained a blue protein which absorbed at 600–630 mμ. from *Pseudomonas aeruginosa* during the isolation of the cytochrome concerned in nitrate reduction; but Verhoeven's pigment is clearly different from desulphoviridin since it has little absorption in the region of 411 mμ., where desulphoviridin absorbs strongly. The chromophoric group of desulphoviridin is clearly a porphyrin-like compound since it survives contact with conc. H$_2$SO$_4$; a fluorescent metallo-porphyrin such as chlorophyll, or a metallo-bile pigment such as the red fluorescent zinc derivatives, would lose their metal in these conditions. The character of the chromophore has not been established; the type of spectrum in aqueous media was reminiscent of that of a chlorin, but the high solubility in water, which prevented a neutral spectrum being obtained, is quite uncharacteristic, because the HCl numbers of chlorin lie in the region of 15–20 %. The properties so far established would not be inconsistent with a highly carboxylated chlorin structure but are insufficient to allow a definite conclusion.

The author wishes to record his indebtedness to the very large number of authorities who have discussed this work with him and made helpful suggestions. Particularly is he grateful to Professor D. D. Woods; Dr June Lascelles (who first observed cytochrome c_3); Professor Keilin and Dr Hartree; Dr N. K. Boardman; Dr J. E. Falk; Dr K. G. Paul; Dr R. Barer; Dr Lucile Smith; Dr A. G. Ogston, all of whom spared him considerable time to discuss various points. Errors and misinterpretations are, however, the author's own. He is also indebted to Dr M. Ishimoto, Dr Jacqueline Millet and Dr W. Verhoeven for giving him access to unpublished material, and to Mr P. S. S. Dawson and his colleagues in the author's laboratory for supplying large quantities of centrifuged bacteria. This paper is published by permission of the Director, Chemical Research Laboratory.

REFERENCES

ALLEN, M. B. & VAN NIEL, C. B. (1952). Experiments on bacterial denitrification. *J. Bact.* **64**, 397.

APPLEBY, C. A. & MORTON, R. K. (1954). Crystalline cytochrome b_2 and lactic dehydrogenase of yeast. *Nature, Lond.* **175**, 749.

BAALSRUD, K. & BAALSRUD, K. S. (1954). Studies on *Thiobacillus denitrificans. Arch. Mikrobiol.* **20**, 41.

BARER, R. (1955). Spectrophotometry of clarified cell suspensions. *Science,* **121**, 709.

BOARDMAN, N. K. & PARTRIDGE, S. M. (1955). Separation of neutral proteins on ion-exchange resins. *Biochem. J.* **59**, 543.

BUTLIN, K. R., ADAMS, M. E. & THOMAS, M. (1949). The isolation and cultivation of sulphate-reducing bacteria. *J. gen. Microbiol.* **3**, 46.

BUTLIN, K. R. & POSTGATE, J. R. (1953). Microbial formation of sulphide and sulphur. *Microbial Metabolism, Symp. 6th Congr. int. Microbiol.* p. 126.

CHANCE, B. (1954). Spectrophotometry of intercellular respiratory pigments. *Science*, 120, 767.

DARBY, R. T. & GODDARD, D. R. (1950). The effects of cytochrome oxidase inhibition on the cytochrome oxidase and respiration of the fungus *Myrothrecium verrucaria*. *Physiol. Plant.* 3, 453.

DAVENPORT, H. E. (1952). Reductive cleavage of cytochrome *c*. *Nature, Lond.* 169, 75.

DAVENPORT, H. E. & HILL, R. (1952). The preparation and some properties of cytochrome *f*. *Proc. roy. Soc.* B, 139, 327.

EGAMI, F., ITAHASHI, M., SATO, R. & MORI, T. (1953). A cytochrome from halotolerant bacteria. *J. Biochem., Tokyo*, 40, 527.

GIBSON, J. & LARSEN, H. (1955). Cytochromes from *Chlorobium thiosulphatophilum*. *Biochem. J.* 60, 27.

GROSSMAN, J. P. & POSTGATE, J. R. (1953a). The cultivation of sulphate-reducing bacteria. *Nature, Lond.* 171, 600.

GROSSMAN, J. P. & POSTGATE, J. R. (1953b). The estimation of sulphate-reducing bacteria. *Proc. Soc. appl. Bact.* 16, 1.

GROSSMAN, J. P. & POSTGATE, J. R. (1955). The metabolism of malate and certain other compounds by *Desulphovibrio desulphuricans*. *J. gen. Microbiol.* 12, 429.

HODGMAN, C. D. (1949). *Handbook of Chemistry and Physics.* Chemical Rubber Publishing Co., Cleveland, Ohio, U.S.A.

HÜBSCHER, G., KIESE, M., NICOLAS, R. (1954). Untersuchungen über Cytochrome. III. Cytochrom *b* aus Rinderherzen. *Biochem. Z.* 325, 223.

HUGHES, D. E. & WILLIAMSON, D. H. (1951). Removal of acids by trioctylamine from samples for microbiology assay. *Biochem. J.* 48, 487.

ISHIMOTO, M. & KOYAMA, J. (1955). On the role of a cytochrome in thiosulfate reduction by sulphate-reducing bacteria. *Bull. chem. Soc. Japan*, 28, 231.

ISHIMOTO, M., KOYAMA, J. & NAGAI, Y. (1954a). A cytochrome and a green pigment of sulfate-reducing bacteria. *Bull. chem. Soc. Japan*, 27, 565.

ISHIMOTO, M., KOYAMA, J. & NAGAI, Y. (1954b). Biochemical studies on sulfate-reducing bacteria. IV. *J. Biochem., Tokyo*, 41, 763.

ISHIMOTO, M., KOYAMA, J. & NAGAI, Y. (1955). Biochemical studies on sulfate-reducing bacteria. V. *J. Biochem., Tokyo*, 42, 41.

JEBB, W. H. H. (1949). The use of Nile blue in the study of tetrathionase activity. *J. gen. Microbiol.* 3, 112.

KAMEN, M. D. & VERNON, L. P. (1954a). Existence of haem compounds in a photosynthetic obligate anaerobe. *J. Bact.* 67, 617.

KAMEN, M. D. & VERNON, L. P. (1954b). Enzymatic activities affecting cytochromes in photosynthetic bacteria. *J. biol. Chem.* 211, 663.

KEILIN, D. (1933). Cytochrome and intracellular respiratory enzymes. *Ergebn. Enzymforsch.* 2, 239.

KEILIN, D. & HARTREE, E. F. (1945). The purification and properties of cytochrome *c*. *Biochem. J.* 39, 289.

KEILIN, D. & HARTREE, E. F. (1955). Relationship between certain components of the cytochrome system. *Nature, Lond.* 176, 200.

KEILIN, D. & SLATER, E. C. (1953). Cytochrome. *Brit. med. Bull.* 9, 89.

KLUYVER, A. J. & MANTEN, A. A. (1942). Some observations on the metabolism of bacteria oxidizing molecular hydrogen. *Leeuwenhoek J. Microbiol. Serol.* 8, 71.

LASCELLES, J. & STILL, J. L. (1946). Utilization of molecular hydrogen by bacteria. *Aust. J. exp. Biol. med. Sci.* 24, 37.

LEES, H. & SIMPSON, J. R. (1955). The use of cyanate and chlorate in studies on the relation between the nitrite oxidation and the reduction of a cytochrome system in *Nitrobacter*. *Biochem. J.* 59, 16.

LEMBERG, R. & LEGGE, J. W. (1949). *Hematin Compounds and Bile Pigments*. New York, U.S.A.: Interscience Publishers Inc.

LEWIS, H. J. (1954). Acid cleavage of heme proteins. *J. biol. Chem.* **206**, 109.

MEL, H. C. (1954). Chemical thermodynamics of aqueous thiosulfate and bromate ions. *Chem. Abstr.* **48**, 6228.

MILLET, J. (1955). Le sulphite comme intermédiaire dans la réduction du sulfate par *Desulphovibrio desulphuricans*. *C.R. Acad. Sci., Paris*, **240**, 253.

NEWTON, J. W. & KAMEN, M. (1955). *Chromatium* cytochrome. *Arch. Biochem. Biophys.* **58**, 247.

PAUL, K.-G. (1950). The splitting with silver salts of the cysteine and porphyrin bonds in cytochrome *c*. *Acta chem. scand.* **4**, 239.

PAUL, K.-G. (1952). Iron-containing enzymes. A. Cytochromes. In *The Enzymes* (ed. Summer, J. B. & Myrbäck, K.) **2**, 357. New York: Academic Press.

PEEL, J. L. (1955). The flavins of some micro-organisms. *J. gen. Microbiol.* **12**, ii.

POSTGATE, J. R. (1949). Competitive inhibition of sulphate reduction by selenate. *Nature, Lond.* **164**, 670.

POSTGATE, J. R. (1951*a*). On the nutrition of *Desulphovibrio desulphuricans*. *J. gen. Microbiol.* **5**, 714.

POSTGATE, J. R. (1951*b*). The reduction of sulphur compounds by *Desulphovibrio desulphuricans*. *J. gen. Microbiol.* **5**, 725.

POSTGATE, J. R. (1952). Competitive and non-competitive inhibitors of bacterial sulphate reduction. *J. gen. Microbiol.* **6**, 128.

POSTGATE, J. R. (1953). On the nutrition of *Desulphovibrio desulphuricans*: a correction. *J. gen. Microbiol.* **9**, 440.

POSTGATE, J. R. (1954*a*). Presence of cytochrome in an obligate anaerobe. *Biochem. J.* **56**, xi.

POSTGATE, J. R. (1954*b*). Dependence of sulphate reduction and oxygen utilization on a cytochrome in *Desulphovibrio*. *Biochem. J.* **58**, ix.

POSTGATE, J. R. (1955*a*). Cytochrome-linked bacterial reduction of sulphite and related ions. *Abs. 3rd Int. Congr. Biochem.* (10–39), p. 94.

POSTGATE, J. R. (1955*b*). Cytochrome c_3, a bifunctional haematohaematin. *Biochim. biophys. Acta*, **18**, 427.

REPORT (1953). *Chemistry Research 1952. Rep. Chem. Res. Bd. Lond.*

REPORT (1954). *Chemistry Research 1953. Rep. Chem. Res. Bd. Lond.*

ROSSINI, F. D., WAGMAN, D. D., EVANS, W. H., LEVINE, S. & JAFFE, I. (1952). Selected values of chemical thermodynamic properties. *Circ. U.S. Bur. Stand.* no. 500.

SADANA, J. C. & JAGANNATHAN, V. (1954). Purification of hydrogenase from *Desulphovibrio desulphuricans*. *Biochim. biophys. Acta*, **14**, 287.

SALTON, M. R. J. (1951). The adsorption of cetyltrimethylammonium bromide by bacteria, its action in releasing cellular constituents and its bactericidal effects. *J. gen. Microbiol.* **5**, 391.

SANDELL, E. B. (1944). *Colorimetric Determination of Traces of Metals*. New York, U.S.A.: Interscience Publishers, Inc.

SATO, R. & EGAMI, F. (1949). Nitrate reductase, III. *Bull. chem. Soc., Japan*, **22**, 137.

SCARISBRICK, R. (1947). Haematin compounds in plants. *Rep. Progr. Chem.* **44**, 226.

SCHAEFFER, P. & NISMAN, B. (1952). Recherches sur le métabolisme des cytochromes et des porphyrines. Cas des bactéries anaérobies strictes. *Ann. Inst. Pasteur*, **82**, 109.

SCHLEGEL, H-G. (1953). Physiologische Untersuchungen an Wasserstoffoxydierenden Bakterien. *Arch. Mikrobiol.* **18**, 362.

SMITH, L. (1954). Bacterial cytochromes. Difference Spectra. *Arch. Biochem. Biophys.* **50**, 299.

STÁRKA, J. (1951). Nové poznatky o mikrobiálni redukci sulfátů při vzniku léčivého bahna. *Biol. listy*, **32**, 108.

STARKEY, R. L. & WIGHT, K. M. (1945). *Anaerobic Corrosion of Iron in Soil.* New York, U.S.A.: Amer. Gas Assoc.

TAGER, J. M. & RAUTANEN, N. (1955). Sulphite oxidation by a plant mitochondrial system. *Biochim. biophys. Acta*, **18**, 111.

THEORELL, H. (1936). Reines Cytochrom *c*. II. *Biochem. Z.* **285**, 207.

THEORELL, H. (1948). A comment on the absorption bands of ferricytochrome *c*. *Arch. Biochem.* **17**, 359.

THEORELL, H. & AKESSON, A. (1941). Studies on cytochrome *c*. II. The optical properties of pure cytochrome *c* and some of its derivatives. *J. Amer. chem. Soc.* **63**, 1812.

VERHOEVEN, W. & TAKEDA, Y. (1956). Bacterial cytochrome *c* and denitrification. *J. Bact.* (in the Press).

VERNON, D. & KAMEN, M. D. (1954). Hematin compounds in photosynthetic bacteria. *J. biol. Chem.* **211**, 643.

WIDMER, C., CLARK, H. W., NEUFELD, H. A. & STOTZ, E. (1954). Components of the soluble SC factor preparation. *J. biol. Chem.* **210**, 861.

WILSON, J. P., LEE, S. B. & WILSON, P. W. (1942). Mechanism of biological nitrogen fixation. IX. *J. biol. Chem.* **144**, 265.

ZOBELL, C. E. & RITTENBERG, S. C. (1948). Sulphate-reducing bacteria in marine sediments. *J. mar. Res.* **7**, 602.

5

Reprinted from *J. Biol. Chem.* **230**:41–64 (1958)

ON THE NEW HEME PROTEIN OF FACULTATIVE
PHOTOHETEROTROPHS*

By ROBERT G. BARTSCH[†][‡] AND MARTIN D. KAMEN[‡]

(From the Edward Mallinckrodt Institute of Radiology, Washington University School of Medicine, St. Louis, Missouri)

(Received for publication, June 24, 1957)

Vernon and Kamen (1, 2) demonstrated the existence of a new type of heme protein in TCA[1] extracts prepared from cell suspensions of the facultative photoheterotrophs, *Rhodospirillum rubrum* and *Rhodopseudomonas spheroides*. They noted that this new heme protein presented an anomaly in exhibiting spectrochemical properties of a myoglobin-like protein on the one hand and the thermal stability and hemochromogen reactions of a cytochrome *c* on the other. They also showed that the purified protein could be reduced by mammalian, DPNH-linked, cytochrome *c* reductase as prepared by Mahler *et al.* (3). This property, together with its autoxidizability and reactivity with carbon monoxide, suggested that it might function as a terminal oxidase.

Hill and Kamen[2] confirmed and extended these observations and ascribed to the new protein a structure in which the prosthetic heme group was bound by thio ether linkages to alkyl side chains as in cytochrome *c*, although possessing a free or loose linkage at the central iron as in myoglobin. They also showed that it had the peculiar property of reversibly binding *only* carbon monoxide and not at all any of the other usually effective reagents, such as azide, cyanide, hydrosulfide, oxygen, 4-methylimidazole, etc. They proposed that the new protein be called "RHP" (abbreviation for *Rhodospirillum*, or *Rhodopseudomonas*, heme protein). This name will be used in the present paper, although it appears that similar proteins exist in a number of bacterial species other than the facultative photoheterotrophs (1, 2, 4).

In none of the researches described was it possible to work with prepara-

* This work was supported by grants from the Charles F. Kettering Foundation, the National Science Foundation, and the Linde Air Products Company. One of us (M. D. K.) gratefully acknowledges tenure of a fellowship awarded by the John Simon Guggenheim Memorial Foundation during 1956.

† Research Associate, Linde Air Products Company.

‡ Present address, Graduate Department of Biochemistry, Brandeis University, Waltham, Massachusetts.

[1] The following abbreviations are used throughout: TCA, trichloroacetic acid; DPN, DPNH, oxidized and reduced diphosphopyridine nucleotide; Tris, tris(hydroxymethyl)aminomethane.

[2] R. Hill and M. D. Kamen, unpublished observations. See also footnote 8.

tions completely free from traces of the bacterial cytochrome c, nor could the purity of the samples used be determined precisely. Recently, we have developed new methods of extraction and purification. These, together with large scale production of *R. rubrum*, have made available sufficient crude proteins (approximately 250 to 500 mg.) so that highly purified samples, electrophoretically homogeneous and free from cytochrome c, could be obtained in amounts up to 50 mg. With this material we have investigated in more detail some of the important physicochemical properties of RHP.

Methods

Bacterial Culture—The medium[3] used for the photoheterotrophic growth of *R. rubrum* contained the following: malic acid 2.7 gm., L-glutamic acid 1.0 gm., sodium acetate·3H$_2$O 1.0 gm., ammonium sulfate 1.0 gm., dipotassium phosphate 3.5 gm., magnesium chloride·7H$_2$O 0.2 gm., calcium chloride 0.05 gm., nicotinic acid 1 mg., thiamine·HCl 0.5 mg., biotin 0.01 mg., neutral red indicator 0.1 mg., metal solution[4] 0.25 ml., tap water 1000 ml.

The acidic medium contained in Pyrex bottles (9 to 20 liter capacity) was autoclaved, cooled, and neutralized to neutral red end point by the addition of sterile 4 M sodium hydroxide solution, of which approximately 12 ml. per liter were required. Approximately 10 per cent (v/v) inoculum of a 24 to 48 hour-old culture was then added and any remaining space in the bottles was filled with sterile tap water. The culture bottles were finally sealed with rubber stoppers which were tied in place with strips of cloth.

The cultures were illuminated by a bank of 200 watt incandescent lamps which provided about 300 foot candles at the nearest surface of the culture bottles. Electric fans were used for cooling. After 7 to 10 days of incubation in the light, the bacteria were collected by centrifugation in a Sharples supercentrifuge. The cell mass was frozen and stored at −15°. After sufficient material was collected, it was thawed, suspended in an equal volume of water to make a thick cream, distributed into flasks, frozen, and dried by lyophilization. The dried bacterial mass was then fragmented into a powder with the aid of a high speed blender and the powder was stored at room temperature in tightly covered polyethylene containers. Usually 200 to 300 liters of culture were grown at one time

[3] The procedure used is essentially the same as one suggested to us by Dr. R. Y. Stanier.

[4] The metal stock solution contained per liter of final volume the following: disodium ethylenediaminetetraacetate (25 gm.), ZnSO$_4$·7H$_2$O (21 gm.), FeSO$_4$·7H$_2$O (28 gm.), MnSO$_4$·1H$_2$O (3 gm.), CuSO$_4$·5H$_2$O (0.8 gm.), Co(NO$_3$)$_2$·6H$_2$O (0.5 gm.), Na$_2$B$_4$O$_7$·10H$_2$O (0.34 gm.), (NH$_4$)$_6$Mo$_7$O$_{24}$·4H$_2$O (0.4 gm.).

and from these mass cultures about 1 gm. of dry bacteria per liter of culture medium was routinely obtained.

Physical Measurements[5]—The sedimentation velocity constant s was determined in the Spinco analytical centrifuge with the procedure and calibrations described by Taylor (5). A synthetic boundary cell was used. The diffusion constant D was measured in a Klett electrophoresis apparatus by the procedure of Taylor and Lowry (6). All measurements of s and D were corrected for temperature and viscosity of medium (6) to give $s_{20,w}$ and $D_{20,w}$. The partial specific volume was found by a modification (6) of the original gradient tube procedure (7).

Electrometric titrations were performed by using the ferric-ferrous oxalate system, as described in the literature (8, 9).

The iron content of the protein was determined with 1,10-phenanthroline after wet ashing with nitric acid as described by Sandell (10). The well known procedure based on wet ashing with alkaline hydrogen peroxide (11) did not appear to be applicable to RHP. The reason for this is not known.

Spectra were obtained with either the Beckman DU spectrophotometer or the Cary spectrophotometers, model 11 or 14. All spectra shown in this report were recorded with model 14.

Isolation and Purification Procedures
General Remarks

The original method involving the classical Keilin-Hartree extraction with warm TCA of washed tissue was employed in early studies (1) before the existence of RHP was suspected and when a rapid extraction of cytochrome c only was desired. It was known, however, that TCA extraction was characterized by frequent low yields and excessive denaturation of both cytochrome c and RHP. Hence, it was quickly abandoned in favor of less drastic procedures, such as sonic disintegration combined with phosphate extraction in the cold, cold extraction of acetone powders with various buffers, mechanical disruption with blenders, etc. In all these procedures, RHP invariably was found associated with the bacterial cytochrome c in the soluble phase.

Further experience showed that, while the two heme proteins differed appreciably in electrophoretic and solubility characteristics, their separation from each other on a bulk scale was tedious. Hence, there appeared to be considerable advantage accruing to methods by which one or the

[5] We are indebted to Miss Carmelita Lowry, Department of Biochemistry, Washington University School of Medicine, for performing experiments on the electrophoretic, sedimentation, and diffusion properties of RHP. A Cary spectrophotometer, model 11, in the Department of Chemistry, was made available by Professor S. I. Weissman. A Cary spectrophotometer, model 14, in the Department of Microbiology, was placed at our disposal by Professor Arthur Kornberg.

other was extracted preferentially so as to yield material enriched in RHP relative to cytochrome c. The simplest procedure was found to be preliminary, exhaustive, cold extraction of the lyophilized bacterial powder at pH 4.0, a method employed frequently (12) for extraction of cytochrome from mammalian tissues. This procedure removed practically all of the cytochrome c, leaving RHP quantitatively in the residue.[6]

Although several procedures could be used for the extraction of RHP from the residual powder, the simplest one appeared to be incubation in a minimal volume of 1 per cent citric acid at 50° for 10 minutes, followed by cooling to room temperature, neutralization, and recovery of the liquid phase. Other extraction procedures at low temperatures, while more tedious, gave neither better yields nor preparations differing in degree of denaturation or other detectable properties from those obtained with warm citric acid. The use of this reagent was suggested by a number of successes attending its use, in place of TCA, in the isolation of cytochrome c from bacterial sources (13, 14).

Notwithstanding many attempts, it was not found possible to arrive at a precise procedure for isolation and purification of RHP. Many factors difficult to control appeared to affect ultimate recoveries, notably the previous history of the cultures, delays in procedure schedule occasioned by the need to accumulate material, etc. Once a certain degree of purity was achieved, it appeared that any of a number of procedures was effective in arriving at comparable degrees of purity and yield. With the exceptions as noted, the procedure given in the next section was found to be quite reproducible when adhered to.

Extraction and Purification of RHP

Procedure for RHP Optical Assay—The concentration of RHP in test solutions was monitored by measuring the reduced Soret absorption at 424 mμ for which ϵ (mg. per ml.) $= 4$. Because the reduced Soret absorption of the bacterial cytochrome c had its maximum at 415 mμ, and could contribute to light absorption at 424 mμ, this practice could be misleading when a crude preparation containing the cytochrome was examined. Hence, the ratio between optical densities at 415 and 424 mμ was used as a rough qualitative index for cytochrome c contamination of RHP, $R_{415/424}$ for the purest preparation being 0.84. The optical density ratio at 275 mμ (oxidized) to 424 mμ (reduced) ($R_{275/424}$) was used as a qualitative index of RHP purity. This ratio varied from more than 30 in certain crude extracts to 0.274 in the purest preparations reported here.

[6] One of us (M. D. K.) is indebted to Professor H. Theorell, whose hospitality and cooperation made possible researches sponsored by the John Simon Guggenheim Memorial Foundation during the course of which these observations were first noted.

In crude preparations both protein and nucleic acid contributed to the light absorption at 275 mμ; in purified RHP protein absorption was maximal at 275 mμ (see the spectral data below).

When $R_{275/424}$ was less than 0.3, the preparation appeared homogeneous upon electrophoresis at pH values from 5.8 to 7.8. No visible additional peaks could be seen unless the value of $R_{275/424}$ was ≥ 0.33, when a very small colorless component, migrating anodically and at a speed much less than the main RHP peak, appeared. This peak was less than 2 per cent of the total protein present as estimated by the relative areas of the peak patterns. It could be concluded that RHP with an $R_{275/424}$ less than 0.3 possessed a spectroscopic purity greater than 98 per cent. Crude preparations of RHP ($R_{275/424}$ greater than 2) usually showed at least one, and more often several, colorless components equal to, or greater in amount than, the RHP component and migrating faster anodically. These impurities could be correlated spectroscopically with nucleic acid-containing proteins or peptides or nucleic acid fragments. The small amount of residual protein contaminant remaining after removal of nucleic acid ($R_{275/424} = 0.33$ to 0.6) was spectroscopically identical with RHP protein and may have been denatured RHP.

Extraction of RHP—Proportions for the complete procedure are described in terms of 100 gm. of starting bacterial powder.

100 gm. of dry *R. rubrum* were suspended in 1.5 liters of cold water and the pH was adjusted to 4 by the addition of 1 M sulfuric acid. The suspension was then stirred in the cold, the pH being checked occasionally and adjusted to 4 as necessary. After 1 hour the suspension was centrifuged, the supernatant solution containing mostly cytochrome *c* was set aside, and the residue was resuspended in 1 liter of cold water. The pH was again adjusted to 4; the suspension was stirred for 1 hour and centrifuged. The two supernatant solutions were combined and neutralized with 6 N sodium hydroxide and the flocculent precipitate which formed was centrifuged. If the second extract contained more than one-tenth as much cytochrome *c* as the first extract, the residue was washed again with 1 liter of water at pH 4 and this supernatant solution was discarded.

The residue from the cytochrome *c* extraction was suspended in 1 liter of 1 per cent (w/v) citric acid solution; the suspension was heated rapidly to 50–60° and then maintained at this temperature for 10 minutes. The suspension was then rapidly cooled to room temperature and the pH was adjusted to 7 by the addition of 6 N sodium hydroxide. After the preparation had stood in the cold (5°) overnight, the solids were centrifuged at 20,000 $\times$ *g* for 30 minutes in the Lourdes large capacity centrifuge. The nearly clear yellow-brown supernatant solution was set aside. The gummy dark brown residue was resuspended in 500 ml. of 10 per cent (w/v) ammonium sulfate solution and stirred for 1 hour and the suspension was centrifuged. A clear extract was obtained only with prolonged centrifugation if the salt was omitted from the wash solution. The initial extract was combined with this second yellow-brown supernatant solution which contained about one-tenth as much RHP as the first. The solid residue was discarded.

For each 100 ml. of combined crude RHP extract, 20 gm. of solid ammonium sulfate were stirred into solution and the suspension was stirred in the cold for 1 hour. The precipitate (P-1) was centrifuged and then dissolved in a minimal amount of M/15 phosphate buffer, pH 7, and the solution was dialyzed free of salt and lyophilized.

To the supernatant solution were added 40 gm. of solid ammonium sulfate for each initial 100 ml. of extract and the suspension was left overnight in the cold. The crude RHP precipitate (P-2) was centrifuged, dissolved in M/15 phosphate, pH 7, dialyzed, and lyophilized. The supernatant solution contained a small amount of cytochrome c which was readily precipitated when one-tenth volume of cold 10 per cent (w/v) TCA was added. This precipitate was added to the crude cytochrome c obtained above.

Isoelectric Precipitation and Extraction of RHP—The crude dry RHP (P-2) was dissolved in 20 ml. of cold water for each gm. of powder to give a clear brown solution. To this solution 1 M citric acid was added to reduce the pH from an initial value of approximately 6 to about 5, at which pH the first trace of precipitate appeared. This reddish brown precipitate which contained traces of bacterial pigments such as carotenoids was centrifuged and discarded. The clear supernatant solution was adjusted to pH 4.6 by the further addition of 1 M citric acid, the suspension was stirred for 1 hour in the cold, and then the relatively small gray-brown precipitate was centrifuged. This precipitate (P-3) was taken up in 0.1 M citrate-Tris buffer, pH 5.0, and the solution was clarified by centrifugation and set aside. The residue which contained some crude RHP was dissolved in M/15 phosphate, pH 7, dialyzed, lyophilized, and set aside to be reworked with a later batch of crude starting material.

The pH of the supernatant solution from the precipitation at pH 4.6 was adjusted to pH 3.6 and the suspension was stirred for 1 hour in the cold. The precipitate (P-4) was centrifuged. The precipitate was washed twice to remove soluble nucleic acid-containing material by suspending it as well as possible in cold 0.1 M citrate-Tris buffer, pH 3.6, equal to one-half the volume of the first supernatant solution of pH 3.6, stirring in the cold for 20 minutes, and then centrifuging. The two wash solutions were added to the supernatant solution at pH 3.6 and the small amount of heme compounds present was precipitated by the addition of 60 gm. of solid ammonium sulfate for each 100 ml. of solution. The precipitate was centrifuged, dissolved in M/15 phosphate, pH 7, dialyzed, lyophilized, and set aside to be reworked as crude RHP.

The washed RHP precipitate (P-4) was washed successively with 0.1 M citrate-Tris buffer of pH 3.8, 4.0, 4.25, 4.5, 4.75, and 5.0. At each step the supernatant wash solutions were checked for RHP concentration and relative purity. Any step that appeared to aid the purification was repeated until it was obvious that further repetition was valueless. At the lower pH values, nucleic acid was usually dissolved preferentially and the reverse held above pH 4. However, this finding was not invariably the case. In different preparations the best RHP fraction appeared between pH 3.5 and pH 4.75. Finally, the residue was suspended in water, neutralized by the addition of M Tris, clarified by centrifugation, dialyzed, lyophilized, and set aside to be reprocessed as crude RHP.

Supernatant wash solutions of comparable purity were combined and the RHP was precipitated by the addition of M citric acid to adjust the pH to 3.5. Each precipitate was dissolved in 0.1 M citrate-Tris, pH 5.0, dialyzed, and lyophilized.

It was noted that the cytochrome c initially present in the crude RHP tended to concentrate in the precipitates which were insoluble at pH 5.0. After repetition of the precipitation and extraction process, the RHP was free of any spectroscopically detectable contamination by the cytochrome c. By repeating the isoelectric precipitation and extraction process once or twice on a given preparation, and by reworking the various tailing fractions, several hundred mg. of the purest material reported here were prepared. Best results were obtained when the RHP from the first precipitation-extraction step was stored for several weeks in the cold, either in solution or as a dried powder, before the process was repeated. Apparently the nucleic acid-like material that was the chief contaminant at that stage was degraded to such an extent as to become soluble at pH 3.6 to 4.

Purified RHP was ordinarily stored in the cold, preferably at $-15°$, although no spectroscopic change was noted in dry material stored at room temperature for as long as 30 days. In Table I are given results selected from typical runs.

Alternative procedures in which are employed either continuous paper electrophoresis, batch paper electrophoresis, or percolation through carboxymethylcellulose columns have been examined.[7] All of these methods have effected good purifications of RHP. Continuous paper

[7] We are indebted to Dr. G. Zweig of the Charles F. Kettering Foundation, Yellow Springs, Ohio, for his cooperation in testing various continuous electrophoresis procedures using facilities at the Kettering Foundation laboratories, kindly made available to us by Dr. H. A. Tanner.

electrophoresis at pH 7 has appeared well suited to the processing of crude RHP, especially in regard to removal of cytochrome c contamination. To bring samples of intermediate purity to a degree of purity shown in Step 5 the isoelectric extraction procedure is most convenient. Purification beyond Step 5 is readily achieved invariably by paper electrophoresis at pH 7.

It is conceivable that enzymic degradation of nucleic acid could be combined with the precipitation and extraction steps to effect savings in

TABLE I

RHP Extraction and Purification*

Step No.	Fraction	$R_{275/260}$	$R_{275/424}$	$R_{415/424}$	Dry weight	RHP or cyto-chrome c[†]
	Extraction of cytochrome c and RHP					
					mg.	*mg.*
1	Cytochrome c	1.17	1.23	1.55	1050	256
2	RHP (P-1)	0.89	5.9	1.02	567	27
3	" (P-2)	0.57	25.5	0.98	2660	190
	Purification of RHP (P-2)					
					mg.	
4	Combined pH 4.25, 4.5, 4.75 washings	0.75	3.6	0.92	438	141
5	Combined pH 4.25, 4.5, 4.75 washings (from Step 4)	0.75	1.9	0.87	161	96

* Based on 100 gm. of starting *R. rubrum* powder.

† Based on Soret absorption peaks; ϵ (mg. per ml.) = 4.0 for RHP; and mg. per ml. = 10.9 for cytochrome c (calculated from ϵ (micromoles per ml.) = 142 (Paléus and Neilands (15)).

time and total number of operations, but this possibility remains to be investigated.

Results

General Physical and Chemical Properties of RHP[8]—RHP is soluble in water or buffers above pH 5. Below pH 5 it exhibits minimal solubility, in accord with its isoelectric point which lies close to this pH (see below). It possesses a thermal stability much like that of bacterial cytochrome c. Thus, it can be boiled for 1 to 2 minutes at 100° with little irreversible

[8] Many of the observations described in this section were made originally in previously published researches (1, 2), or in unpublished observations by R. Hill and M. D. Kamen, and confirmed in the present studies.

denaturation. Heating for 10 to 15 minutes at 50–60° in 1 per cent citric acid is without effect. However, prolonged boiling at neutral pH will result in irreversible denaturation, as evidenced by a typical acid hematin spectrum with absorption maxima at 400 and 530 mμ.

RHP is stable in the cold in the range pH 2 to 11. RHP at pH > 11 appears to undergo a transition to a reversibly denatured form which upon reduction exhibits a hemochromogen spectrum which is identical with that of the bacterial cytochrome c at neutral pH (see below). The oxidized form is spectroscopically similar to that of an alkali hematin, with absorption maxima at approximately 415 mμ and approximately 540 mμ. When the pH is brought back to 7, RHP reappears in its original spectral form. Treatment with glacial acetic acid results in a compound with a spectrum like that obtained by prolonged boiling.

RHP can be oxidized and reduced reversibly with reagents commonly employed for this purpose in chemical manipulation of hematin compounds. It is reduced completely at neutral pH by hydrogen-palladium, ferrous oxalate, dithionite, and hydrogen sulfide. Reduction by ascorbate is incomplete even when the ascorbate is present in 100-fold molar excess. RHP is reduced enzymically by DPNH when incubated with the mammalian DPNH-linked cytochrome c reductase (1) but not by DPNH alone. The specific cytochrome b_5 reductase of liver microsomes (16) fails to catalyze reduction with DPNH.[9]

RHP was found to be rapidly autoxidizable. No precise determination of the oxidation kinetics was attempted, but a semiquantitative estimate was made on the basis of the following observations. RHP (18 mg.) dissolved in 4 ml. of M/15 phosphate buffer at pH 7.0 was reduced with hydrogen-palladium. The solution was filtered free of the reductant under helium and then exposed to air and shaken vigorously at room temperature. The disappearance of the characteristic α-band at 550 to 560 mμ (see below) was observed visually with a Hartridge reversion spectroscope. It could be estimated that the half life of the reduced form was approximately 3 seconds.

If RHP is brought to pH > 11 in the presence of lauryl sulfate and then subjected to several cycles of reduction with dithionite and oxidation with air, it is observed that the heme moiety disappears. This behavior is not observed with the bacterial cytochrome c and is much like the well known degradation of hemoglobin and similar hematin compounds when subjected to oxidative denaturation (17). Presumably the products of degradation of RHP are bile salts, as in the case of myoglobin.

RHP does not bind reversibly many reagents which form addition compounds with hemoglobin or myoglobin. Thus, it fails to react at

[9] P. Strittmatter, private communication (1957).

neutral pH to form stable addition compounds, either in the oxidized or reduced form, with hydrogen sulfide, oxygen, nitric oxide, sodium azide, sodium cyanide, and 4-methylimidazole. On the other hand, reduced RHP reversibly binds carbon monoxide, the resultant compound showing a typical hemochromogen spectrum (see below). The carbon monoxide compound is extremely sensitive to light at pH 7, but appears quite stable at pH $\leq$ 4.0. This anomalous behavior is unique to RHP, as far as we are aware. The half life of the carbon monoxide compound at pH 7 and at light intensities in the range of 100 to 200 foot candles is of the order of 10^{-1} second.

If RHP is partially denatured by treatment with lauryl sulfate in dilute alkali, it appears to be able to form a complex with 4-methylimidazole, as assayed by the appearance of a typical hemochromogen spectrum. However, reaction with cyanide or pyridine requires complete denaturation by heating in strong alkali (6 N sodium hydroxide). When this is done, the derivative hemochromogens are identical with those obtained in the same manner from pure beef heart cytochrome c or bacterial cytochrome c (1, 2).

The prosthetic heme of RHP cannot be split off, as in hemoglobin, by treatment with cold dilute acid-acetone mixtures. Reductive cleavage with sodium amalgam (18) produces a mixture of mesoporphyn and chlorin spectroscopically absolutely identical with that obtained from pure cytochrome c, either mammalian or bacterial. No other method, such as the silver-salt cleavage (19), or strong acid cleavage (20), has been attempted.

Analytic Data

Electrophoretic Measurements—The combined results of all electrophoretic determinations are presented in Table II. Unfortunately, insufficient amounts of the purest preparation were available to determine mobilities at the various pH values shown, so less pure samples ($R_{275/424}$ = 0.35 to 0.50) were used for pH 5.8 and pH 7.8. In these cases, however, impurity peaks which were visible were colorless and only one colored peak could be seen. The colored component was used in determining mobilities at these pH values.

Another difficulty arose in the inadvertent use of buffers with different ionic strengths. While corrections for ionic strength effects are uncertain, an attempt was made to reduce all mobility μ values to a constant ionic strength of $\tau = 0.2$. This was done by using the two values at pH 6.0 and 6.8 to establish a linear relation of mobility and pH. Then, the value at pH 5.8 was corrected downward to fall on the same line. By this procedure, it was possible to obtain a factor by which to increase the observed mobility at pH 7.8 so as to arrive at a mobility for RHP at pH 7.8 and ionic strength of $\tau = 0.2$. The predicted value was -7.5×10^{-5} e.s.u. The value determined by extrapolation of the line based on the experimental points at pH 6.0 and 6.8 was -7.35×10^{-5} e.s.u.

Another procedure was based on correction of mobilities, assuming that these depended on the square root of the ionic strength, all values being normalized to $\tau = 0.2$.

By using either of these procedures, it was found by extrapolation to $\mu = 0$ that the isoelectric point was at pH 5.0 to 5.1. This value must be considered as tentative until sufficient pure material is available to make possible enough determinations under proper conditions, but it is reasonable in view of the observed tendency of RHP to precipitate at pH < 5.

TABLE II

Electrophoretic Mobilities (μ) of RHP

pH	Ionic strength*	μ (cm.^{2} sec.$^{-1}$ volt^{-1}) $\times 10^5$ (observed)	μ (cm.^{2} sec.$^{-1}$ volt^{-1}) $\times 10^5$ † (corrected)
5.8	0.1156	−2.54	−1.6
6.0	0.2000	−2.2	−2.2
6.8	0.2000	−4.39	−4.39
7.8	0.2888	−5.1	−7.5

* Phosphate buffers of the following composition were used: pH 5.8, 78 ml. of M Na_2HPO_4 and 922 ml. of M KH_2PO_4 per 10 liters; pH 6.8, 500 ml. each of M Na_2HPO_4 and M KH_2PO_4 per 10 liters; pH 7.8, 944 ml. of M Na_2HPO_4 and 56 ml. of M KH_2PO_4 per 10 liters.

† See the text.

As noted from the sign of the mobility coefficient, RHP is an acidic protein, migrating anodically at pH > 5.

Sedimentation and Diffusion Constants—The sedimentation velocity constant of RHP was determined with a sample of RHP approximately 98 per cent pure ($R_{275/424} = 0.33$) which displayed only one major colored peak and a barely detectable minor colorless peak in the schlieren picture. The average value obtained from several runs (concentration of RHP, 0.9 per cent (w/v)) in phosphate buffer at pH 7.0 (ionic strength (τ) = 0.2) and 20° was 2.66 Svedberg units (S). Corrected to pure water solvent, the value ($s_{20,w}$) was 2.76 S. This value could be estimated to have a standard deviation of approximately ±2 per cent. Systematic errors noted occasionally (5) in this procedure could increase the estimated error to ±5 per cent.

The diffusion constant for the same RHP preparation was determined by measuring the rate of area broadening of the peak in the electrophoretic pattern at pH 6.8 (6). Corrected to 20° and pure water solvent, the value $(D_{20,w})$ was 8.65×10^{-7} c.g.s. unit, with an uncertainty estimated from previous experience (5) of ±5 per cent.

Partial Specific Volume—The density of the protein solution, ρ, and the density of the solvent, ρ_0, for a given concentration of RHP in water containing a trace of Tris buffer sufficient to maintain the pH at 7 and at 20° (±0.01°) were determined by the gradient tube method (6). The partial specific volume, $\bar{v}_{20}$, then was calculated according to the formula

$$\bar{v} = \left(1 - \frac{100(\rho - \rho_0)}{c}\right) \Big/ \rho_0$$

The value obtained was 0.731.

TABLE III

Spectral Properties of RHP

	Extinction coefficients of absorption peaks at					
	275 mμ*	390 mμ*	424 mμ	500 mμ*	550 mμ	640 mμ*
ϵ, mg. per ml........	1.09	3.63	4.00	0.452	0.464	0.132
E μmoles per ml.....	30.7	101.6	112.0	12.7	13.0	3.70

Characteristic ratios of extinction coefficients as follows: $\epsilon_{275}/\epsilon_{424} = 0.274$, $\epsilon_{424}/\epsilon_{550} = 8.62$, $\epsilon_{275}/\epsilon_{640} = 8.3$.

* Oxidized.

Molecular Weight (M)—By substituting the values for the various parameters determined as described previously in the well known formula

$$M = \frac{RTS_{20,w}}{D_{20,w}(1 - \bar{v}\rho)}$$

the value of 27,740 was determined for the molecular weight of RHP. The systematic errors could be estimated as ±5 per cent; hence a value of 28,000 ± 1000 was taken for calculation of millimolar extinction coefficients of Table III. The frictional ratio (21) was calculated as 1.33.

Determination of the heme content as the pyridine hemochromogen according to the procedure of Drabkin (22) gave a value of $M = 25,000$, assuming one heme per mole.

The agreement between these two independent procedures can be considered satisfactory.

The iron content of the same highly purified RHP preparation used for the ultracentrifugal and electrophoretic and gradient measurements was found to be 0.18 per cent. This indicated a molecular weight of 31,000, assuming one iron per mole. Because the iron analysis is likely to be low rather than high, leading to a high estimate of the molecular weight, it was assumed that the molecular weight was close to 28,000 and that all iron was accounted for as heme iron, of which there was 1 mole per mole of protein.

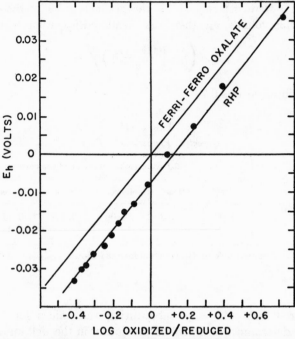

Fig. 1. Oxidation-reduction equilibrium of RHP with the iron-oxalate system at pH 7 and 30°. The reaction mixture contained initially 5×10^{-3} M potassium phosphate, pH 7, 0.5 M potassium oxalate, pH 7, 10^{-3} M ferric-ammonium sulfate, and 0.36 mg. of RHP (approximately 1.3×10^{-2} μmole) in 2.0 ml. and was titrated anaerobically by the addition of increments of 0.02 M ferrous-ammonium sulfate.

Electrochemical Potential—The oxidation-reduction equilibria between RHP and ferric-ferrous oxalate at pH 7 were measured in the manner described by Velick and Strittmatter (9), except that the equilibrium concentrations of RHP were determined from optical densities at 550 and 640 mμ rather than at the Soret absorption peak. The calculated results were identical at the two wave lengths.

The reversibility of the equilibrium was indicated by the ready reoxidation of ferrous oxalate-reduced RHP by the ferric salt. In Fig. 1 the results of an electrometric titration are represented in the manner described by Hill (8). It is apparent that the ferric-ferrous oxalate and RHP curves are

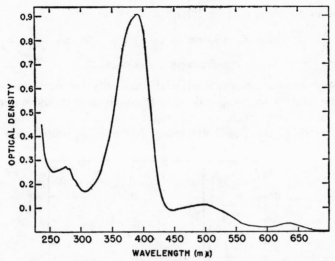

FIG. 2. Spectrum of oxidized RHP (0.25 mg. per ml. of RHP, approximately 0.93 $\times$ 10^{-2} μmole per ml.) in M/15 phosphate, pH 7.

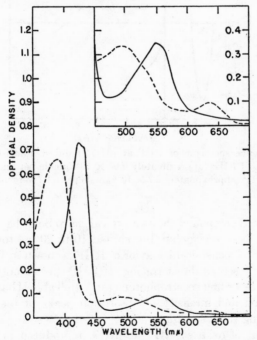

FIG. 3. Spectrum of oxidized (broken line) and reduced (solid line) RHP at pH 7. For the main curves 0.186 mg. per ml. of RHP (approximately 0.66 $\times$ 10^{-2} μmole per ml.) and for the inset curves 0.745 mg. per ml. of RHP (approximately 2.7 $\times$ 10^{-2} μmole per ml.) were used in M/15 phosphate, pH 7.

almost coincident and that for RHP

$$E_0' = E_h \ (0.5 \ \text{reduced, pH 7}) \ = \ -0.008 \ \text{volt}$$

Spectroscopic Observations

The spectroscopic properties of RHP exemplify the novel character of this heme protein as compared with those commonly encountered. It exhibits a spectrum such as one might expect from a myoglobin-like protein in which the prosthetic group possesses saturated side chains.

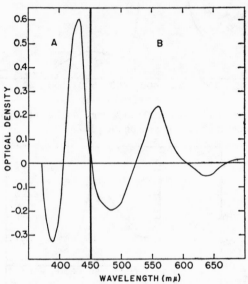

FIG. 4. Difference spectrum of RHP at pH 7, reduced minus oxidized. In A 0.186 mg. per ml. of RHP (approximately 0.66×10^{-2} μmole per ml.) and in B 0.745 mg. per ml. of RHP (approximately 2.7×10^{-2} μmole per ml.) were used in M/15 phosphate, pH 7.

Thus, the reduced compound shows a typical sharp Soret band and a rather diffuse α-band, as in myoglobin, but shifted 10 to 20 mμ toward the blue. The complex spectrochemical behavior of RHP is shown in Figs. 2 through 8, wherein are presented direct tracings of RHP spectra obtained with the Cary model 14 recording spectrophotometer. In Table III are summarized data on location and intensity of absorption peaks of the RHP sample used in obtaining these spectra.

The spectrum of oxidized RHP at pH 7, reproduced in Fig. 2, shows the protein absorption band with a maximum at 275 mμ and a shoulder at 280 mμ, the Soret band at 390 mμ, another band at 500 mμ, and the hematin band at 640 mμ.

The reduced RHP spectrum is shown in Fig. 3. There is a broad α-band extending from 550 to 560 mμ. The Soret band is sharp with a maximum at 424 mμ and a shoulder at approximately 431 mμ. The significance of this shoulder is not known. The spectrum of the oxidized

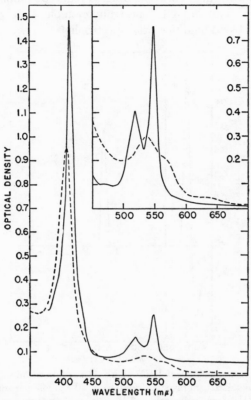

FIG. 5. Spectrum of oxidized (broken line) and reduced (solid line) RHP at pH 11.8. For the main curves 0.186 mg. per ml. of RHP (approximately 0.66×10^{-2} μmole per ml.) and for the inset curves 0.745 mg. per ml. of RHP (approximately 2.7×10^{-2} μmole per ml.) were used in 0.1 M trisodium phosphate buffer adjusted to pH 11.8.

form is included for comparison, demonstrating the shift in absorption maxima toward the red for both the Soret and α-bands, as well as the loss of the hematin band that accompanies reduction of RHP. The reduced pigment possesses no β absorption band. It may be that the unsymmetric nature of the reduced α-band conceals fine structure that could be revealed by examination at low temperature. Alternatively, the presence of traces of contaminating cytochrome c may be betrayed by the slightly skewed α-band and the hint of a slightly high absorption in the regions of 520 to 525 mμ.

The RHP difference spectrum at pH 7 is given in Fig. 4. Minimal absorption peaks, corresponding to oxidized components, fall at 388, 485, and 640 mμ and maxima, corresponding to reduced components, occur at 432 and 510 mμ. This difference spectrum resembles closely that of Chance and Smith (23), based on differential spectrophotometry of cultures *in vivo*,

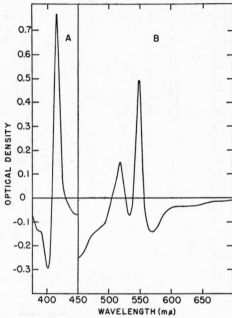

FIG. 6. Difference spectrum of RHP at pH 11.8, reduced minus oxidized. In A 0.186 mg. per ml. of RHP (approximately 0.66×10^{-2} μmole per ml.) and in B 0.745 mg. per ml. of RHP (approximately 2.7×10^{-2} μmole per ml.) were used in 0.1 M trisodium phosphate, pH 11.8.

in which a heme compound showing a difference Soret absorption peak at 430 mμ has been suggested as identical with RHP.

The oxidized and reduced hemochromogen type spectra of RHP at pH 11.8 are presented in Fig. 5. Major absorption maxima for the oxidized spectrum occur at 407 and 537 mμ and for the reduced spectrum at 413, 518, and 549 mμ. In the reduced spectrum the values of optical densities at 413, 518, and 549 mμ are 1.48, 0.11, and 0.205, respectively. These values give ratios for Soret to α and β absorption not identical to, but somewhat higher than, those found for the hemochromogen-like spectrum of *R. rubrum* cytochrome c (1).

Fig. 6 represents RHP difference spectra (reduced minus oxidized) at pH 11.8, of which the structure and orders of magnitude are very similar to those of cytochrome c. Minimal absorption peaks occur at 402, 450, 534, and 569 mμ and maxima occur at 415, 532, and 549 mμ.

The absorption spectrum of the reduced RHP-carbon monoxide complex is given in Fig. 7. Formation of the complex appears to shift the Soret absorption band from 424 to 415 mμ, to intensify the absorption (ε (mg.

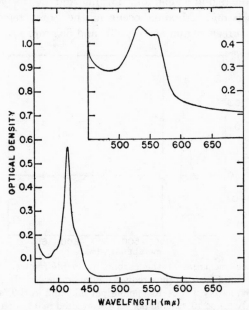

FIG. 7. Spectrum of the carbon monoxide-reduced RHP compound at pH 4.75. For the main curve 0.0745 mg. per ml. of RHP (approximately 0.27×10^{-2} μmole per ml.) and for the inset curve 0.745 mg. per ml. of RHP (approximately 2.7×10^{-2} μmole per ml.) were used in 0.1 M citrate-Tris buffer, pH 4.75, with pure carbon monoxide in the gas phase.

per ml.) changes from 4 to 7.65), and almost to obliterate the shoulder seen in the absence of carbon monoxide. However, the remnant of that shoulder may be responsible for the inflection near the base of the carbon monoxide Soret peak. The α-peak of the carbon monoxide complex is a composite of two peaks with maxima at 534 and 560 mμ. When the RHP-carbon monoxide complex is examined at pH 4 or less with the Hartridge reversion spectroscope, two sharp bands are seen at 535 and 560 mμ, whereas at pH 7 only one broad band over the range 540 to 560 mμ is noted. At the lower pH much of the protein is insoluble, making it difficult to obtain a satisfactory spectrum. For the spectrum in Fig. 7, pH 4.75

was chosen as the lowest pH value which would permit an indication of the splitting of the α-band without undue protein precipitation; however, as is indicated by the inset tracing, sufficient protein precipitation occurred at the protein concentration used for the α-band spectrum to move the base line upward from zero to approximately 0.1 optical density.

Finally, in Fig. 8 is presented the difference spectrum for reduced RHP-carbon monoxide minus reduced RHP at pH 4.75. Minimal absorption occurs in the Soret region at 396 and 432 mμ and in the yellow-green at 407, 550, and 586 mμ. Maxima occur in the Soret region at 413 mμ and in the yellow-green region at 477, 531, and 565 mμ.

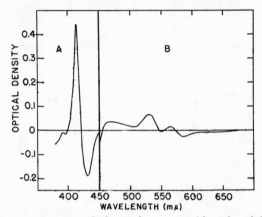

Fig. 8. Difference spectrum of the carbon monoxide-reduced RHP compound at pH 4.75 and carbon monoxide plus reduced minus reduced. In A 0.0745 mg. per ml. of RHP (approximately 0.27×10^{-2} μmole per ml.) and in B 0.745 mg. per ml. of RHP (approximately 2.7×10^{-2} μmole per ml.) were used in 0.1 M citrate-Tris buffer, pH 4.75, with pure carbon monoxide as the gas phase in the experimental cuvette.

DISCUSSION

All of the spectroscopic and chemical observations on RHP described in this report can be rationalized in so far as the prosthetic group and its relation to the apoprotein are concerned by assuming that RHP represents a variant of cytochrome c (note (24) for brief summary of present concepts of cytochrome c structure) in which one (or both) of the extraplanar protein links to the central iron atom is loose or missing. Such a structure would account for the myoglobin-like spectra and at the same time explain the characteristic shift in absorption maxima of some 10 mμ toward the blue, as compared with myoglobin. In this respect, the compound can be thought of as a myoglobin type of protein with a meso- or hematoheme prosthetic group like those reported by Hill and Holden (25). RHP appears to share with cytochrome c and cytochrome f (Davenport and Hill (25)) the property of being the only naturally occurring heme protein compound containing these stable linkages between side chains and protein.

The failure to observe fission of the heme from protein by the classical cold acid-acetone treatment effective for myoglobin shows that the prosthetic group is linked stably to the protein through the heme side chains. The fact that reductive cleavage with sodium gives both qualitatively and quantitatively identical mixtures of mesoheme and chlorin strongly supports the notion that the binding of the heme in RHP is identical with that in cytochrome c. It is known that hematoheme is also reduced to mesoheme under the conditions of the cleavage procedure (18). However, it would not be expected that quantitative agreement in nature and yield of products from RHP compared to cytochrome c would result if the linkage in RHP were, say, an ether linkage to a hydroxyamino acid rather than a thio ether linkage to cysteine. The proof of the identity of the heme and its binding in RHP and cytochrome c must await accumulation of sufficient pure material to enable isolation of iron peptides after tryptic digestion, as done in the cytochrome c studies. From such peptides it may be possible to ascertain the nature of the linkage between the heme side chains and the moiety involved in the protein.

It is of interest that reduced RHP exhibits a true cytochrome c spectrum when brought to pH > 11. This behavior is opposite to that of cytochrome c at high pH. In other words, RHP can be "changed" into a hemochromogen almost identical with cytochrome c spectroscopically by going to high alkaline pH. The change is strictly reversible, however, for on lowering the pH to 7 the original acid hematin spectrum is restored.

While RHP can be changed in this fashion to exhibit a spectrum similar to that of cytochrome c at neutral pH, it is not possible to effect a similar change in cytochrome c whereby it resembles RHP other than superficially. If cytochrome c is brought to pH 4 in the presence of lauryl sulfate, it exhibits a characteristic acid hematin type spectrum, a fact well known for some time (26). However, the resultant spectrum, while resembling RHP in general appearance, is quite different quantitatively. The oxidized form of the acidified cytochrome c has maxima at 405 and 630 mμ, the ratio of the Soret to red bands being 12.5. The corresponding Soret and α-band maxima for oxidized RHP either at pH 4 or 7 are at 395 and 640 mμ, the ratio being 23.6.

These changes in RHP at high pH may result from a reversible twisting of the protein in which a group hindering chelation of the iron to a nitrogenous residue in the protein moves aside and a nitrogen atom from the protein moves in, thus forming a cytochrome c-like hemochromogen.

RHP is unusual among heme proteins in that, although it exhibits an acid hematin spectrum, it is incapable of forming stable addition complexes with any of the usual reagents (cyanide, azide, 4-methylimidazole, oxygen, hydrogen sulfide, nitric oxide). This fact would argue for some form of steric hindrance, as postulated to explain the spectrochemical behavior during reversible alkaline denaturation. However, more than this is needed to understand the remarkable reaction of reduced RHP with carbon monoxide to form a typical hemochromogen addition complex. Furthermore, the RHP-carbon monoxide complex appears to be the first instance reported of a light-sensitive heme-carbon monoxide compound in which the photodissociation rate depends on pH. Thus, the remarkable chemical properties of RHP require further elaboration before any attempt can be made to rationalize them in terms of structure.

The possibility that RHP is an artifact of the extraction procedure may be dismissed as most unlikely on the following grounds: (1) RHP is localized in bacterial chromatophores along with cytochrome c, cytochrome b, and all the photoactive pigments. It can be seen in these chromatophores directly when they are treated with acetone to remove the photoactive pigments. (2) RHP is obtained in the same yields relative to cytochrome c, regardless of the manner of extraction, except when TCA is used. With TCA, yields of RHP are too erratic from one culture to the next to determine a relative yield. (3) Isolated RHP is not formed from bacterial cytochrome c, or any other components of the chromatophores, by treatment with reagents used in the extraction procedures. (4) Difference spectra of actively metabolizing cells determined under a variety of conditions (anaerobic with and without carbon monoxide and other inhibitors, aerobic with and without inhibitors) can all be correlated with known spectroscopic characteristics of a mixture of RHP and cytochrome c (23). (5) RHP is one of the most abundant proteins in the bacteria. It can be obtained in yields as high as 3 mg. per gm. dry weight, thus constituting 0.6 per cent of all the cellular protein. This amount is comparable to that of the cytochrome c component in $R.$ $rubrum$ on a molar basis. The relative amounts of RHP and cytochrome c are in accord with those estimated visually in the experiment with acetone-treated chromatophores.

The identity of RHP with the terminal oxidase of $R.$ $rubrum$ is suggested by the following considerations. First, the difference spectra (reduced minus oxidized and carbon monoxide reduced minus reduced) are identical with those for a component in the oxidation chain of the intact cell suspensions actively metabolizing under a variety of conditions (23). The major portion of the differences in absorption in the visible light region when $R.$ $rubrum$ suspensions are shifted from light anaerobic to dark anaerobic, or dark anaerobic to dark aerobic conditions (23), can be accounted for by assuming RHP as the active reagent. Similarly, the shift in Soret absorption seen when the cells are subjected to carbon monoxide in the dark (23) is precisely that to be expected for RHP. Secondly, RHP is reversibly oxidized and reduced readily by DPNH-linked cytochrome c reductases, such as those found in bacterial or mammalian tissue, although it is not coupled with DPNH-linked cytochrome b_5 reductase as found in mammalian liver microsomes. Thirdly, RHP is rapidly oxidized in air.

The rate of autoxidation is of an order of magnitude consistent with the respiratory rate observed in the weakly aerobic photoheterotrophically grown cells from which RHP is isolated. In a typical manometric experiment, 200 c.mm. cells suspended in 2 ml. of buffer will take up 60 c.mm. (approximately 2.5 μmoles) of oxygen per hour in dark aerobic metabolism of a substrate such as acetate. This quantity of cells corresponds to at least 90 γ of RHP or 3×10^{-3} μmole of RHP. The minimal rate of oxidation, assuming first order kinetics and the observed half life of RHP of 3 seconds, is approximately 1.5×10^{-3} μmole in 3 seconds or approximately 2 μmoles per hour. This corresponds to a rate of oxygen uptake of at least 0.50 μmole per hour.

If RHP is an integral portion of the respiratory chain in $R.$ $rubrum$, functioning as a terminal oxidase, it may be possible to use it for monitoring oxidase and reductase activities in cell-free extracts, thereby leading perhaps to isolation and characterization of other components in the electron transport systems supporting both light and dark metabolism. It is also interesting in this regard that RHP is a major constituent of the chromatophores, which have been demonstrated to support light-catalyzed anaerobic phosphorylation (27). The possibility of RHP as a prototype for bacterial oxidases in general remains to be explored.

Spectrophotometry of metabolizing cell suspensions has revealed the presence in a variety of bacteria of moieties with spectroscopic properties like RHP which appear to function as terminal oxidases (4). However, at least one strict anaerobe, the photosynthetic bacterium $Chromatium$, also contains an RHP type of pigment (1, 2). The isolation of this compound from $Chromatium$ has been accomplished on a mg. basis recently.[10]

Further research on these heme proteins directed toward clarification of their chemistry and structure should help to solve the problem of how they function in the richly variegated metabolism of the photosynthetic bacteria and by extension how analogous proteins act in other photosynthetic tissues, as well as related non-photosynthetic systems, such as facultative anaerobes which are chemosynthetic.

SUMMARY

1. The isolation and purification of a new heme protein from the facultative photoheterotroph, $Rhodospirillum$ $rubrum$, are described.

[10] M. D. Kamen, unpublished observations.

2. The new protein, termed a "pseudohemoglobin" in previous studies and renamed "*Rhodospirillum* heme protein" (RHP) in these studies, is characterized on the basis of its spectroscopic and chemical properties as an autoxidizable variant of cytochrome *c*, in which one of the extraplanar protein bonds to the central heme iron is missing or hindered.

3. RHP is a soluble acidic protein, with an isoelectric point at pH 5.0 to 5.1 and with one heme per molecular weight of 25,000. Measurements of sedimentation velocity, diffusion, and partial specific volume lead to a calculated molecular weight of 28,000. Total iron analysis yields a somewhat higher figure. There appears to be no iron in excess of that accounted for as heme.

4. A function as a terminal oxidase for *R. rubrum* is suggested for RHP and evidence for this suggestion is presented. The possible significance of RHP as a prototype for bacterial oxidases in general is noted. The circumstance of its presence in the strict anaerobe *Chromatium* is confirmed.

BIBLIOGRAPHY

1. Vernon, L. P., and Kamen, M. D., *J. Biol. Chem.*, **211**, 643 (1954).
2. Kamen, M. D., and Vernon, L. P., *Biochim. et biophys. acta*, **17**, 10 (1955).
3. Mahler, H. R., Sarkar, N. K., Vernon, L. P., and Alberty, R. A., *J. Biol. Chem.*, **199**, 585 (1952).
4. Smith, L., *Bact. Rev.*, **18**, 106 (1954).
5. Taylor, J. F., *Arch. Biochem. and Biophys.*, **36**, 357 (1952).
6. Taylor, J. F., and Lowry, C., *Biochim. et biophys. acta*, **20**, 109 (1956).
7. Linderstrøm-Lang, K., and Lanz, H., Jr., *Compt.-rend. trav. Lab. Carlsberg, Série chim.*, **21**, 315 (1938).
8. Hill, R., *Nature*, **174**, 501 (1954).
9. Velick, S. F., and Strittmatter, P., *J. Biol. Chem.*, **221**, 265 (1956).
10. Sandell, E. B., Colorimetric determination of traces of metals, New York (1944).
11. Drabkin, D. L., *J. Biol. Chem.*, **140**, 387 (1941).
12. Paléus, S., *Acta chem. Scand.*, **8**, 971 (1954).
13. Verhoeven, W., and Takeda, Y., in McElroy, W. D., and Glass, B., Inorganic nitrogen metabolism, Baltimore, 159 (1956).
14. Kamen, M. D., and Takeda, Y., *Biochim. et biophys. acta*, **21**, 518 (1956).
15. Paléus, S., and Neilands, J. B., *Acta chem. Scand.*, **4**, 1024 (1950).
16. Strittmatter, P., and Velick, S. F., *J. Biol. Chem.*, **221**, 277 (1956).
17. Lemberg, R., and Legge, J. W., Hematin compounds and bile pigments, New York, chapter 10 (1949).
18. Davenport, H. E., *Nature*, **169**, 75 (1952).
19. Paul, K. G., *Acta chem. Scand.*, **5**, 389 (1951).
20. Theorell, H., *Enzymologia*, **4**, 102 (1937).
21. Svedberg, T., and Pedersen, K. O., The ultracentrifuge, Oxford (1940).
22. Drabkin, D. L., *J. Biol. Chem.*, **146**, 605 (1942).
23. Chance, B., and Smith, L., *Nature*, **175**, 803 (1955).
24. Ehrenberg, A., and Theorell, H., *Nature*, **175**, 158 (1955).
25. Hill, R., and Holden, H. F., *Biochem. J.*, **20**, 1326 (1926). Davenport, H. E., and Hill, R., *Proc. Roy. Soc. London, Series B*, **139**, 327 (1952).
26. Keilin, D., and Hartree, E. F., *Nature*, **145**, 934 (1940).
27. Frenkel, A. W., *J. Biol. Chem.*, **222**, 823 (1956).

6

Copyright © 1962 by the American Society for Microbiology
Reprinted from *J. Bact.* **84**:822–828 (1962)

CYTOCHROME-LINKED FERMENTATION IN *BACTEROIDES RUMINICOLA*

D. C. WHITE,[1] M. P. BRYANT, AND D. R. CALDWELL

Rockefeller Institute, New York, New York, and Animal Husbandry Research Division, Agricultural Research Service, Beltsville, Maryland

Received for publication May 21, 1962

ABSTRACT

WHITE, D. C. (Rockefeller Institute, New York, N.Y.), M. P. BRYANT, AND D. R. CALDWELL. Cytochrome-linked fermentation in *Bacteroides ruminicola*. J. Bacteriol. **84**:822–828. 1962—Previous studies showed that *Bacteroides ruminicola*, an anaerobic, saccharolytic, ruminal bacterium, ferments glucose with the production of succinic, acetic, and formic acids, requires a large amount of CO_2, and most strains require heme for growth. Difference spectra of cell suspensions of both heme-requiring strain 23, *B. ruminicola* subsp. *ruminicola*, and heme-independent strain GA33, *B. ruminicola* subsp. *brevis*, showed the presence of a cytochrome (absorption maxima at 560 mµ, near 530 mµ, and 428 mµ) similar to cytochrome *b*. This cytochrome and flavoprotein (trough at 450 mµ) in the cells, reduced by endogenous metabolism, were oxidized on addition of air, CO_2, oxalacetate, malate, or fumarate but no oxidation occurred in the presence of succinate, malonate, lactate, pyruvate, aspartate, citrate, NO_3^-, $SO_4^=$, 2-*n*-heptyl or hydroxyquinoline-N-oxide (HOQNO), amytal or azide. The oxidation of these cellular pigments by fumarate was not inhibited by CN^-, CO, malonate, succinate, amytal, or HOQNO. Glucose and reduced diphosphopyridine nucleotide (DPNH), but not succinate, reduced the pigments in frozen-thawed cells previously exposed to air for 4 hr at room temperature. The results suggest that this cytochrome and flavoprotein form an electron transport system for fumarate reduction to succinate by DPNH generated by glycolysis, and that succinate is produced via CO_2 condensation with pyruvate or phosphoenolpyruvate and with oxalacetate, malate, and fumarate as intermediates. A pigment similar to cytochrome *o* (absorption maxima at 570, 555, and 416 mµ) was observed when reduced cells were treated with CO and compared to reduced cells, but there was no detectable cytochrome oxidase activity. The function of this pigment is obscure. No peroxidase or catalase activity was detected in either strain. Pyridine hemochromogens of both strains indicate one major heme, a protoheme-like pigment, with absorption in the α region maximum at 556 mµ. As *B. ruminicola* is one of the most numerous of rumen bacteria and ferments a wide variety of carbohydrates of importance in ruminant rations, cytochrome must be of importance in electron transport in rumen contents, a highly anaerobic environment.

Bacteroides ruminicola appears to be one of the most important species of ruminal bacteria, as indicated by the wide range of carbohydrates fermented and by its presence among the predominant culturable bacteria in the rumen of animals fed a variety of rations (Bryant, 1959). It ferments glucose with the production of a large amount of succinate and requires a large amount of CO_2 for good growth (Bryant et al., 1958). The fact that a majority of strains require hemin for growth (Bryant and Robinson, *unpublished data*) led to the study of the hemoprotein in these bacteria.

MATERIALS AND METHODS

The strains studied included type strain 23 of *B. ruminicola* subsp. *ruminicola*, which requires hemin for growth, and type strain GA33 of *B. ruminicola* subsp. *brevis*, which does not require hemin. The methods of isolation and culture and descriptions of characteristics of the strains have been described (Bryant et al., 1958).

Media from which cells were harvested were similar to that of Bryant and Robinson (1961) except that 3×10^{-6} M hemin, 0.3% glucose, 1.0% Trypticase (BBL), and 3.6×10^{-5} M $FeSO_4$ were added and the other casein hydrolysate, vitamins, cellobiose, Na_2S, and $(NH_4)_2SO_4$ were deleted. Hemin was deleted from the medium

[1] Present address: Department of Biochemistry, University of Kentucky, School of Medicine, Lexington.

used to culture strain GA33. In culture vessels similar to that of Allison et al. (1962), 1,500 or 3,000 ml of medium were inoculated with about 0.5% (v/v) of a culture of the strain incubated for about 24 hr at 37 C in the same medium.

After 15 to 20 hr of incubation at 37 C, the cells were harvested by centrifugation and were washed twice with ½ volume of 0.05 M phosphate buffer (pH 7.0). They were then resuspended in the buffer, made 30% (v/v) with glycerol, and kept under N_2 at 4 C or frozen at −70 C in the broken-cell preparations.

Spectra were measured using the difference spectra methods described by Chance (1954). In this technique, the absorption spectrum of the reduced respiratory pigments is measured against a similar cell suspension containing the oxidized pigments. A Cary model 14 spectrophotometer modified to utilize a more intense light source was used. Bacteria were measured at a cell density of between 10 and 30 mg of protein per ml. At these densities, the band width is less than 20 A at 560 mμ. The 0.1 to 0.2 optical density (OD) slide wire has an inherent noise level of $\pm 7 \times 10^{-4}$ OD and the spectra were traced by drawing a line through the middle of the recording error.

The contents of cuvettes were kept anaerobic by passing a stream of prepurified N_2 into the gaseous phase whenever the stoppers were removed, using the anaerobic techniques for culture transfer of the bacterium. The N_2 was passed through a column of hot reduced copper filings to remove traces of O_2. Solutions added to a cuvette were equilibrated with and kept under a gaseous phase of N_2. When substrate solutions were added to a cuvette, a similar volume of 0.05 M phosphate buffer (pH 7.0) was added to the balancing cuvette and both transfers were done under a stream of N_2.

Substrate solutions were adjusted to pH 7.0 and molar concentration. Reagent grade materials were used, except for sodium oxalacetate which was a gift from Chas. Pfizer & Co., Inc. (Brooklyn, N.Y.) to S. Granick and 2-n-heptyl-4-hydroxyquinoline-N-oxide (HOQNO), a gift from J. W. Lightbown.

Protein determinations were made by the biuret method (Gornall, Bardawill, and David, 1949) in the presence of 0.06% sodium deoxycholate.

Pyridine hemochromogens of the bacteria were measured in 50% pyridine plus 50% 0.09 M KOH containing 0.03% sodium deoxycholate, and a

few mg of $Na_2S_2O_4$ were then added and the solution was stirred by bubbling with N_2.

Peroxidase assays were done utilizing the guaiacol reaction of Maehly and Chance (1954). Bacterial cells were shattered by pounding, after freezing with liquid nitrogen, and used on rewarming (Moses, 1955).

Catalase was assayed by the iodometric titrations of Herbert (1955) on whole cells or cells treated with toluene as described by Clayton (1959). The conditions for the assay were those of White (1962).

RESULTS

Difference spectra. Figure 1 gives some difference spectra of strain GA33, the hemin-independent strain. It contains a cytochrome with a difference spectrum similar to cytochromes of the *b* type and henceforth referred to as the *b*-like cytochrome. The *b*-like cytochrome has absorption maxima at 560 mμ, near 530 mμ, and at 428 mμ, and a flavoprotein can be detected as the

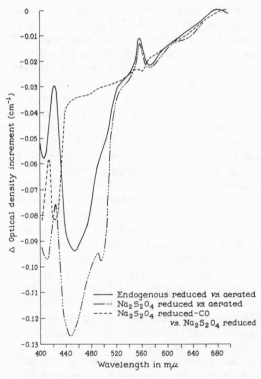

FIG. 1. *Difference spectra of a cell suspension of Bacteroides ruminicola, strain GA33, at room temperature and with cells representing 15 mg of protein per ml.*

trough at 450 mμ. Addition of dithionite to cells already reduced by their endogenous metabolism reduces more of the flavoproteins, yet does not significantly increase the b-like cytochrome absorption. If reduced cells are treated with CO and compared with reduced cells, the spectrum of an "oxidase" with absorption similar to that of cytochrome o (maxima at about 570 mμ, about 555 mμ, 416 mμ, and minima at 425 mμ) becomes evident. While the maxima at about 570 and 555 mμ were small, they were always found in cells of both strains and the soret peak at 416 mμ was more definite. The absorption maximum at 500 mμ may represent an unknown pigment first described by Lindenmeyer and Smith (1957) and since reported in other species. The conventions for naming these respiratory pigments are those of Smith (1961).

That these are indeed respiratory pigments can be demonstrated by the ability to oxidize the b-like cytochrome and flavoprotein with air, then reversibly reduce them by treating the same sample with N_2. The 500-mμ pigment likewise can be oxidized with air and then reduced by displacing the air with N_2. The oxidase-like pigment can be demonstrated by bubbling with CO (treated to remove O_2 and CO_2) and then by removing the CO by bubbling with N_2. It will lose its characteristic absorption maxima. The hemin-independent strain GA33 and hemin-requiring strain 23 have identical respiratory pigments.

If the frozen-thawed bacteria are allowed to partially equilibrate with air, glucose and reduced diphosphopyridine nucleotide (DPNH), but not succinate, can increase the level of reduction of the b-like cytochrome and flavoprotein. To demonstrate this, the cells were held at room temperature and exposed to air for 4 hr. Presumably, by this time they exhaust their endogenous metabolic stores. Some lysis appears to have occurred by this time, as evidenced by an increased viscosity. Similar cells kept at 4 C under N_2 for 4 hr maintained the pigments in the reduced state and do not increase in viscosity.

Pyridine hemochromogens of both strains of bacteria indicate one major heme, a protoheme-like pigment with maximal absorption in the α region at 556 mμ. The hemin-independent strain contained about 5×10^{-7} moles of protoheme per 10 mg of bacterial protein. The hemin-requiring strain, grown in medium containing excess hemin, contains about twice this amount.

Cytochrome oxidase activity. The presence of cytochrome o (a cytochrome oxidase)-like pigment in these obligate anaerobes is puzzling and no cytochrome oxidase activity could be detected. By use of a vibrating platinum electrode similar to that described by Chance (1954) in a chamber maintained at 30 C by circulating water and stirred with a 5-mm magnetic flea, measurements of the effect of the bacteria on the O_2 level of the suspending buffer were made. If 0.5 ml of cell suspension (150 mg of bacterial protein) were added to 4.5 ml of 0.05 M phosphate buffer (pH 7.0), no change in the O_2 level (220 μmole of O_2 per ml) could be detected after 20 min. Addition of glucose, malate, fumarate, succinate, citrate (0.1 M final concentration), or DPNH (2×10^{-4} M final concentration) had no effect on the O_2 tension. If the buffer was saturated with O_2 rather than air, there was a very slow O_2 concentration-dependent decrease in O_2 tension produced by the bacteria. This is typical of the behavior of flavoprotein and not of cytochrome oxidase (Chance, 1957). Again, both strains behaved similarly.

Neither NO_3^- nor $SO_4^=$ oxidized the cytochromes reduced by endogenous metabolism, and incorporation of 1×10^{-3} M KCN, azide, or amytal into growth medium resulted in little, if any, inhibition of growth of strain 23. These findings add further weight to the probability that cytochrome oxidase-like activity is not present in *B. ruminicola.*

Peroxidase activity. There was no detectable peroxidase activity as measured by the optical density change at 470 mμ with guaiacol (final concentration: 0.02 M) incubated for 5 min at 25 C in 0.05 M phosphate buffer (pH 7.0) with 24 mg of bacterial protein per ml and H_2O_2 concentrations of between 60 and 600 μmoles. Cells of both strains were shattered at liquid nitrogen temperature before addition to the guaiacol solution.

Catalase activity. Using the iodometric titration of Herbert (1955) on whole cells suspended in 0.01 M phosphate buffer (pH 6.8), *Katalase-fahigkeit* (protein) values of 0.01 and 0.20 were measured for strains 23 and GA33, respectively. Identical values were obtained with cells treated with toluene as described by Clayton (1959). Toluene would destroy any permeability barrier to H_2O_2. This low level of catalase activity probably represents nonspecific catalase activity of the hemoproteins of the cell.

Cytochrome-linked fermentation. Figure 2 shows

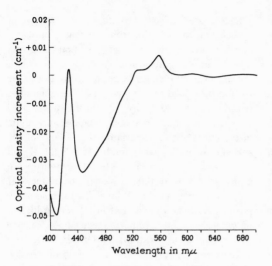

FIG. 2. *Difference spectrum of a cell suspension of Bacteroides ruminicola, strain 23 (15 mg protein per ml), oxidized by malate (0.05 M final concentration) compared with cells reduced by endogenous metabolism.*

TABLE 1. *Oxidation of endogenously reduced pigments in cell suspensions of Bacteroides ruminicola by addition of substrates**

Substrate	Strain	$\alpha \Delta$ OD (560 to 580 mμ)	$\gamma \Delta$ OD (428 to 455 mμ)
Fumarate	23	0.007	0.037
	GA33	0.009	0.049
Malate	23	0.007	0.036
	GA33	0.006	0.033
Oxalacetate	23	0.009	0.045
HCO_3^-, CO_2	23	0.004	0.034
	GA33	0.005	0.039
CO + fumarate	GA33	0.004	0.025
Fumarate + KCN	23	0.004	0.035
Succinate	23	<0.0008	0.0008
Succinate + fumarate	23	0.007	0.032
Malonate	23	<0.0008	0.0008
Malonate + fumarate	23	0.007	0.057
HOQNO	GA33	<0.0008	0.0008
HOQNO + fumarate	GA33	0.006	0.039
Amytal	GA33	<0.0008	0.0008
Amytal + fumarate	GA33	0.004	0.037

* The change in OD measured at the α maximum of cytochrome b (560 mμ) and between the γ maximum (428 mμ) and trough of flavoprotein (455 mμ). This represents the change produced in 15 mg of bacterial protein after anaerobic addition of substrate to one cuvette and a similar amount of phosphate buffer to the other, as described in Materials and Methods. In each case, a base line of reduced cells vs. reduced cells was run to establish that the pigments were not oxidized during addition of the cell suspension to the cuvettes. The reactions were complete within 5 min. All substrates were at a final concentration of 0.05 M except for HOQNO (2-n-heptyl-4-hydroxyquinoline-N-oxide) which was at 3×10^{-5} M and amytal at 3×10^{-3} M, and HCO_3^- and CO_2 indicates the addition of 0.05 M final concentration of $NaHCO_3$ and saturation of the suspension with CO_2.

the difference spectrum produced by adding malate anaerobically to cells reduced by their endogenous metabolism. The b-like cytochrome maxima and flavoprotein trough can be seen. The changes in OD measured at the α maximum (the difference between OD at 560 mμ and at 580 mμ) and at the γ maximum (the difference between OD at 428 mμ and 455 mμ) were almost as large as those obtained by reducing cells in one cuvette with $Na_2S_2O_4$ and shaking the cells in the other cuvette vigorously in air. In this experiment, the cells were added as anaerobically as possible to stoppered cuvettes, and a base line was run to be sure that no oxidation had occurred. Substrate (0.1 ml of a 1 M solution) was then added anaerobically to one cuvette and 0.1 ml of buffer was added anaerobically to the other. Adding buffer to each cuvette as described produced no detectable change in OD (less than 0.0008 OD units). If a cuvette with 2 ml of cell suspension and with 1 ml of air as the gas phase was tipped as was done to mix the substrates, no detectable oxidation occurred in the 560-mμ region and a change of less than 0.004 OD was detected at 428 mμ.

Data in Table 1 show the effect of certain substrates and inhibitors of oxidation of the reduced b-like cytochrome; CO_2, oxalacetate, malate, and fumarate oxidized the reduced flavoprotein and

cytochrome in the bacterial suspensions. Compounds that failed to produce oxidation of these pigments included succinate, malonate, HOQNO, amytal, lactate, pyruvate, aspartate, citrate,

NO_3^-, $SO_4^=$, and azide. The fumarate oxidation of the pigments was not inhibited by CN^-, CO, malonate, succinate, amytal, or HOQNO. In some bacteria, HOQNO inhibits oxidation of cytochrome b (Lightbown and Jackson, 1956).

DISCUSSION

Anaerobic bacteria have been known for some time to contain cytochrome pigments (reviewed by Newton and Kamen, 1961); however, strictly fermentative, saccharolytic, obligate anaerobes were not known to contain these pigments. This might very well be due to the fact that very little effort has been made to look for cytochromes in fermentative anaerobes other than in spore-formers of the genus *Clostridium*. Chaix and Fromageot (1942) showed that *Propionibacterium pentosaceum* contains cytochromes, including a cytochrome b, but this organism produces catalase, shows considerable oxygen uptake during catabolism of various substrates, and shows only a tendency toward anaerobiosis in growth.

The fact that *B. ruminicola* subsp. *ruminicola*, a saccharolytic, nonsporeforming anaerobe functioning in the rumen fermentation, requires hemin for growth led us to look for functional hemoproteins in the cells. In this bacterium and in *B. ruminicola* subsp. *brevis*, the subspecies not requiring exogenous hemin for growth, two cytochromes were detected having the characteristic absorption maxima of cytochrome b and one similar to cytochrome o.

Cytochrome o behaves as an oxidase in a number of bacterial species (Castor and Chance, 1959). In *Hemophilus* species, it reacts with O_2 and NO_3^- (White and Smith, 1962). The function of the similar pigment in this obligate anaerobe is obscure, since no cytochrome oxidase activity could be detected and growth occurs readily in fairly high concentrations of CN^-, azide, and amytal. Growth of *B. ruminicola* requires an E_h at which resorufin, the pink reduction product of resazurin added to media, is reduced to colorless. At pH 6.9, the E_h of resorufin is -0.042 v (Twigg, 1945). The cytochrome o-like pigment has not been detected by means other than its CO complex, and CO does not interfere with activity of the b-like cytochrome. At present we can assign no functional activity to this pigment.

On the other hand, the b-like cytochrome and flavoprotein are reversibly oxidized and reduced in such a manner as to suggest that they are involved in an electron transport system which couples DPNH oxidation with fumarate reduction. Addition of DPNH to cell suspensions resulted in reduction of these pigments, while addition of fumarate resulted in their oxidation.

The facts that CO_2, oxalacetate, and malate also oxidize the b-like cytochrome and flavoprotein of *B. ruminicola* seem best explained on the basis of the probable mechanisms involved in its glucose fermentation. *B. ruminicola* requires a large amount of CO_2 and produces mainly succinic, acetic, and formic acids during growth in media containing glucose (Bryant et al., 1958). In studies on *Cytophaga succinicans*, which requires substrate amounts of CO_2 for fermentation of glucose and produces proportions of succinic, acetic, and formic acids similar to those of *B. ruminicola*, Anderson and Ordal (1961a, b) concluded that CO_2 was essential because it provided, through condensation with phosphoenolpyruvate, oxalacetic acid which is reduced to succinic acid using available hydrogen generated in glucose degradation. They suggested that *B. ruminicola* and other ruminal anaerobes producing similar fermentation products carry out a similar CO_2-dependent fermentation of glucose. The present results (that addition of CO_2, oxalacetate, malate, and fumarate to cells in which the b-like cytochrome and flavoprotein are reduced by endogenous metabolism results in oxidation of the pigments) further suggest that *B. ruminicola* and *C. succinicans* ferment glucose via similar mechanisms. It seems probable that CO_2, oxalacetate, and malate are precursors of fumarate, which accepts electrons from the flavoprotein b-like cytochrome system. It seems probable that the cytochrome and flavoprotein would not be involved in reduction of oxalacetate by DPNH.

Anderson and Ordal (1961b) suggested that 3 moles of adenosine triphosphate (ATP) could be generated per mole of glucose fermented by *C. succinicans* when only substrate-linked phosphorylations were considered. It is possible that electron transport between DPNH and fumarate, involving flavoprotein and the b-like cytochrome, is coupled with a high-energy phosphate generating system, and this could result in production of an additional mole of ATP per mole of glucose fermented. Elsden (*see* Gunsalus and Shuster, 1961) considered this as a possibility in *Propionibacterium* and *Veillonella* fermentations.

B. ruminicola appears to be one of the most important species of ruminal bacteria (Bryant et al., 1958); therefore, cytochrome-linked electron transport must be of importance in the highly anaerobic ruminal environment. It would be of interest to determine whether the many other species of predominant anaerobic ruminal bacteria, which produce fermentation products similar to *B. ruminicola*, also contain a cytochrome that is involved in fumarate reduction. These species include *Bacteroides succinogenes*, *B. amylophilus*, *Borrelia* sp., *Succinimonas amylolytica*, *Succinivibrio dextrinosolvens*, and *Ruminococcus flavefaciens* (see Bryant, 1959, for references). Wolin et al. (1960) isolated, via enrichment cultures of rumen contents, an anaerobic vibrio that contains a cytochrome *c* and a cytochrome *b* which are oxidized by malate, fumarate, or nitrate (Jacobs and Wolin, 1961). However, this organism does not ferment carbohydrates, and its functional significance in the rumen is not known.

The results suggest that *B. ruminicola* may have a fumaric reductase (succinic dehydrogenase) similar to that of the anaerobe *Veillonella alcalescens* (*Micrococcus lactilyticus*) and different from that of certain aerobically grown bacteria and mitochondria, because succinate and malonate did not inhibit oxidation of the pigments by fumarate and succinate did not reduce the pigments. Peck, Smith, and Gest (1957) showed that the fumaric reductase in cell-free extracts of *V. alcalescens* catalyzed the reduction of fumarate to succinate far faster than the reverse reaction, and fumarate reduction was not inhibited by succinate and was only slightly inhibited by malonate. It should be emphasized that the present study involved washed cells of *B. ruminicola*, and studies of its fumaric reductase using cell-free extracts might yield different results. It is of interest that studies of the purified fumaric reductase of *V. alcalescens* indicate that it is a flavoprotein and it does not contain heme (Warringa and Giuditta, 1958).

ACKNOWLEDGMENT

The authors are greatly indebted to S. Granick, in whose laboratory the experiments were conducted and whose guidance contributed greatly to our understanding of the problem.

LITERATURE CITED

ALLISON, M. J., M. P. BRYANT, I. KATZ, AND M. KEENEY. 1962. Studies on the metabolic function of branched-chain volatile fatty acids, growth factors for ruminococci. II. Biosynthesis of higher branched-chain fatty acids and aldehydes. J. Bacteriol. **83**:1084–1093.

ANDERSON, R. L., AND E. J. ORDAL. 1961*a*. *Cytophaga succinicans* sp. n., a facultatively anaerobic, aquatic myxobacterium. J. Bacteriol. **81**:130–138.

ANDERSON, R. L., AND E. J. ORDAL. 1961*b*. CO_2-dependent fermentation of glucose by *Cytophaga succinicans*. J. Bacteriol. **81**:139–146.

BRYANT, M. P. 1959. Bacteral species of the rumen. Bacteriol. Rev. **23**:125–153.

BRYANT, M. P., AND I. M. ROBINSON. 1961. Some nutritional requirements of the genus *Ruminococcus*. Appl. Microbiol. **9**:91–95.

BRYANT, M. P., N. SMALL, C. BOUMA, AND H. CHU. 1958. *Bacteroides ruminicola*, sp. nov. and *Succinimonas amylolytica*, gen. nov.—species of succinic acid-producing anaerobic bacteria of the bovine rumen. J. Bacteriol. **76**:15–23.

CASTOR, L. N., AND B. CHANCE. 1959. Photochemical determinations of the oxidases of bacteria. J. Biol. Chem. **234**:1587–1592.

CHAIX, P., AND C. FROMAGEOT. 1942. Les cytochromes de *Propionibacterium pentosaceum*. Bull. soc. chim. biol. **24**:1125–1127.

CHANCE, B. 1954. Spectrophotometry of intracellular respiratory pigments. Science **120**:767–776.

CHANCE, B. 1957. Cellular oxygen requirements. Federation Proc. **16**:671–680.

CLAYTON, R. K. 1959. Permeability barriers and the assay of catalase in intact cells. Biochim. et Biophys. Acta **36**:35–39.

GORNALL, A. G., C. J. BARDAWILL, AND M. M. DAVID. 1949. Determination of serum proteins by means of the biuret reaction. J. Biol. Chem. **177**:751–766.

GUNSALUS, I. C., AND C. W. SHUSTER. 1961. Energy-yielding metabolism in bacteria, p. 1–58. *In* I. C. Gunsalus and R. Y. Stanier [ed.], The bacteria, vol. II: Metabolism. Academic Press, Inc., New York.

HERBERT, D. 1955. Catalase from bacteria (*Micrococcus lysodeikticus*), p. 784–788. *In* S. P. Colowick and N. O. Kaplan [ed.], Methods in enzymology, vol. II. Academic Press, Inc., New York.

JACOBS, N. J., AND M. J. WOLIN. 1961. The cytochrome content of an anaerobic vibrio. Bacteriol. Proc., p. 166.

LIGHTBOWN, J. W., AND F. W. JACKSON. 1956. Inhibition of cytochrome systems of heart muscle and certain bacteria by the antagonists of dihydro-streptomycin 2-alkyl-4-

hydroxy quinoline N-oxide. Biochem. J. **63:** 130-137.

LINDENMEYER, A., AND L. SMITH. 1957. Some oxidative enzymes of anaerobically grown yeast. Federation Proc. **16:**212.

MAEHLY, A. C., AND B. CHANCE. 1954. The assay of catalases and peroxidases, p. 357–424. *In* D. Glick [ed.], Methods of biochemical analysis, vol. I. Interscience Press, New York.

MOSES, V. 1955. Tricarboxylic acid cycle reactions in the fungus *Zygorrhynchus moelleri*. J. Gen. Microbiol. **13:**235–251.

NEWTON, J. W., AND M. D. KAMEN. 1961. Cytochrome systems in anaerobic electron transport, p. 397–423. *In* I. C. Gunsalus and R. Y. Stanier [ed.], The bacteria, vol. II: Metabolism. Academic Press, Inc., New York.

PECK, H. D., JR., H. O. SMITH, AND H. GEST. 1957. Comparative biochemistry of the biological reduction of fumaric acid. Biochim. et Biophys. Acta **25:**142–147.

SMITH, L. 1961. Cytochrome systems in aerobic electron transport, p. 365–396. *In* I. C. Gunsalus and R. Y. Stanier [ed.], The bacteria, vol. II: Metabolism. Academic Press, Inc., New York.

TWIGG, R. S. 1945. Oxidation-reduction aspects of resazurin. Nature **155:**401–402.

WARRINGA, M. G., AND GIUDITTA, A. 1958. Studies on succinic dehydrogenase. IX. Characterization of the enzyme from *Micrococcus lactilyticus*. J. Biol. Chem. **230:**111–123.

WHITE, D. C. 1962. Cytochrome and catalase patterns during the growth of *Haemophilus parainfluenzae*. J. Bacteriol. **83:**851–859.

WHITE, D. C., AND L. SMITH. 1962. Hematin enzymes of *Haemophilus parainfluenzae*. J. Biol. Chem. **237:**1332–1336.

WOLIN, M. J., E. A. WOLIN, N. JACOBS, AND G. WEINBERG. 1960. A new cytochrome-producing anaerobic vibrio. Bacteriol. Proc., p. 77.

91

Editor's Comments
on Papers 7 and 8

7   **CHANCE**
     Spectra and Reaction Kinetics of Respiratory Pigments of Homogenized and Intact Cells

8   **ASANO and BRODIE**
     Oxidative Phosphorylation in Fractionated Bacterial Systems. XIV. Respiratory Chains of Mycobacterium phlei

DYNAMICS OF ELECTRON TRANSPORT

Previous selections utilize methods that do not permit examination of dynamic interactions of the carriers studied, since only steady-state values of the extent of carrier reduction are employed to infer kinetic positions. During the course of investigation of the kinetics of formation and disappearance of the intermediate peroxide compounds of catalase and peroxidase, Britton Chance and his associates developed procedures allowing the surveillance of time-dependent absorbance changes in those chromophores over very short time intervals.[1] Chance went on to improve these techniques so as to permit their application to the study of the respiratory pigments in mitochondria, submitochondrial particles, and microorganisms. The light-scattering properties of these preparations, which change according to the metabolic state of mitochondria or bacteria, produce difficulty in interpretation of the data. Chance overcame this source of error by simultaneously measuring absorbance at the absorption maximum of the pigment and at an "isosbestic" point (Gr. "equally extinguished"), using the difference of absorbance at the two wavelengths as the quantitative estimate of the reduction level of the carrier. Careful design of the optical configuration of the system further enhanced the power of observation.

The array of techniques brought to a high state of utility by Britton Chance ranks in importance with the other indispensable instruments of biochemistry. Paper 7 is an early summary of much of that work.

As described in Paper 8, Akira Asano and Arnold F. Brodie used these procedures to study the compounds participating in respiration in subcellular particulate preparations of *Mycobacterium phlei,* an organism studied by Brodie and his associates for more than a decade. This study was carried out and reported with care, and is an outstanding example of the use of Chance's techniques in the examination of a microbial respiratory system. The paper also illustrates Brodie's extensive study of the participation of quinones in bacterial respiration.

REFERENCE

1. Chance, B. Enzyme-substrate compounds and electron transfer. In D. Green, ed. *Currents in Biochemical Research.* Interscience, New York, 1956, pp. 308–337.

7

Copyright © 1952 by Macmillan (Journals) Ltd

Reprinted from *Nature* (London) **169**:215–221 (1952)

SPECTRA AND REACTION KINETICS OF RESPIRATORY PIGMENTS OF HOMOGENIZED AND INTACT CELLS

By Dr. BRITTON CHANCE

Johnson Research Foundation, University of Pennsylvania

THE pioneer studies of MacMunn[1], later followed by those of Keilin[2] and Warburg and his co-workers[3], have demonstrated the existence of absorption bands of oxidized and reduced forms of respiratory pigments of muscle tissues, yeasts, bacteria, etc., by means of visual spectroscopy. A quantitative study of only one component of the respiratory system has so far been obtained, and that is the carbon monoxide compound of *Atmungsferment*, measured by means of its photochemical action spectrum by Warburg and Negelein[4]. On the other hand, Keilin and Hartree's incisive chemical studies have revealed much information on the nature of cytochrome action and have indicated their sequential action from oxygen to succinate[5]; and Slater has added more detail to the cytochrome sequence and has clarified the reactions with reduced coenzyme-I[6].

As a consequence of the development of rapid and sensitive spectrophotometric techniques, it is now possible to record in a quantitative manner the changes in optical density that occur upon the reduction of the cytochrome and pyridine nucleotide enzymes of muscle homogenates or intact cells upon addition of their natural substrates[7]. The 'difference spectra' that are obtained in this manner are very useful for the identification of the various cytochrome components, for the comparison of the cytochromes of different cellular material, for the quantitative estimation of relative and absolute cytochrome content of various systems, and for studies of the dynamics of cytochrome action in various physical and chemical environments. The results of such studies lead to a quantitative evaluation of the properties of the succinic oxidase system and to a formulation of a physical chemical explanation of the action of insoluble enzymes of the respiratory pathway in either homogenates or intact cells.

This study does not represent the first attempt to measure photoelectrically the absorption bands of cytochrome. In 1934, Haas[8] measured the appearance of the ferrocytochrome-c band in yeast cells, as did Baumberger in 1938[9]; Arvanitaki and Chalazonitis measured spectra of nerve fibres[10]; and Lundegårdh has obtained curves for maize and wheat roots[11]. But little of this material is useful in an incisive study of the mechanism of cytochrome action.

Method. According to our studies, a respiratory enzyme is identified by the fact that its reduction coincides with the termination of the oxidase activity as the oxygen concentration falls to zero. As shown in Fig. 1, the linear decline of the concentration of dissolved oxygen caused by the oxidase reaction is followed continuously by a platinum microelectrode (Davies and Brink[11]), and the termination of the oxidase activity caused by the exhaustion of the oxygen supply is marked by the reduction of the cytochrome (in this case, component a_3 is measured at 445 mμ). This change in optical density is clearly synchronized with the oxidase activity. Such simultaneous recording techniques largely eliminate artefacts that might otherwise be mistaken for cytochrome reduction.

A very steady beam of intense monochromatic light illuminates an absorption cell (or a rapid-flow apparatus) containing the turbid cell suspension, which transmits less than 10 per cent of the incident light. Nevertheless, a photocurrent of 10^{-10}–10^{-11} amp. is obtained in an especially selected electron multiplier phototube when the spectral interval is 2 mμ or less at 550 mμ. This current is measured with an error limited only by shot noise, which corresponds to an error of optical density of 2×10^{-4}. The apparatus is arranged to record the changes in optical density at two wave-lengths of light simultaneously by means of two monochromators, a vibrating mirror, and related electronic circuits[7].

Difference spectra of the cytochromes of heart muscle preparations. (Most of the heart muscle preparations were carried out by Mrs. Helen Conrad and Mr. T. M. Devlin, to whom our thanks are due.) Upon addition of succinate to the oxidized cytochromes of a heart-muscle homogenate prepared according to the method of Keilin and Hartree[12], changes in optical density are measured at various wave-lengths upon reduction of the cytochromes, and the clear

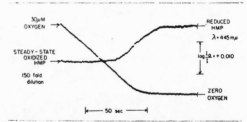

Fig. 1. Correlation between the termination of the oxidase activity and the reduction of cytochrome component-a_3 of the succinic oxidase system. The experiments were carried out in an open cuvette of the recording spectrophotometer with 150-fold dilution of the heart-muscle preparation. The oxidase activity is measured by means of a platinum micro-electrode inserted into the suspension. The time of addition of succinate is not shown and occurs some seconds before the record begins. (Expt. 589b4)

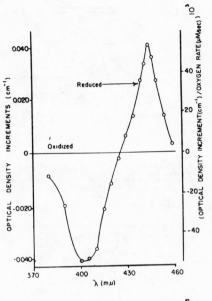

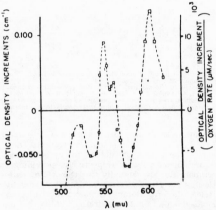

Fig. 2. Difference spectra corresponding to the optical density changes from oxidized to reduced heart-muscle preparation. The spectra in the region of the Soret band and in the visible region were obtained with different heart-muscle preparations, but the scale on the right-hand ordinate permits a comparison of the absorption spectra on the basis of the oxidase activity. (Expts. 643e, 701b)

absorption bands shown in Fig. 2 are obtained. The wave-lengths of the maxima are 444, 551, 561 and 604 mμ, not far from the positions observed by visual means[5], and are thereby identified with cytochromes-a_3, c, b and a respectively. In studies of the Soret bands, preparations having a very low hæmoglobin content are used. In this region the absorption bands of cytochromes-b and c appear only as a slight shoulder on the short-wave side of the band of cytochrome-a_3, but they are more distinct in yeast cells (see Fig. 5a later).

In accordance with the work of Keilin and Hartree[5] on the effect of cyanide and carbon monoxide upon

cytochromes-a and a_3, we find that they may be independently measured at 604 and 444 mμ respectively, although there may be some contribution of cytochrome-a at 444 mμ. By measuring from the peak of the cytochrome-c band at 551 mμ to its isosbestic point at 541 mμ, the contribution of cytochrome-c to the spectrum is evaluated. The cytochrome-b band is similarly estimated from its peak at 561 mμ to the trough at 575 mμ. Thus much of the interaction of the absorption bands is avoided and quantitative estimates of the relative amounts of the cytochromes may be obtained: average values of the relative changes in optical density for six preparations are 6·2, 1·0, 1·0 and 0·7 for cytochromes-a_3, a, c and b respectively.

Effects of light scattering. Light scattering by the turbid material could cause errors in the changes in measured optical density, and therefore the absorption of cytochrome-c has been remeasured in the presence of two substances that diminish the light scattering[5]. First, the addition of 67 per cent glucose greatly increases the refractive index of the medium surrounding the particles, but does not measurably decrease the change in optical density at 551 mμ. Secondly, a decrease of only 25 per cent in the change in optical density at 551 mμ occurs upon addition of 2 per cent cholate, which allows the cytochrome-c to leave the particles. No large error can be attributed to light scattering under the conditions of our experiments, and we shall proceed to estimate the cytochrome content with no correction for light scattering.

Cytochrome content of the succinic oxidase system. The concentrations of a solution of these cytochromes spectrophotometrically equivalent to the insoluble material is termed the 'cytochrome content' and is calculated from the estimated changes of molecular extinction coefficients ($\Delta \varepsilon$) as follows. In the case of cytochrome-c, the content is computed directly from known data on the soluble material,

$$[c] = \frac{\Delta D_{551} - \Delta D_{541}}{19 \cdot 1} \ mM \ {}^{13}.$$

For cytochrome-b, two values of the value of $\Delta \varepsilon$ are available, one for cytochrome-b_2 [14] and one for cytochrome-b from diphtheria bacteria[15]. Both these data give results very close to 20 cm.$^{-1}$ × mM^{-1}, and

$$[b] = \frac{\Delta D_{561} - \Delta D_{575}}{20} \ mM.$$

In the case of *Atmungsferment* of yeast cells the photochemical absorption spectrum of the carbon monoxide compound[4] gives a value of $\varepsilon_{431} = 161$ cm.$^{-1}$ × mM^{-1}. We have observed the absorption peak of ferrocytochrome-a_3 to shift from 444 to 430 mμ in respiring yeast cells in the presence of carbon monoxide, and Keilin and Hartree previously found the same shift in heart muscle[5] which we have verified by our spectrophotometric method. None of these data agrees with the result of Ball *et al.*, who find the a_3·CO band at 423 mμ in a desoxycholate-treated preparation that was probably contaminated with hæmoglobin[16]. Thus it appears justifiable to identify Warburg's data on *Atmungsferment* with our data on heart muscle. By a comparison of the Soret spectra of the oxidized and reduced forms of the pure dichroic-hæmin enzyme, lactoperoxidase[17], and its carbon monoxide compound with the corresponding spectrum of cytochrome-a_3, proportionality constants are derived, and a value of $\Delta\epsilon_{444} = 180$ cm.$^{-1} \times$ mM^{-1} is computed for cytochrome-a_3 :

$$[a_3] = \frac{\Delta D_{444}}{180} \text{ mM.}$$

(According to Lemberg[18], the analogy between the hæmins of these verdoperoxidases and that of the respiratory enzyme is not as close as might be desired, but the chemical and spectroscopic properties of the intact enzymes are rather similar.) In the case of cytochrome-a, no carbon monoxide compound is known at pH 7, and this is a point in common with verdoperoxidase[19], which is a non-autoxidizable green hæmin enzyme with a single band in the red (at 630 mμ) in the difference spectrum of the oxidized and reduced forms. We thus assume that the values of $\Delta\epsilon_{630}$ for verdoperoxidase (14 cm.$^{-1} \times$ mM^{-1}) is identical with the value for cytochrome-a at 605 mμ. Thus

$$[a] = \frac{\Delta D_{605}}{14} \text{ mM.}$$

On the basis of these data, the relative content of these four cytochrome components in an average preparation is 1, 2, 1·6, 1·0 for cytochromes-a_3, a, c and b respectively ; and on the basis of a titration of heart muscle preparation with antimycin-a[20], we find the relative content of Slater's factor to be 1·2 (assuming antimycin binds two iron equivalents). Thus there is remarkable similarity in the content of five components of the succinic oxidase system, sufficient similarity to allow the suggestion that the 'succinic oxidase assembly' consists of roughly one each of the components. A more exact stoichiometry has not yet been proved.

Studies of the cytochrome content of the giant mitochondria of the flight muscle of the blow-fly[21] give a rather similar content for cytochromes-a and a_3, the relative values being 1, 1·6, 3·7, 3·5 respectively for cytochromes-a_3, a, c and b. The content of cytochromes-c and b exceeds that of the heart muscle homogenates.

Turnover numbers of the cytochrome components. On the basis of the relative concentrations of the cytochrome components, their turnover number in succinic oxidase activity at 26° is readily calculated as the quotient

$$\frac{\mu M \text{ O}_2/\text{sec.}}{\Delta D_{444}} = K_4,$$

and has values ranging over 80 for a very active preparation. By converting from oxygen to iron equivalents (4 ×) and from ΔD_{444} to concentration

$$\text{in } \mu M \left(\times \frac{10^3}{180} \right),$$

Source	$K_4 = \dfrac{\mu M \text{ O}_2/\text{sec.}}{\Delta D_{444}}$	Turnover numbers				
		a_3	a	c	b	'factor'
Heart muscle (horse or pig)	80 (max.)	58	29	36	58	48
Pea seedlings	35	25	—	—	—	—
Flight muscle (mitochondria)	25	18	11	5	5	—
Yeast cells (baker's)	220	160	58	18	46	—

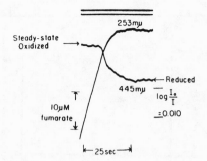

Fig. 3*A*. Correlation between the rate of production of fumarate and the extent of reduction of cytochrome-a_3 as measured by the double-beam spectrophotometer. 50-fold dilution of heart-muscle preparation

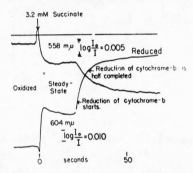

Fig. 3*B*. Correlation between the kinetics of reduction of cytochrome-a and cytochrome-b. The moment at which succinate is added to the oxidized heart-muscle preparation is indicated and is followed by the steady-state operation of these enzymes. Reduction occurs when the dissolved oxygen is exhausted. An inward deflexion of these traces corresponds to an increase of optical density. (Expt. 763)

the turnover number of cytochrome-a_3 is 0·72K_4, or 58 sec.$^{-1}$ for the highly active preparation. The other values are 29, 36, 58 and 48 for cytochromes-a, c, b, and Slater's factor respectively, providing these components are actually in the main pathway. Results for plant succinic oxidase (prepared by Dr. Helen Stafford, Botany Department, University of Pennsylvania), mitochondria of blow-fly muscle (prepared by Dr. L. Levenbook, Biological Laboratories, Harvard University) and yeast cells are summarized in Table 1.

Percentage oxidation of the cytochromes in the steady state. Upon addition of a few microlitres of saturated succinate ($\sim 2 M$) to aerated heart muscle preparation, the partially reduced spectrum of cytochromes-a, b and c appears, remains in a steady state and is about doubled in intensity when the oxygen is used up (see Fig. 3*B*). This is interpreted to mean that the cytochromes are only partially oxidized in the presence of excess oxygen and succinate. (This dynamic phenomenon must not be confused with an oxidation-reduction potential effect[9], which will only set the limits of reduction following the steady state.) By measuring at the appropriate wave-lengths, described above, the percentages of steady-state oxidation for six preparations are 87, 69, 64, 68 for cytochromes-a_3, a, c and b. These percentages are sensitive to inhibitors and other factors as described below and are, in fact, indicators of the level of activity of the cytochromes.

A steady-state analysis of the kinetics of cytochrome action. By means of a simple theory which assumes that reactions of the bound cytochromes occur in accordance with the law of mass action, for example, by collision with one another with thermal vibrations, the velocity constants for the following sequence of reactions are readily computed if it is assumed that the reverse reactions proceed at a negligible rate :

$$O_2 \xrightarrow{k_1} a_3 \xrightarrow{k_2} a \xrightarrow{k_5} c \xrightarrow{k_7} s \xrightarrow{k_9} \text{succinate.} \quad (1)$$

s represents succinic dehydrogenase plus Slater's factor, and the oxidized and reduced forms of the enzymes are appropriately identified (for example, a_2'', a_3'''). The oxygen and succinate concentrations at any time are x and y respectively.

$$k_3 = \frac{a'''}{a_3'''} \cdot \frac{c''}{a''} k_5, \quad k_5 = \frac{c'''}{a''} \cdot \frac{a''}{c'i} k_7, \quad k_7 = \frac{s'''y}{c'''s''} k_9,$$

$$k_9 = \frac{1}{s'''y} \left(-\frac{dy}{dt} \right).$$

Since the overall activity at a given succinate concentration $(- dy/dt)$, the total concentrations of the components, and their percentage oxidation are known, k_3, k_5, k_7 and k_9 are readily calculated and represent the reaction velocity constants that would obtain in a solution spectrophotometrically equivalent to the insoluble system. (Since there is a question of the role of cytochrome-b, the value of s is based on the content of Slater's factor, and the steady-state oxidation is estimated to be 50 per cent.)

In the case of the reaction with oxygen, cytochrome-a_3 is so largely oxidized in the steady-state that non-steady-state conditions must be used. The velocity constant is calculated from oxidase activity data at low oxygen concentrations as in Fig. 1 from the equation

$$k_1 = \frac{1}{xa_3''} \left(-\frac{dx}{dt} \right),$$

which applies to any portion of the traces of Fig. 1. The experimental results and the tentative values of the reaction velocity constants for the equivalent system are summarized :

Reaction velocity constant
$\times 10^{-6}$ ($M^{-1} \times$ sec.$^{-1}$)

$$\qquad\qquad\quad \overset{10}{O_2} \xrightarrow{} \overset{30}{a_3} \xrightarrow{} \overset{30}{a} \xrightarrow{} \overset{40}{c} \xrightarrow{} \overset{0 \cdot 01}{s} \xrightarrow{} \text{succinate (2)}$$

Relative content	1·0	2·0	1·6	1·2
Per cent oxidation	87	69	64	(50)

The magnitudes of these velocity constants are quite reasonable in view of the measured rates of reactions of peroxidases, catalases[22], and myoglobin[23].

The extent to which the data on the spectrophotometrically equivalent soluble system apply to the actual insoluble system has been considered in detail. The velocity constants for the external reactions (those with oxygen and succinate) are probably about the same for the insoluble system, because the diffusibility of the soluble enzyme molecule is already almost negligible compared to that of the substrate molecule. If the internal enzymes react with each other by collision and are physically bound to the heart muscle particles, their spacing would be of the order of a molecular diameter, and consequently their effective concentration would be very large. On the other hand, a sequential arrangement of these bound cytochromes in 'succinic oxidase assemblies' containing roughly one each of the components may occur, and interaction between the corresponding members of different assemblies may not be possible. This consideration would reduce the effective concentration of closely packed cytochromes, since an internal enzyme would react only with its neighbours in the sequence. The best estimate of the effective concentration of the internal enzymes is based on kinetic data : soluble cytochrome-c and 'solubilized cytochrome oxidase'[24] react in solution with very nearly the same velocity constant as that computed above for the equivalent soluble system of heart muscle preparation ($\sim 10^7 M^{-1} \times$ sec.$^{-1}$). Thus the effective concentration of the internal enzymes may be of the same order as that of the spectrophotometrically equivalent system. The values of relative content given above may then be regarded as preliminary estimates of the micromolar concentrations of the internal enzymes.

Kinetic studies of the reduction of the cytochromes. The kinetics of reduction of the cytochromes have been examined with respect to one another and with respect to the termination of the overall enzymatic activity as the oxygen concentration falls to zero as shown in Figs. 3A and B respectively. These records were obtained with a double-beam spectrophotometer which permits simultaneous recording at two wave-lengths in the visible and ultra-violet[7]. Fig. 3A shows that the reduction of cytochrome-a_3 and the decrease of fumarate production occur at the same time (the equivalent oxygen affinity corresponds to $2 \times 10^{-6} M$ from this record). Similar simultaneous studies of cytochromes-a_3, a and c show that their reduction also occurs at very nearly the same time, even when studied at 4°. In detail, the initiation of the reduction of cytochrome-c lags behind that of cytochromes-a and a_3, but then runs faster and is about 10 per cent ahead at the half-way point. The reduction of cytochrome-b lags considerably, as is shown by Fig. 3B ; its reduction does not start until that of cytochrome-a has proceeded appreciably, and is only half completed when that of cytochrome-a has reached 80 per cent. Thus the reduction of cytochrome-b is prolonged not only after that of the other cytochromes but also continues after the production of fumarate has ceased. An electric analogue computer study of the reaction mechanism of equation 2 shows that this behaviour is inconsistent ; cytochrome-b does not participate in the pathway of electron transfer provided by this simple mechanism. (A general theorem applicable to enzyme systems of this type is that the time derivatives of the concentrations of the intermediate compounds must be zero when the time derivatives of the substrate concentrations are zero.)

No evidence of time separation in the oxidation of the cytochromes has yet been obtained (4°, $\sim 1 \times 10^{-4} M$ oxygen, time resolution $\sim 0 \cdot 5$ sec.).

Kinetics of reduction of cytochromes-a, b and c in cyanide-inhibited systems. In a cyanide-inhibited system, it is possible to measure the speed with which the various cytochromes are reduced by succinate and to compare these rates with the values of oxidase activity that are obtained in the uninhibited system. This procedure was used in 1934 by Haas, who studied the cytochrome-c band of yeast cells[8]. Again, these studies are most effectively carried out at low temperatures (4°), and the data of Table 2 have been so obtained. The uninhibited oxidase activity is cal-

Table 2. COMPARISON OF THE RATES OF SUCCINATE REDUCTION OF CYTOCHROMES-*a*, *b* AND *c*, WITH THE ESTIMATED VALUES OF TURNOVER OF THESE COMPONENTS REQUIRED BY . THE MEASURED OXIDASE ACTIVITY. (4° C.) (EXPTS. 774 AND 775.)

Estimated concentration of cytochromes-*a*, *c* and *b*, 4, 2·7 and 1·7 μM respectively

	32	320	800	3,200
Succinate (μM)	32	320	800	3,200
Oxidase activity (μM O$_2$/sec.)	0·06	0·12	0·19	0·26
Estimated turnover numbers (sec.$^{-1}$)				
for cytochrome-*a*	0·06	0·12	0·19	0·26
for cytochrome-*c*	0·09	0·18	0·28	0·38
for cytochrome-*b*	0·14	0·28	0·44	0·61
Measured rates of reduction in cyanide-inhibited heart-muscle preparation (sec.$^{-1}$)				
for cytochrome-*a*	0·034	0·090	0·18	0·39
for cytochrome-*c*	—	0·17	0·28	0·28
for cytochrome-*b*	—	0·004	0·0140	0·009

culated from the time interval between the addition of substrate and the exhaustion of dissolved oxygen, and the rates are computed for various initial succinate concentrations. These values are converted into turnover numbers by means of the estimated cytochrome concentrations, and may be compared with the velocity constants for the reduction of the cyanide-inhibited material. It can be seen that there is reasonable agreement for cytochromes-*a* and *c*, and therefore the rate of reduction of these cytochromes is sufficiently rapid to explain the measured oxidase activity (not only at 4° but also at 26°). But the rate of reduction of cytochrome-*b* by succinate is so slow that only 2 per cent of the oxidase activity could be carried through this cytochrome component. Our cyanide concentrations and reaction times are much too small to cause the inhibition of succinic dehydrogenase observed by Tsou[25]. It is proposed that cytochrome-*b* is linked to succinic dehydrogenase as follows :

$$O_2 \xrightarrow{} a_3 \xrightarrow{} a \xrightarrow{} c \xrightarrow{} s \xrightarrow{} \text{succinate.} \quad (3)$$

$$\underset{\text{oxidation}}{\overset{\text{fast}}{\Big\uparrow}} \underset{\text{reduction}}{\overset{\text{slow}}{\Big\downarrow}}$$
$$b$$

Effect of physical and chemical factors upon the steady state of cytochrome action. The steady-state oxidation of the cytochromes may be varied over wide ranges by selective inhibitors in a manner that indicates the point of action of the inhibitor. This is clearly illustrated by the effect of antimycin-*a* (Ahmad, Schneider and Strong[26]) upon the cytochrome components as shown in Fig. 4. According to equation 2, representing the mechanism of action

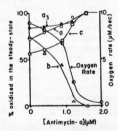

Fig. 4. Effect of antimycin-*a* upon the oxidase activity and the steady-state oxidation of the cytochrome components. The steady-state oxidation of cytochromes is measured as in experiments similar to those of Fig. 3*B* for various concentrations of antimycin-*a*. The antimycin-*a* sample was kindly given by Dr. F. M. Strong and the stock solution was made up in ethanol. (Expt. 793)

of the cytochromes, one would expect an increase in the steady-state concentrations of the oxidized form of those cytochromes on the oxygen side of the inhibited component and a decrease for those on the succinate side. Also a larger inflexion of the curves for the components nearer the inhibited component would be expected. Thus the traces of Fig. 4 represent the effect of the inhibitor upon a component acting between cytochrome-*c* and succinic dehydrogenase, Slater's factor, in agreement with Potter and Rief[20]. No change in optical density in the region 530–565 mμ is observed on adding this inhibitor to the oxidized cytochromes. But the absorption band in the region of 555–570 mμ upon succinate reduction of heart-muscle preparation inhibited by antimycin-*a* is somewhat stronger than the 561-mμ band in the uninhibited enzyme. This modification of the absorption band may be caused specifically by Slater's factor or by a compound of cytochrome-*b* and the inhibitor.

The cyanide inhibition of heart-muscle preparation is much more complicated than would be expected on the basis of analogies with soluble hæmoproteins. Although the disappearance of the absorption band of ferrocytochrome-a_3 at 444 mμ upon the addition of cyanide (and some oxygen) is a rapid reaction and is presumably caused by a binding of ferricytochrome-a_3 by cyanide[5], the inhibition of the oxidase activity upon adding cyanide to the oxidized enzyme, preliminary studies on which were carried out in collaboration with Dr. E. C. Slater, occurs very slowly (over several minutes). The results of these studies suggest that the form of cytochrome oxidase inhibited by cyanide is present in large concentrations in the reduced system, in low concentrations in the steady-state oxidized system, and in very low concentrations in the fully oxidized system. Some reconsideration of the mechanism of cyanide inhibition of the succinic oxidase system is required, but a full explanation is difficult in the absence of any evidence for competition between oxygen and cyanide.

Whereas the effect of temperature upon the succinic oxidase activity is very large (μ ~ 11,000 cal.), the steady-state oxidation of the cytochromes varies but little over the temperature range 4°–40° and corresponds to less than 1,000 cal. On the basis of the mechanism of equation 2, the velocity constants for the reactions of the cytochromes with one another have about the same temperature dependence as those that react with oxygen and succinate.

Studies of the respiratory enzymes of intact yeast cells. The methods that have been used for heart-muscle particles are also suitable for studies of five of the respiratory enzymes of baker's yeast cells, cytochromes-a_3, *a*, *c*, *b*, and the pyridine nucleotide enzymes. The difference spectra of the components have been obtained as shown in Fig. 5*a* and correspond to a sequence of optical densities of 4·5, 1, 4·2, 1·8 and 29, giving a relative content of 1, 2, 8·9, 3·6 and 200 respectively. (Euler *et al.*[27] found 250 μgm. of coenzyme-I in 1 gm. of yeast. Our data give 300 μgm. of total pyridine nucleotides per gram of our yeast.) The value of turnover numbers of the cytochrome components is 160, 58, 18 and 46 at 26°, assuming that they are in the main pathway of electron transfer. The pyridine nucleotide content of the yeast cells is relatively enormous compared with that of the cytochromes ; and the content of cytochromes-*c* and *b* is larger than in the heart-muscle preparations.

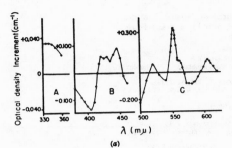

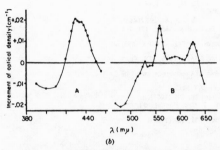

Fig. 5. Difference spectra of the cytochrome components of a yeast and a bacterial culture

Fig. 5a shows the changes in optical density from the steady-state to reduced for baker's yeast in the ultra-violet, violet, and visible regions of the spectrum. The dilutions of the yeast cells were 22·5, 4·5 and 1 for *A*, *B* and *C* respectively, and the changes in optical density are computed per cm. The value of the oxygen rate for the 4·5-fold dilution was 100 μM O_2/sec. at 25°, corresponding to $K_4 = \mu M$ O_2/sec./$\Delta D_{444} = 110$. (Expt. 719a, b and 791)

Fig. 5b shows the difference spectrum of *Aerobacter aerogenes* reduced in the presence of 3·3 mM glucose. In *A*, the dilution of the cells is 6-fold, and in *B*, 1·5-fold. $K_4 = \dfrac{\mu M\ O_2/sec.}{\Delta D433} = 150$ at 25°

The reduced pyridine nucleotides (DPNH) are not stable under anaerobic conditions; at the end of a minute their concentration has fallen to half the maximum value, presumably because of the delayed initiation of anaerobic glycolytic reactions. The (DPNH) band is shifted towards 325 mμ, presumably by binding to protein in the manner of alcohol dehydrogenase[28]. Such bound reduced pyridine nucleotide is more closely associated with the cytochromes than the free reduced pyridine nucleo-tides.

The yeast cells also contain a peroxidase[29] which, in common with other peroxidases[30], rapidly oxidizes ferrocytochrome-c in the presence of peroxide. By adding methyl hydrogen peroxide (that is, not decomposed into oxygen by catalase[31]) to the reduced cytochromes of yeast cells, oxidation of not only cytochrome-c but also the pyridine nucleotide enzymes is obtained to the extent of 75 and 65 per cent respectively. This is the first direct evidence for the intracellular oxidation of respiratory enzymes via the peroxidase – peroxide system, but the function of this system with endogenous peroxide is not proved.

In the presence of peroxide, cytochrome-a_2 is bound in what appears to be a peroxide complex and remains so bound until the peroxide is used up; only then may the oxidized form of cytochrome-a_2 be obtained.

Difference spectra of some bacterial cytochromes (Dr. Lucile Smith has collaborated in these studies). The

visible and ultra-violet absorption spectra of a few bacterial strains have been measured and the result for *Aerobacter aerogenes* (a culture kindly given by Dr. A. Tissières, Molteno Institute, University of Cambridge) is shown in Fig. 5b. The peak of the cytochrome-a_2 lies at 628 mμ and cytochrome-b_1 at 561 mμ. A small peak is also found at about 590 mμ in accordance with Tissières[32]. In the region of the Soret band there is a single peak at 430 mμ, presumably the γ-band of cytochrome-b_1. The shoulder in this Soret band is unidentified, since it is well removed from 444 mμ, where the γ-band of cytochrome-a_2 would have been expected in view of the photochemical data of Kubowitz and Haas on *Acetobacter*[33], and in view of the high respiration of these cells (μM O_2/sec./$\Delta D_{430} = 150$ at 25°). But carbon monoxide does not reveal the characteristic cytochrome a_2-CO absorption bands, and those attributable to a_2-CO differ markedly from those of hæmoproteins : the Soret band (437 mμ) is less than one-third as large as the visible band (645 mμ). The earlier view that cytochrome-a_2 is a bile pigment hæmochromogen[17] is supported.

Summary. Effective spectrophotometric methods for the study of spectra and kinetics of the respiratory pigments of muscle homogenates or intact cells have been developed. At present, an intensive and detailed study of the four cytochrome components of heart-muscle homogenates has clearly defined the spectra representing the difference between their oxidized and reduced states, has led to estimates of the relative and absolute amounts of these cytochromes, and has permitted an estimate of the velocity constants with which such insoluble cytochromes may react with each other and with their substrates. The latter calculations are made on the basis of a simple hypothesis that requires only that the bound cytochromes collide with each other by thermal vibrations about the point of their attachment to the particle. The kinetics of reduction of these cytochromes by succinate in uninhibited and in cyanide-inhibited systems has been measured. In the uninhibited systems, the reduction of cytochrome-b lags considerably behind the nearly simultaneous reduction of cytochromes-a_3, a and c and the cessation of the overall activity. In the inhibited system, the velocity constant for the reduction of cytochrome-b is so small that only 2–10 per cent of the measured oxidase activity (in the uninhibited system) could be accounted for. Thus cytochrome-b is regarded more as an indicator of succinic dehydrogenase activity than as a component in the main pathway of electron transfer of heart muscle preparations.

In respiring yeast cells, the kinetics and spectra of not only the four cytochrome components, but also the pyridine nucleotide enzymes may be studied in detail. In the anaerobic yeast, direct evidence for the intracellular oxidation of respiratory enzymes via the peroxidase – peroxide system has been obtained, but no proof of the functions of this system with endogenous peroxide can yet be given.

In a bacterial strain that contains cytochrome-a_2, there was no evidence of the characteristic absorption band of cytochrome-a_2 in the region of the Soret band, and the behaviour with carbon monoxide differs considerably from that of cytochrome-a_3. This finding may require a revision of our views on the uniformity of the properties of the 'oxygen transporting enzyme'.

This investigation has been supported in part by a grant from the Division of Research Grants and

Fellowships, National Institutes of Health, United States Public Health Service, and by a grant from the Office of Naval Research.

[1] MacMunn, C. A., *J. Physiol.*, **6**, 22 (1885).

[2] Keilin, D., *Proc. Roy. Soc.*, B, **98**, 312 (1925).

[3] Warburg, O., for a summary, see "Schwermetalle ...", chapter 14 (Freiburg, 1949).

[4] Warburg, O., and Negelein, E., *Biochem. Z.*, **214**, 64 (1929).

[5] Keilin, D., and Hartree, E. F., *Proc. Roy. Soc.*, B, **127**, 167 (1939).

[6] Slater, E. C., *Biochem. J.*, **45**, 14 (1949).

[7] Chance, B., *Rev. Sci. Instr.*, **22**, 619 (1951).

[8] Haas, E., *Naturwiss.*, **22**, 207 (1934).

[9] Baumberger, J. P., Cold Spring Harbor Symposia, **7**, 195 (1939).

[10] Arvanitaki, A., and Chalazonitis, N., *Arch. Internat. Physiol.*, **54**, 441 (1947).

[11] Davies, P. W., and Brink, F., *Rev. Sci. Instr.*, **13**, 524 (1942).

[12] Keilin, D., and Hartree, E. F., *Biochem. J.*, **41**, 503 (1947).

[13] Theorell, H., *Biochem. Z.*, **285**, 207 (1936).

[14] Bach, S. J., Dixon, M., and Zerfas, L. G., *Biochem. J.*, **40**, 229 (1946).

[15] Pappenheimer, A. M., and Hendee, E. D., *J. Biol. Chem.*, **171**, 701 (1947) (and personal communication).

[16] Ball, E. G., Strittmatter, C. F., and Cooper, O., *J. Biol. Chem.*, **193**, 635 (1951).

[17] Theorell, H., and Akesson, A., *Ark. Kemi, Min. o. Geol.*, **17B**, No. 7 (1943).

[18] Lemberg, R., and Legge, J. W., "Hematin Compounds and Bile Pigments" (Interscience, 1939).

[19] Agner, K., *Acta Physiol. Scand.*, **2**, Supp. 8 (1941).

[20] Potter, V. R., and Rief, A. C., *Fed. Proc.*, **10**, 234 (1951).

[21] Watanabe, M. I., and Williams, C. M., *J. Gen. Physiol.*, **34**, 675 (1951).

[22] Chance, B., in "Advances in Enzymology", **12**, 153 (1951).

[23] Millikan, G. A., *Physiol. Rev.*, **19**, 503 (1939).

[24] Smith, L., *Fed. Proc.*, **10**, 249 (1951).

[25] Tsou, C. I., *Biochem. J.*, **49**, 512 (1951).

[26] Ahmad, K., Schneider, H. G., and Strong, F. M., *Arch. Biochem.*, **28**, 281 (1950).

[27] Euler, H. v., Schlenk, F., Heiwinkel, H., and Hogberg, B., *Z. physiol. Chem.*, **256**, 208 (1938).

[28] Theorell, H., and Bonnichsen, R. K., *Acta Chem. Scand.*, **5**, 1105 (1951).

[29] Altschul, A. M., Abrams, R., and Hogness, T. R., *J. Biol. Chem.*, **136**, 777 (1940).

[30] Chance, B., in "Enzymes and Enzyme Systems" (Harvard Univ. Press, 1951).

[31] Stern, K. G., *J. Biol. Chem.*, **114**, 473 (1936).

[32] Tissières, A., *Biochem. J.*, **50**, 279 (1951)

[33] Kubowitz, F., and Haas, E., *Biochem. Z.*, **255**, 247 (1932).

8

Reprinted from J. Biol. Chem. **239**:4280–4291 (1964)

Oxidative Phosphorylation in Fractionated Bacterial Systems

XIV. RESPIRATORY CHAINS OF *MYCOBACTERIUM PHLEI**

Akira Asano† and Arnold F. Brodie

From the Department of Microbiology, University of Southern California School of Medicine and Los Angeles County General Hospital, Los Angeles, California 90033

(Received for publication, May 4, 1964)

Bacterial and mammalian systems capable of oxidative phosphorylation require the presence of a highly organized particulate structure. Although the methods required for the isolation of particles from bacteria (1) are more vigorous than the procedures used for the isolation of mitochondria from animal tissues, the bacterial particles remain relatively intact and contain the terminal respiratory carriers necessary for coupled oxidative phosphorylation (2). Nevertheless, the particles alone fail to carry out coupled activity unless supplemented with soluble protein factors (2–8). The soluble fraction from *Mycobacterium phlei* contains both oxidative components and coupling factors (4, 6).

Phosphorylation with a cell-free system from *M. phlei* was shown to be inextricably associated with oxidation. Thus, an understanding of the mechanisms of oxidative phosphorylation requires detailed knowledge of the respiratory chains. Earlier studies of the electron transport chain (2, 9) suggested broad areas associated with the phosphorylative process; however, more detailed analysis was necessary in order to locate the phosphorylative sites precisely. The respiratory chains of *M. phlei* appear to be similar to those described for mammalian mitochondria (10). In many respects, this bacterial system resembles the system observed with disrupted mitochondrial preparations. Differences between the *M. phlei* and the mitochondrial system were found in quinone composition (11–14) and in the presence of an additional respiratory chain for malate. In the bacterial system, oxidative phosphorylation with malate can occur by a pathway independent of nicotinamide adenine dinucleotide (15). The flavin adenine dinucleotide-linked malate and NAD+-linked chains converge at the naphthoquinone (vitamin K_9H) level and utilize the same terminal respiratory carriers. The succinate chain in *M. phlei* enters the terminal respiratory chain at the cytochrome *b* level. The properties of these three respiratory chains in *M. phlei* will be described in this paper.

EXPERIMENTAL PROCEDURE

Vitamin K_1 used in these experiments was a gift from Dr. K. Folkers of Merck Sharp and Dohme, Rahway, New Jersey, or was purchased from Mann Research Laboratories. This vitamin was further purified by column chromatography on Permutit

* This work was supported by Grant AI-05637 from the National Institutes of Health, United States Public Health Service, and by the Hastings Foundation of the University of Southern California School of Medicine.

† On leave of absence from the Institute for Protein Research, Osaka University, Osaka, Japan.

before use. The purified vitamin K_1 (10 mg) was suspended in 2 ml of 0.05 M Tris, pH 7.4, containing 50 mg of Asolectin with sonic oscillation for 5 minutes.

Asolectin (plant phospholipid mixture) was purchased from Associated Concentrates, Woodside, New York. Oligomycin was obtained from the Wisconsin Alumni Foundation, Madison. 2-*n*-Nonylhydroxyquinoline *N*-oxide was obtained from Sigma Chemical Company. Yeast hexokinase was obtained from Pabst Laboratories. All of the other chemicals used were commercially available and of reagent grade.

Inhibitors such as 2-*n*-nonylhydroxyquinoline *N*-oxide, Dicumarol, carbonyl cyanide *m*-chlorophenylhydrazone, pentachlorophenol, and sodium Amytal were suspended in 8 ml of water, and 3 N KOH or 1 N HCl was added dropwise with vigorous stirring until a clear solution was obtained. The pH was adjusted to 7.2 or 7.4, and the mixture was brought to a final volume of 10 ml. 2-*n*-Nonylhydroxyquinoline *N*-oxide was adjusted to pH 8.5 before dilution. Other relatively insoluble compounds such as rotenone, oligomycin, or thienyltrifluorobutanedione were dissolved in a small amount of acetone (0.1 to 1.0 ml) and then diluted 100 times with distilled water. Many of the solutions, ascorbate, phenazine methosulfate, 2-*n*-nonylhydroxyquinoline *N*-oxide, Dicumarol, and carbonyl cyanide *m*-chlorophenylhydrazone were prepared fresh daily. In addition, the concentration was checked by spectrophotometric means when possible.

Preparation of Particles and Soluble Components—*M. phlei* ATCC 354 cells were grown and harvested by procedures previously described (16). Sonically disrupted cells were separated into particulate and supernatant fractions by differential centrifugation in the Spinco preparative centrifuge (6). The particles obtained following centrifugation were washed with 0.15 M KCl containing 0.01 M $MgCl_2$ and adjusted to pH 7.4 with Tris buffer (0.01 M). Two types of particles were used in these studies: (*a*) washed particles freshly prepared and (*b*) particles stored at −15°, which are referred to as aged particles (2). The supernatant fraction was dialyzed with distilled water for 2 or 3 days with several changes of water. Dialysis was carried out at 4° with constant stirring. The crude supernatant either was used directly or was further fractionated with ammonium sulfate and chromatographed on DEAE-cellulose (17).

Measurement of Oxidation and Coupled Phosphorylation—Respiration was measured by conventional manometric techniques at 30°. The main compartment of each vessel contained washed particles (5 to 10 mg of protein), dialyzed supernatant (5 to 15 mg of protein), 15 µmoles of $MgCl_2$, 5 to 12 µmoles of inorganic phosphate, 3 mg of yeast hexokinase, and 10 μmoles of glucose. The cofactors or inhibitors indicated were added to the main compartment and allowed to incubate with the particulate and supernatant fractions for at least 10 minutes before addition of substrate. The side arm of the vessels contained 25 μmoles of KF, 2.5 μmoles of ADP, and substrate. The total volume was adjusted to 1.5 ml with water. Inorganic phosphate esterification was determined by the method of Fiske and SubbaRow (18). Protein was determined by the turbidmetric method of Stadtman, Novelli, and Lipmann (19) or by the method of Lowry *et al.* (20).

Measurement of Difference Spectra—The reduced minus oxidized difference spectrum of the particulate preparation was measured following substrate addition with a split beam spectrophotometer (21). A cuvette with a 1- or 0.2-cm light path was used at room temperature; however, at the temperature of liquid nitrogen, a cuvette with a 0.2-cm light path was employed (22). The difference spectrum between a CO-treated reduced preparation and a reduced preparation was measured by the method described by Chance (23) with a Cary model 11 recording spectrophotometer. A gentle stream of carbon monoxide was added to the anaerobic sample for about 1 minute. The inability to change the difference spectrum by the further addition of carbon monoxide was taken to indicate saturation of the binding capacity of this agent.

The double beam spectrophotometer with a vibrating platinum oxygen electrode was used for measurement of the rate of cytochrome reduction. These experiments were carried out in the laboratory of Dr. B. Chance. The dual wave length spectrophotometer (American Instrument Company) was also used to measure the rate of reduction of the terminal respiratory pigments.

Artificial electron acceptors were used to measure malate-vitamin K reductase (15) activity or NADH oxidation. These reactions were followed spectrophotometrically with the Cary model 11 recording spectrophotometer or Gilford automatic recording attachment for the Beckman spectrophotometer.

RESULTS

Respiratory Chain Components—The distribution of respiratory carriers differs in the particulate and supernatant fractions. The particulate fraction contains all of the known respiratory carriers (bound NAD^+, flavins, vitamin K_9H, and the cytochromes), whereas the supernatant fraction contains NAD^+, flavins, and small amounts of vitamin K_9H. The particulate fraction appears to contain sufficient quantities of the respiratory carriers, since oxidative phosphorylation with generated NADH or succinate can be carried out with the particles alone. Stimulation of both oxidation and phosphorylation occurs on the addition of soluble protein components found in the supernatant fraction (6, 17, 24). Oxidation with β-hydroxybutyrate or malate as electron donor requires the addition of cofactors (NAD^+ or FAD) and the solubilized dehydrogenases for these substrates.

Evidence for participation of the terminal respiratory chain of the particulate fraction was obtained by examining the difference spectrum with various substrates as electron donors. The reduced minus oxidized difference spectrum of the particulate fraction or particulate and supernatant fractions of *M. phlei* was measured after substrate, or substrate and inhibitor, was added and the system allowed to achieve the anaerobic state.

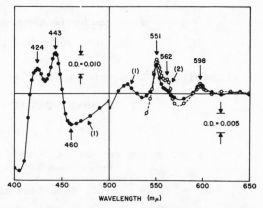

Fig. 1. Reduced minus oxidized difference spectrum of particles from *M. phlei*. The system consisted of 32 μmoles of $MgCl_2$, 107 μmoles of KCl, 3 μmoles of inorganic phosphate, 5.3 μmoles of ADP, 2.5 mμmoles of FAD, 6.0 mg of washed particles, 8.6 mg of dialyzed supernatant fluid, 36 μmoles of Tris-HCl buffer (pH 7.4), and water to a final volume of 3.0 ml. The reaction was carried out at room temperature (24°) in a 1-cm cuvette. *Curve 1*, spectrum obtained following incubation of the system with succinate for 10 minutes (the time necessary to reach the anaerobic state). The reference system was kept in the oxidized state by supplying a stream of oxygen. *Curve 2*, spectrum obtained following the addition of 2-*n*-nonylhydroxyquinoline *N*-oxide (9.0 μg) and sodium dithionite.

Following the addition of succinate, absorption bands appear at 598, 562, and 550 mμ (Fig. 1). These peaks are characteristic of the α-bands of cytochrome types *a*, *b*, and *c*, respectively. Examination of the Soret region revealed a trough characteristic of flavoprotein (460 mμ). The Soret band of cytochrome *b* was found at 430 mμ, while those of cytochromes *c* and *a* + *a₃* were distinguished as shoulders at 420 and 445 mμ, respectively. In the presence of 2-*n*-nonylhydroxyquinoline *N*-oxide the Soret band of cytochrome *b* was shifted from 430 to 433 mμ. The difference spectrum of the particulate fraction with succinate as substrate was independent of the addition of the supernatant fraction; however, stimulation of the rate of reduction of cytochromes *b*, c,[1] and *a* + *a₃* occurred on the addition of the soluble fraction. Reduction of the terminal respiratory pigments with malate or β-hydroxybutyrate, in contrast to succinate, required the addition of supernatant components.

Quantitative differences in reduction of the terminal respiratory pigments were observed with substrates that utilize different pathways of oxidation. The reduced bands of cytochrome *b* (562 and 430 mμ) with succinate or malate as electron donor were less prominent than those observed with β-hydroxybutyrate as substrate. Reduction with sodium dithionite resulted in a difference spectrum which was qualitatively similar to that observed on the addition of substrate and which differed only in that a greater reduction of cytochrome *b* was observed following chemi-

---

[1] Cytochrome c_1 contributes to the absorption in the *c* region and cannot be distinguished at room temperature; from low temperature studies it would appear that the absorption due to this component at 551 mμ is small when compared with that of cytochrome *c*. Nevertheless, the values reported for the enzymatically reducible cytochrome *c* represent the absorption of cytochrome $c + c_1$.

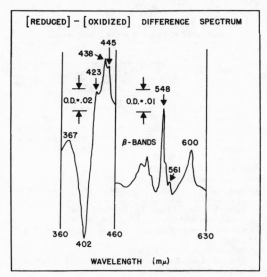

FIG. 2. Reduced minus oxidized difference spectrum of *M. phlei* particles at the temperature of liquid nitrogen. The system contained 2 μmoles of MgCl₂, 32 μmoles of KCl, 4.1 mg of washed particles, 4 μmoles of Tris-HCl buffer (pH 7.4), and water to a final volume of 0.6 ml. In addition, one of the cuvettes contained 20 μmoles of succinate and 1.0 μmole of sodium sulfide. The reaction was carried out in a 0.2-cm cuvette at room temperature and brought to 77° K.

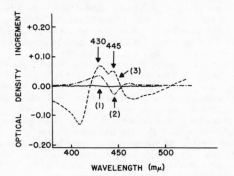

FIG. 3. Carbon monoxide difference spectrum. The system consisted of 15 μmoles of MgCl₂, 23 μmoles of KCl, 1.4 μmoles of NAD⁺, 11.8 mg of washed particles, 11.1 mg of ammonium sulfate-fractionated supernatant fluid, 100 μmoles of Tris-HCl buffer (pH 7.4), and water to a final volume of 3.0 ml. Reduction of the cytochromes was accomplished following incubation for 10 minutes with 30 μmoles of succinate and 30 μmoles of β-hydroxybutyrate. *Curve 1,* reduced minus reduced spectrum; *Curve 2,* carbon monoxide-treated reduced minus reduced spectrum; *Curve 3,* reduced minus oxidized spectrum.

cal reduction (*Curve 2,* Fig. 1). In contrast to differences in cytochrome *b* reduction, cytochromes *c* and *a* were reduced to the same extent by all three substrates. Inhibitors of cytochrome oxidase (cyanide or sulfide up to 3 mM) did not qualitatively alter the difference spectrum in the visible region.

Examination of the pigments of the bacterial particle preparations at low temperature (liquid nitrogen) revealed absorption bands at 600 and 561 mμ, indicative of cytochromes *a* and *b* (Fig. 2). The α-bands of cytochrome *c* components were further resolved by low temperature spectroscopy. Under these conditions a cytochrome of the c_1 type appeared as a shoulder at about 554 mμ, while cytochrome *c* was evident at 548 mμ. At low temperature the absorption bands in the Soret region revealed the presence of cytochromes $a + a_3$ (445 mμ) and *c* (423 mμ). The band at 438 mμ may be due to cytochromes *b* and a_3.

Carbon monoxide-binding pigments were also observed with the particulate fraction from *M. phlei* (Fig. 3). A gentle stream of carbon monoxide was added to the enzymatically or chemically reduced (sodium dithionite) sample, and the rapid change in absorption was followed. The reference cuvette contained the preparation that was reduced enzymatically. Chemical reduction with dithionite resulted in an increased reduction of the cytochrome *b* of the particles; however, the carbon monoxide difference spectrum was identical with that obtained by enzymatic reduction. The carbon monoxide difference spectrum exhibited a trough at 445 mμ and a peak at 430 mμ. These results are qualitatively similar to those obtained by Chance with mammalian mitochondria, yeast, and *Bacillus subtilis* (23).

The concentration of the respiratory pigments was determined spectrophotometrically by the method of Chance and Williams (25) and is shown in Table I. The concentration of the respiratory carriers was calculated on the assumption that the cytochromes from this microorganism have molar extinction coefficients similar to those found in mammalian mitochondria. The molar extinction coefficients for pure cytochromes isolated from other microorganisms are in close agreement with those obtained from mitochondria even though the absorption peaks of the cytochromes may differ (28–34). The major absorption peaks of the various cytochromes in *M. phlei* are similar to those of the homologous cytochromes of mitochondria. The relative concentrations of the respiratory pigments in *M. phlei* are similar to those found for rat liver (25) and pigeon heart mitochondria determined by a similar method (26). The absolute concentrations of the bacterial respiratory pigments were calculated and expressed as millimicromoles per mg of protein (Table II). The value for cytochrome *b* in this table was obtained following enzymatic reduction with a combination of succinate, malate, and β-hydroxybutyrate, since addition of a single substrate resulted in only partial reduction of cytochrome *b*. The further addition of dithionite increased the total amount of cytochrome *b* reduction by 27%. The amounts of enzymatically or chemically reducible carriers of *M. phlei* were compared with the amounts of reducible carriers found in different mitochondrial preparations (Table II). The amount of cytochromes *b,* $a + a_3,$ and a_3 in the bacterial particles was found to be lower than observed in mammalian particles, whereas the amount of cytochrome *c* was almost the same. The concentration of pyridine nucleotides in *M. phlei* particles (35) is also substantially lower than the corresponding levels in intact mitochondria.

The reduced steady state level of the terminal respiratory components was studied with substrates that utilize different respiratory pathways (Table III). The individual substrates differed in their capacity to reduce cytochrome *b*. The highest reduced steady state level of cytochrome *b* was observed with β-hydroxybutyrate, and the lowest with succinate. The values recorded in this table represent the average of eight determinations for each substrate, since the amount of enzymatically reducible cytochrome b varied from preparation to preparation. Although the system from $M.$ $phlei$ does not exhibit respiratory control, the electron transport sequence was ascertained from studies with respiratory inhibitors and from the reduced steady state level of the carriers following the addition of substrate (Table III). Thus, the electron transfer sequence of the terminal respiratory chain of this microorganism, like the mitochondrial system, flows from cytochrome b to c to $a + a_3$ to oxygen.

Simultaneous determination of oxygen consumption and spectrophotometric changes as described by Chance and Williams (40) revealed that the cytochrome reached a steady state level which was maintained until the oxygen concentration reached about 10 mμmoles per ml. The rate of oxygen disappearance

TABLE I

Relative concentration of respiratory carriers in particles from M. phlei

The concentration of the particulate respiratory carriers was measured with either the split beam or double beam spectrophotometer. The system contained 30 μmoles of MgCl$_2$, 80 μmoles of KCl, 200 μmoles of Tris-HCl buffer (pH 7.2 to 7.4), particulate fraction (1.3 to 4.0 mg of protein per ml), and water to a final volume of 3 ml. Succinate (30 μmoles) or β-hydroxybutyrate (30 μmoles) was used as an electron donor to reduce the particulate respiratory carriers. The concentration of the carriers was determined following exhaustion of oxygen or following the addition of a respiratory inhibitor such as sodium sulfide (9 μmoles). Cytochrome b was determined after reduction by succinate, β-hydroxybutyrate, and malate; the system included NAD$^+$ (0.3 μmole), FAD (0.1 μmole), and dialyzed supernatant fraction (4.0 mg of protein). In contrast to reduction of cytochrome b, cytochromes $a + a_3$ and c were reduced to the same level by individual substrates as was observed with the three substrates and cofactors. Each value represents the average of at least four determinations.

Component	Wave length pair	E_{mM} used (10)	Relative concentration		
			$M.$ $phlei$	Mitochondria	
				Rat liver[a]	Pigeon heart[b]
	$m\mu$	mM^{-1} cm^{-1}			
Cytochrome a $(+ a_3)$	598, 623	16	1.00	1.00	1.00
Cytochrome b	562, 574	20	0.68	0.9	0.64
			0.86[c]		
Cytochrome c $(+ c_1)$	551, 540	19	2.26	1.7	1.28
Flavoprotein	455, 510	11	2.47	3.6	3.00
			1.37[d]		
Cytochrome a_3[e]	430, 445	91	0.82		
Vitamin K$_9$H			43.7[f]		9.30[g]

[a] From data of Chance and Williams (25).

[b] From data of Chance and Hagihara (26).

[c] Chemically reducible cytochrome b.

[d] Acid-extractable flavin (27).

[e] Calculated from carbon monoxide difference spectrum. The millimolar extinction coefficient was assumed to be similar to that of heart muscle (28).

[f] From data of Kashket and Brodie (27). The concentration of the naphthoquinone was revised since the molar extinction coefficient of vitamin K$_9$H has been determined (12).

[g] Coenzyme Q.

TABLE II

Comparison of enzymatically reducible respiratory carriers of M. phlei with those of mitochondrial systems

Components	Concentration				
	Enzymatic reduction	Chemical determinations	Pigeon heart mitochondria[a]	ETP$_H$[b]	Beef KHP[c]
	mμmoles/mg protein				
Cytochrome a $(+ a_3)$	0.27[d]		0.75	1.62	0.85
Cytochrome b	0.18[e]	0.65[f]	0.48	0.85	0.59
Cytochrome c $(+ c_1)$	0.62		0.95	0.63	0.56
Flavoprotein	0.68	0.37[f]	2.2	0.60	0.36
Cytochrome a_3 (CO difference)[g]	0.22				
Pyridine nucleotide		0.33[h]	8.0		
Quinone		12.0[f]	7.0	4.8	4.26

[a] From the data of Chance and Hagihara (26).

[b] From the data of Green and Wharton (36).

[c] Keilin-Hartree preparation. From the data of King, Nickel, and Jensen (37).

[d] Average of eight determinations.

[e] Addition of dithionite increased cytochrome b reduction to 0.25 mμmole per mg of protein.

[f] Kashket and Brodie (27).

[g] Average of four determinations. Difference of millimolar extinction coefficient of CO compound between 445 and 430 mμ was assumed as 82 mM^{-1} cm^{-1} (Chance (28)).

[h] From the data of Weber and Swartz (35).

was constant over the period measured. Following depletion of oxygen, further reduction of the cytochrome occurred at a rapid rate (Fig. 4). With freshly prepared particles the reduced steady state level was achieved rapidly (Fig. 5), whereas with aged particles reduction of the cytochromes occurred continually and at a slower rate. Thus, it was difficult to determine the reduced steady state level with aged particles.

The turnover number for each of the cytochromes (Table III) was determined from the data as presented in Figs. 4 and 5. The turnover numbers of the cytochromes were of the same magnitude as those described for intact mitochondria. The respiratory activities measured by the conventional manometric technique are in good agreement with those obtained by spectrophotometric methods. The Q_{O_2} values obtained with the bacterial particulate preparations are similar to those obtained with intact mitochondria but considerably lower than those obtained with disrupted mitochondria such as ETP$_H$ (41) or the Keilin-Hartree heart muscle preparations (42).

The percentage reduction of the cytochromes was determined at the point of transition from the aerobic to anaerobic state as in Fig. 4. The percentage reduction of cytochromes $a + a_3$, b, and c is shown in Table IV. Reduction of cytochrome b at the transition state was slower than that observed for cytochromes c or $a + a_3$. In addition, the amount of cytochrome b reduced at the transition state was lower than the other cytochromes. The properties of the bacterial particles with respect to the rate and transition state behavior of the enzymatically reduced cytochrome.b appear to place the bacterial system between the fully coupled mitochondrial system (40) and the nonphosphorylative Keilin-Hartree preparation (42). The reduction of cytochromes by substrate, in the presence of inhibitors, or on reaching anaerobiosis, follows first order kinetics.

TABLE III

Respiratory activity and steady state level of cytochromes of *M. phlei*

The K_4 value (millimicromoles of O_2 per second per change in optical density) defined by Chance (38) was determined by the method of Estabrook and Mackler (39). The rate of oxygen consumption was calculated by dividing the protein concentration into the K_4 value, whereas the Q_{O_2} was determined spectrophotometrically and by manometric procedures. The $(K_4)_a$ value was obtained from spectrophotometric studies in which the concentration of cytochrome a was determined. The turnover number was calculated by the formula given by Estabrook and Mackler (39), and is equal to $K_4 \times$ electroequivalents $\times E \times 10^{-3}$, where E represents the millimolar extinction coefficient; the values used in calculating the turnover number for the bacterial system are shown in Table I. The system consisted of 30 μmoles of $MgCl_2$, 80 μmoles of KCl, washed particles (1.3 to 2.5 mg of protein), ammonium sulfate-fractionated supernatant fluid (2.5 to 3.8 mg of protein), 200 μmoles of Tris-HCl buffer (pH 7.2), and water to a final volume of 3.0 ml. The reaction was started by the addition of 50 μmoles of succinate, DL-malate, or DL-β-hydroxybutyrate. In addition, 0.25 μmole of FAD was added to the reaction mixture when malate was employed as substrate, and 1.5 μmoles of NAD^+ were used with β-hydroxybutyrate. The reactions were carried out at 23° in a 1-cm cuvette for the spectrophotometric studies; in the manometric studies the reactions were conducted at 30° for 10 to 15 minutes. The Q_{O_2} values calculated from manometric studies represent the average of 10 experiments, whereas the values obtained from spectrophotometric studies represent the average of 4 experiments.

Substrate	$\Delta O_2{}^a$	$(K_4)a^b$	Turnover No. of cytochromes			Q_O at		Reduction			
			a_2	b	c^c	$23°^d$	$30°^e$	Anaerobiosis, cytochrome b	At steady state,^{f} cytochromes		
									$a + a_2$	$c + c_1$	b
				sec^{-1}				%	%	%	%
Succinate............................	0.73	165	10.2	28.7	5.1	29	39	25	3•	12	45
Malate...............................	0.75	177	12.0	21.5	6.4	30	37	38	4	10	23
β-Hydroxybutyrate...............	1.48	339	22.9	42.6	13.8	60	84	50	6	13	21
All three substrates...............	1.67					67		73			19

^{a} Millimicromoles per second per mg of protein (spectrophotometric determination).

^{b} Millimicromoles of O_2 per second per change in optical density at 598 to 623 mμ.

^{c} Although the absorption of cytochrome c_1 was found to be relatively low at the wave length used to measure cytochrome c (Fig. 2), the values given above for cytochrome c represent a combination of $c + c_1$.

^{d} Spectrophotometric.

^{e} Microliters of O_2 per hour per mg of protein.

^{f} The amount of cytochrome b reduced enzymatically was found to be different with the substrates employed. Thus the percentage of the steady state level for this cytochrome was determined with each substrate from the level obtained following complete anaerobiosis (taken as 100%).

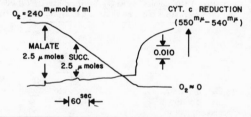

FIG. 4. Simultaneous determination of oxygen consumption and cytochrome reduction. The cuvette contained 2.4 μmoles of $MgCl_2$, 48 μmoles of KCl, 12.0 mg of aged particles, 5.4 mg of ammonium sulfate-fractionated supernatant, 12.5 mμmoles of FAD, 2.5 μmoles of DL-malate, 2.5 μmoles of succinate, and 6 μmoles of Tris-HCl buffer, pH 7.4. Total volume, 1.5 ml; optical path, 0.5 cm; temperature, 24°.

Nature of Respiratory Chains in M. phlei—Three major respiratory pathways have been found in *M. phlei* which are capable of coupling phosphorylation to oxidation. These pathways can be distinguished by their response to added cofactors, to purified supernatant fractions, and to respiratory inhibitors. The requirement for different cofactors for oxidation of substrates utilizing different pathways in the reconstituted system (washed particles and dialyzed supernatant fluid) is shown in Table V. NAD^+-linked substrates such as β-hydroxybutyrate or ethanol required the addition of NAD^+ for activity and were not substantially stimulated by the addition of FAD or FMN.[2] Malate oxidation, however, was stimulated by both FAD and NAD^+.

Fractionation of the supernatant components on DEAE-cellulose (17) resulted in a resolution of two distinct pathways for malate oxidation. One of the purified enzymes exhibited a requirement for FAD for oxidation of malate when added to the particles. Oxidation by this fraction did not occur when FAD was replaced by NAD^+. In the absence of particles, this enzyme can be linked to dye (thiazolyl blue tetrazolium) provided that FAD, vitamin K_1, and phospholipid are added (15). The other purified supernatant fraction exhibited a requirement for NAD^+ for malate oxidation.

Succinate oxidation by the reconstituted system (particles and supernatant fraction) was not affected by the addition of either FAD or FMN. Some inhibition of succinic oxidase by FAD $(3 \times 10^{-4}$ M) was observed with particles alone. Inhibition of other flavin enzymes by a high concentration of FAD has been reported by Ernster *et al.* (43) for mammalian "DT-diaphorase." Succinate oxidation, however, was stimulated by a high concentration of NAD^+ when tested with particles and crude supernatant fluid, but not when tested with particles alone (Table V). The particulate fraction has relatively little fumarase activity. The stimulation of succinate oxidation by NAD^+ exhibited a lag

^{2} The abbreviation used is: FMN, riboflavin phosphate, flavin mononucleotide.

period when tested with particle and supernatant fractions. This lag was presumably due to the time necessary for accumulation of malate, which results in the secondary oxidation via the NAD$^+$-linked pathway.

Differences in the three respiratory chains were also shown by

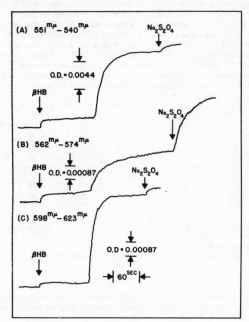

Fig. 5. Anaerobic and steady state levels of the cytochromes of *M. phlei*. The system consisted of 30 μmoles of MgCl$_2$, 80 μmoles of KCl, 6 μmoles of inorganic phosphate, 1.4 μmoles of NAD$^+$, 200 μmoles of Tris-HCl buffer (pH 7.2), washed particles (3.8 mg of protein), and ammonium sulfate-fractionated supernatant fluid (11.3 mg of protein), and water to a final volume of 3.0 ml. The reaction was started by the addition of 5.0 μmoles of β-hydroxybutyrate (βHB).

TABLE IV

Percentage reduction of components of respiratory chain on transition from aerobic to anaerobic state

The system was similar to that described in Table III, except that aged particles (12 mg of protein) were used and the total volume was 1.5 ml. A 0.5-cm cuvette was used, and the reaction was carried out at room temperature (24°). The amount of cytochrome reduced was measured at the transition point, when the oxygen concentration reached zero. The amount of reduction at the transition point was expressed as the percentage of the amount of cytochrome reduced after complete reduction by substrate.

Substrate	Reduction		
	Cytochrome $a + a_3$	Cytochrome $c + c_1$	Cytochrome b
	%	%	%
Malate plus succinate................	75	65	26
β-Hydroxybutyrate...................		77	33

TABLE V

Effect of cofactors on oxidation by different substrates with various fractions from M. phlei

The system consisted of 15 μmoles of MgCl$_2$, 25 μmoles of KF, 45 μmoles of KCl, 2.5 μmoles of ADP, 10 μmoles of glucose, 3 mg of yeast hexokinase, 8 μmoles of inorganic phosphate, washed particles (4.6 to 9.5 mg of protein), ammonium sulfate supernatant ("crude") (6.3 to 8.5 mg of protein) or DEAE-cellulose-fractionated supernatant ("reductase") (3.2 mg of protein), and water to a volume of 1.5 ml. In addition, the vessels indicated contained 40 μmoles of malate, succinate, or β-hydroxybutyrate. The reactions were carried out at 30° for 15 minutes.

Substrate and fraction	Oxygen consumption with various cofactors			
	None	FAD, 1.7×10^{-4} M	NAD$^+$, 10^{-2} M	FAD + NAD$^+$
		μatoms		
Malate				
Particles + supernatant (crude).................	1.08	6.72	5.75	
Particles + supernatant (reductase).............	0.96	4.70	1.40	
β-Hydroxybutyrate				
Particles + supernatant (crude).................	1.36		8.75	9.65
Succinate				
Particles.................	3.2	1.51[a]	3.5	
Particles + supernatant (crude).................	3.6	3.1	11.0	

[a] FAD concentration was 3.3×10^{-4} M.

TABLE VI

Effect of inhibitors on different respiratory chains of M. phlei

The system was similar to that described in Table V. NADH was generated either with yeast alcohol dehydrogenase (0.6 mg) and ethanol (100 μmoles) or with β-hydroxybutyrate (60 μmoles) and the supernatant β-hydroxybutyrate dehydrogenase fraction.

Inhibitor	Inhibition of oxidation		
	Succinate	Malate	NADH (generated)
	%	%	%
Amytal, 10^{-2} M..........................	10	35	35
Atebrin, 3×10^{-3} M...................	85	75	25
Dicumarol, 10^{-4} M......................	5	50	
Dicumarol, 10^{-3} M......................	98	90	50
2-*n*-Nonylhydroxyquinoline *N*-oxide, 2 μg per mg of protein...........	98	80	60
Thienyltrifluorobutanedione, 10^{-3} M.......	60	0	
KCN, 3×10^{-3} M....................	95	95	55
p-Chloromercuribenzoate, 7×10^{-4} M.....	85	95	30
Pentachlorophenol, 10^{-4} M...............	15	75	0
Rotenone, 7×10^{-6} M................	5	0	0
Rotenone, 1.3×10^{-4} M................		5	15

studies with respiratory inhibitors (Table VI). The inhibition of oxidation observed with Amytal occurs only at high concentrations of this agent (10^{-2} M) and is probably nonspecific (44). Rotenone, a specific inhibitor of the NAD$^+$-linked chain (45), failed to inhibit this bacterial system. The inhibition by atebrin of malate and succinate oxidation appears to be a reflection of

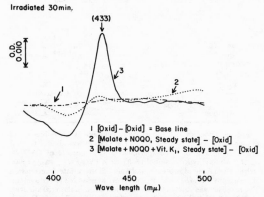

Difference Spectra

Irradiated 30 min,

FIG. 6. Requirement for added vitamin K for reduction of endogenous cytochrome *b* following irradiation. The system consisted of 32 μmoles of $MgCl_2$, 107 μmoles of KCl, 3 μmoles of inorganic phosphate, 4.6 μmoles of ADP, washed particles (8.5 mg of protein) irradiated with light at 360 mμ for 30 minutes, 25 mμmoles of FAD, 92 μmoles of Tris-HCl buffer (pH 7.2), and water to a final volume of 3.0 ml. *NOQNO*, 2-*n*-nonylhydroxyquinoline *N*-oxide.

the flavin nature of these respiratory chains. The inhibition by 2-*n*-nonylhydroxyquinoline *N*-oxide and KCN occurred with all three chains. These observations are in keeping with the findings that all three pathways utilize the terminal respiratory pigments, the succinate chain converging with the malate- and NAD⁺-linked chains at cytochrome *b*. Differences in inhibition of the various pathways were observed with Dicumarol, pentachlorophenol, thienyltrifluorobutanedione, and *p*-chloromercuribenzoate. The insensitivity of the phosphorylative pathway to *p*-chloromercuribenzoate, described earlier (46), can only be applied to the NAD⁺-linked pathway.

Role for Naphthoquinone[3] in Respiratory Chain—The role of vitamin K in the respiratory chain was studied with the double beam spectrophotometer. The bacterial particles were irradiated with light at 360 mμ for 15 to 45 minutes in order to destroy the endogenous vitamin K (K₉H). Particles treated in this manner exhibited little or no oxidative activity with malate, β-hydroxybutyrate, or succinate as electron donors. Irradiation also resulted in an inhibition of the ability to reduce endogenous cytochromes *b* and *c* by these donors (Figs. 6 and 7). Addition of vitamin K₁ suspended in phospholipid restored reduction of cytochrome *b* with malate or β-hydroxybutyrate as substrate, but not with succinate (Fig. 7). Similar results were also obtained with cytochrome *c* reduction. The light-sensitive components of the succinate chain were not replaced by the addition of vitamin K₁, coenzyme Q₆ or Q₁₀, FMN, FAD, or combinations of these cofactors.

The properties of the vitamin K₁-restored system with malate were further examined with inhibitors to determine whether

[3] Vitamin K₁ has been used extensively in studies of the role of the naphthoquinone in oxidative phosphorylation since it is abundantly available and active in this system. This vitamin, however, is not the natural quinone of the *M. phlei* system, which has been identified as vitamin K₉H (12).

the restored activity occurred by an electron transport bypass reaction (Table VII). No significant differences were observed between the untreated and the vitamin K-restored system. In addition to the respiratory inhibitors, uncoupling agents (not shown in Table VII) which affect phosphorylation of the malate chain also uncoupled phosphorylation observed with the vitamin K-restored system.

Sequence of Respiratory Components—Direct measurement of reduction of vitamin K by malate was made with the double beam spectrophotometer (47). The site of participation of FAD on the malate chain was determined with the soluble malate-vitamin K reductase. FAD acts between substrate and vitamin K since it is required for reduction of vitamin K (Fig. 8). The rate of reduction of the naphthoquinone was found to be 9.5 mμmoles per minute per mg of protein with 5.9×10^{-5} M vitamin K₁ added to the system. This activity was 3 times lower than that observed for the reconstituted system (particles and malate reductase fractions) with malate and optimal concentrations of vitamin K₁. The rate of reduction of the quinone was found to be dependent on its concentration; however, it was necessary to carry out the reaction at one-tenth the optimal concentration of vitamin K, owing to the increased turbidity caused by high concentrations of this naphthoquinone in phospholipid. Indirect methods, such as following the rate of reduction of endogenous particulate cytochrome *b* or reduction o

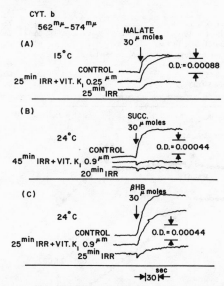

FIG. 7. The restoration of cytochrome *b* reduction by vitamin K₁ with different substrates. The system was similar to that described in the legend of Fig. 5. The particulate fraction was irradiated with light at 360 mμ for the period indicated, whereas the ammonium sulfate-fractionated supernatant fraction was irradiated for 5 hours. The concentration of particles differed: *A*, 5.4 mg of protein; *B*, 4.5 mg of protein; *C*, 4.0 mg of protein. The concentration of the supernatant fraction used was 10.5 mg of protein (*A*), 3.2 mg of protein (*B*), and 7.6 mg of protein (*C*). In addition, NAD⁺ (30 μmoles) was added to the system containing β-hydroxybutyrate (β*HB*), whereas FAD (25 mμmoles) was added with malate as substrate.

dye, reactions dependent on the addition of the naphtoquinone, indicated that reduction and oxidation of the added vitamin K were not rate-limiting when optimal concentrations of vitamin K were added. Reduction of dye was found to occur at 2 to 3 times the rate observed for the over-all oxidation of malate by the complete system.

The soluble reductase required the addition of the particulate fraction for oxidation of malate. Reduction of endogenous cytochromes b and c by malate required the addition of the soluble malate-vitamin K reductase (Fig. 9). The requirement for naphthoquinone was not observed with the particles unless the natural quinone was destroyed by irradiation at 360 mμ. The malate chain converges with the NAD$^+$-linked chain of the

TABLE VII

Effects of respiratory inhibitors on oxidative phosphorylation with vitamin K₁-restored malate chain

The system was similar to that described in Table V. The particulate fraction (4.3 mg of protein) was irradiated with light at 360 mμ for 30 minutes, whereas the ammonium sulfate-fractionated superantant fluid (6.8 mg protein) was irradiated (360 mμ) for 5 hours. Restoration of oxidation and phosphorylation was accomplished by the addition of 2.2 μmoles of vitamin K₁ in Asolectin.

Inhibitors	Inhibition	
	ΔO_2	ΔP_i
	%	%
Amytal, 5 × 10⁻³ M	34	71
Atebrin, 3 × 10⁻³ M	55	75
Dicumarol, 5 × 10⁻⁴ M	66	92
2-n-Nonylhydroxyquinoline N-oxide, 1.4 μg per mg of protein	54	56
KCN, 3 × 10⁻³ M	100	100
Tween 80, 0.33%	55	100

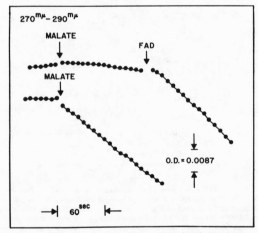

FIG. 8. Reduction of vitamin K by malate-vitamin K reductase. The system consisted of 1.5 mg of protein of purified malate-vitamin K reductase, 1.0 μmole of FAD, 0.20 μmole of vitamin K₁ in Asolectin, 80 μmoles of KCl, 100 μmoles of Tris-HCl buffer (pH 7.4), and water to a final volume of 1.5 ml. The reaction was carried out at 24° in a cuvette with a 0.5-cm optical path. FAD was added at the point indicated on the *upper curve.*

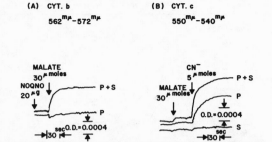

FIG. 9. Effect of the supernatant component on reduction of cytochromes b and c by malate. The system was similar to that described in Fig. 5. In Experiment A, 25 mμmoles of FAD, 20 μg of 2-n-nonylhydroxyquinoline N-oxide (NOQNO), washed particles (P) (4.5 mg of protein), and ammonium sulfate-fractionated supernatant fluid (S) (3.2 mg of protein) were added to the system. The reaction was started by the addition of DL-malate (30 μmoles). Cyanide (5 μmoles) was used as the respiratory inhibitor in Experiment B.

TABLE VIII

Inhibition of succinate chain by metal-chelating compounds

Reduction of cytochrome b was followed by the procedure described in Fig. 7. Reduction of thiazolyl blue tetrazolium was followed spectrophotometrically at 565 mμ. The system contained 15 μmoles of MgCl₂, 40 μmoles of KCl, 0.24 μmole of thiazolyl blue tetrazolium, washed particles (0.8 mg of protein), ammonium sulfate-treated supernatant fraction (1.25 mg of protein), 100 μmoles of Tris-HCl buffer (pH 7.2), and water to a final volume of 1.5 ml. The reaction was started by the addition of succinate (20 μmoles). Reduction of ferricyanide was followed spectrophotometrically at 420 mμ. The system was similar to that used for measuring thiazolyl blue tetrazolium reduction except that 1.5 μmoles of ferricyanide were used instead of the dye.

Inhibitors	Inhibition with reduction of		
	Cytochrome b	Thiazolyl blue tetrazolium	Ferricyanide
	%	%	%
Cyanide, 1.7 × 10⁻³ M	60	60	5
o-Phenanthroline, 5 × 10⁻⁴ M		25	
α,α'-Dipyridyl, 5 × 10⁻⁴ M		27	

particles at the naphthoquinone (K₉H) level of oxidation. Reduction of endogenous cytochrome c by malate was inhibited (50%) by 2-n-nonylhydroxyquinoline N-oxide (1.5 μg per mg of protein).

The site of action of 2-n-nonylhydroxyquinoline N-oxide in low concentrations with this bacterial system is between cytochromes b and c (48). The addition of 2-n-nonylhydroxyquinoline N-oxide and oxygen to a succinate-reduced, anaerobic system resulted in the oxidation of cytochromes a and c and in further reduction of cytochrome b. Although the identity of the light-sensitive component on the succinate chain is unknown, metals appear to participate in succinate oxidation (Table VIII). Reduction of thiazolyl blue tetrazolium was found to be inhibited by KCN when succinate was used as an electron donor, whereas no inhibition occurs with malate. In addition, inhibi-

TABLE IX

Effects of inhibitors on reduction of different electron acceptors

The conditions were similar to those described in Table VIII. Reduction of 2,6-dichlorophenolindophenol (0.15 μmole) was measured spectrophotometrically at 600 mμ, whereas reduction of horse heart cytochrome c (0.16 μmole) was measured at 550 mμ. With malate as substrate, FAD (0.38 μmole) was added.

	Inhibition					
	Malate as substrate			Succinate as substrate		
Inhibitor	2,6-Dichlorophenolindophenol	Cytochrome c	Thiazolyl blue tetrazolium	2,6-Dichlorophenolindophenol	Thiazolyl blue tetrazolium	Ferricyanide
	%	%	%	%	%	%
Amytal, 10^{-2} M..	35	29	36			
Atebrin, 3×10^{-3} M......................................			69		83	
Dicumarol, 10^{-3} M..	67	69				
Irradiation with light at 360 mμ...........................			80		76	
2-n-Nonylhydroxyquinoline N-oxide, 2.5 μg per mg of protein...........	41	81	74	80	90	0
Thienyltrifluorobutanedione, 5×10^{-3} M.................			0		87	

tion of reduction of thiazolyl blue tetrazolium by succinate occurs with o-phenanthroline and α,α'-dipyridyl. Reduction of cytochrome b by succinate was inhibited by cyanide, whereas ferricyanide reduction was not inhibited by this agent.

Dissection of Respiratory Chains—Knowledge of the site of inhibition of several of the inhibitors described in this paper permitted an examination of the sites of interaction of various electron acceptors. The use of exogenous electron acceptors or donors in substrate quantities can afford a means of studying phosphorylative sites in the respiratory chain. A survey of various electron acceptors with the malate and succinate chains is presented in Table IX. Interaction of thiazolyl blue tetrazolium, 2,6-dichlorophenolindophenol, and exogenous cytochrome c with the succinate and malate chains appears to occur in the cytochrome c region. Some interaction of dichlorophenolindophenol occurs before cytochrome b. Addition of NAD+ and malate to the system containing the NAD+-linked malic dehydrogenase appears to alter the interaction of the acceptor, since electrons were channeled off before reaching cytochrome b as in the mitochondrial NAD+-linked chain (49).

DISCUSSION

Systems capable of coupling phosphorylation to oxidation have been obtained from a number of microorganisms (2–8, 16, 50, 51); however, the P:O ratios exhibited by the bacterial systems are consistently lower than those exhibited by the mitochondrial system. Although studies with the bacterial systems have pioneered in the dissection and reconstitution of systems capable of oxidative phosphorylation (3–6), detailed knowledge of the respiratory chains of most of the bacterial system is lacking. Thus, the sites of phosphorylation in most of the microbial systems have not been studied. A detailed examination of the major respiratory pathways of M. phlei was undertaken as a first step in obtaining precise knowledge of the respiratory sites which are coupled to phosphorylation.

The respiratory chain of M. phlei contains bound pyridine nucleotides (35), flavins (27), a naphthoquinone (vitamin K_9H) (11, 12), and cytochromes b, c_1, c, a, and a_3. The cytochromes of this microorganism are both qualitatively and quantitatively similar to those found in mammalian mitochondria. On the assumption that the molar extinction coefficients of the cyto-

chromes are the same as those of mitochondrial origin, the amount of cytochrome $c + c_1$ in the bacterial particles was relatively high compared to cytochromes b, $a + a_3$, and a_3. Although most of the bacterial cytochromes have extinction coefficients similar to those of mitochondrial origin, the exact concentration of the individual cytochromes from M. phlei must await precise determination of these values for this system. Other methods for determining flavins and cytochromes b, c, and c_1 (36, 37) are under investigation. Small amounts of cytochrome were also found in the soluble fraction; however, this chiefly consisted of the cytochrome c type. The lower value for flavin found on acid extraction than that observed enzymatically may be a reflection of the inability to remove flavin associated with succinic dehydrogenase (52), or may in part be due to absorption contributed by nonheme iron proteins (53). The bacterial dehydrogenases which utilize NAD+ (β-hydroxybutyrate and L-malate) are found in the soluble fraction along with the bulk of the NAD+. The ratio of bound pyridine nucleotide to cytochrome $a + a_3$ in washed particles was 1.2, which is significantly lower than that of the mitochondrial system (usually more than 10 (25, 26)). In addition, the ratio of particle-bound NAD+ to the total NAD+ of the cell was only 0.3%, whereas the ratio of mitochondrial bound NAD+ to the total NAD+ is 7% (35). Most of disrupted mitochondrial systems described do not contain bound pyridine nucleotide and require addition of NAD+ (54–58).

Kinetic studies of the respiratory chains of M. phlei indicated a similarity between it and the mitochondrial system. Although cytochrome b undergoes oxidation and reduction, further study is necessary to define precisely the role of this cytochrome in the respiratory pathways. A major difference between this microorganism and the mammalian mitochondrial system was observed in the pathways utilized in malate oxidation. Malate was found to undergo oxidation by two different respiratory chains in M. phlei, one through NAD+ and the other via FAD. The latter pathway corresponds to the α-glycerol phosphate pathway of brain, muscle, and liver mitochondria (59–65), or to the choline chain observed in liver mitochondria (44, 66, 67).

The presence of a pyridine nucleotide-independent pathway for malate oxidation in bacteria has been reported for other microorganisms (68, 69). The two malate enzymes may have

109

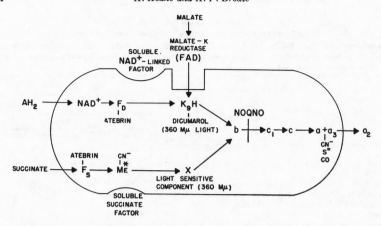

* ORDER OF METAL IN SEQUENCE UNKNOWN

FIG. 10. Schematic representation of the soluble and particulate respiratory chains of *M. phlei*. *K*, vitamin K; *NOQNO*, 2-*n*-nonyl-hydroxyquinoline *N*-oxide.

physiological significance in strictly aerobic microorganisms by providing a means of reoxidizing extraparticulate NADH. Oxaloacetate formed from the bound malate-vitamin K reductase could be reduced to malate by extraparticulate malic dehydrogenase and NADH. This cycle would be analogous to the α-glycerol phosphate cycle of mitochondria suggested by Klingenberg and Bücher (63, 70). The potential of malate/oxaloacetate (E_{M_7}, −0.102 volt at 38°) (71) is higher than that of NADH/NAD⁺ (−0.311 at 25°) (72) or other citric acid cycle intermediates with the exception of succinate. The oxidation-reduction potential of malate/oxaloacetate is similar to that reported for other flavin enzymes.

The role of vitamin K in oxidative phosphorylation has been studied extensively (8, 9, 46, 73, 74). This lipid-soluble respiratory cofactor undergoes oxidation and reduction at a rate consistent with the over-all rate of oxidation of malate by the bacterial system (15). The site of action of this cofactor was postulated to be between the flavoprotein and cytochrome *b* (46). The experiments described in this paper lend further support to the postulated site of interaction of the cofactor. The endogenous naphthoquinone of the particles interacts with both the NAD⁺ and malate chains. It appears to be the site of entrance of electrons from the solubilized malate-vitamin K reductase. Weber and Rosso (76) have suggested that the naphthoquinone-restored respiration with *M. phlei* extracts occurs by a bypass of the normal electron transport pathways. Their results are inconsistent with earlier findings (46, 74, 75) as well as with the data presented in this paper. The differences observed by Weber and Rosso may be due to the use of Tween to suspend the naphtoquinone. This detergent in low concentrations (0.13 to 0.33%) was shown earlier to inhibit the main pathways of oxidation in *M. phlei* and to act as an uncoupling agent in lower concentration (15).

The light-sensitive component (or components) of the succinate chain has been placed between succinic dehydrogenase and cytochrome *b*. The nature of this component(s) has not been elucidated. Studies with 2-*n*-nonylhydroxyquinoline

N-oxide indicate that succinate converges with the NAD⁺ chain at the cytochrome *b* level. Reduction of cytochrome *b* was lost upon irradiation. A metal also appears to be involved in the succinic oxidase pathway, and its site of interaction appears to be before cytochrome *b*. Inhibition by cyanide of cytochrome *b* reduction from succinate with a 2-*n*-nonylhydroxyquinoline *N*-oxide-blocked system occurred at the concentration reported to cause a similar inhibition in the Keilin-Hartree preparation (77); however, with the bacterial system prolonged preincubation was not required. The lack of inhibition of the NAD⁺-linked chain by chelating agents does not rule out the possible involvement of metal in this pathway.

Particles from *M. phlei* isolated by different procedures exhibit differences in their ability to oxidize various substrates (2), in requirements for supernatant factors and cofactors, and in the intactness of their respiratory chains. Particles prepared from cells 1 to 2 days old differ from those obtained from fresh cells in their response to added supernatant factors. In addition, particles stored at −15° (aged particles) differ from freshly prepared particles in the rate of reduction of their terminal respiratory pigments and in their requirement for soluble components. The reduced steady state level of the cytochromes was difficult to achieve with aged particles.

A schematic representation of the three major coupled respiratory pathways of *M. phlei* is shown in Fig. 10. Although the bacterial particles are spherical in shape (2), they are shown elongated. The indentations in the particles indicate the probable sites of interaction of the various soluble protein oxidative factors. Since the particles retain some succinic oxidase activity, it was possible to observe the effect of the supernatant factors on the terminal respiratory chain. The amount of reduction of cytochromes *c*, *b*, and *a* + *a₃* was not influenced by the presence or absence of supernatant fluid; however, with malate the soluble protein components were necessary for reduction of the cytochromes. The malate oxidation factor appears to be malate-vitamin K reductase. In addition, the supernatant contains β-hydroxybutyrate dehydrogenase and another factor necessary for reduction of the naphthoquinone. The crude supernatant fraction also contains a number of nonphosphorylative bypass reactions, which will be described in a later publication.

SUMMARY

The respiratory components in *Mycobacterium phlei* extracts have been determined. The particulate fraction contains bound nicotinamide adenine dinucleotide, flavins, a naphthoquinone (vitamin K_9H), and cytochromes b, c_1, c, a, and a_3. The ratios of the enzymatically reducible cytochromes $a + a_3$, b, $c + c_1$, flavin, and vitamin K_9H were found to be 1.0, 0.68, 2.3, 2.5, and 43.7, respectively. Carbon monoxide binding of cytochrome a_3 was found. The respiratory activity (Q_{O_2}) at 30° with succinate, malate, and β-hydroxybutyrate was 39, 37, and 84, respectively. Studies of the cofactor requirements, effect of inhibitors, and requirement for supernatant components revealed the presence of three distinct respiratory chains, namely, succinic oxidase, malate, and NAD^+-linked chains. The flavin adenine dinucleotide-linked malate pathway was found to be soluble and to converge with the particle-bound NAD^+-linked pathway at the naphthoquinone (K_9H) level, whereas the succinate chain converges at the cytochrome b level. The sequence of respiratory carriers was studied and is described in detail.

The respiratory chains of *M. phlei* were compared with those of mammalian mitochondria and found to be similar, with the exception of the malate pathway and the presence of a naphthoquinone. The naphthoquinone participates in electron transport between flavoprotein and cytochrome b on the NAD^+ and malate chains, but not on the succinate chain. An unidentified light-sensitive compond on the succinic oxidase pathway functions below cytochrome b. The properties of the *M. phlei* system resemble closely the disrupted mammalian mitochondrial system.

Acknowledgments—The authors would like to express their gratitude to Dr. Britton Chance and his colleagues at the Johnson Foundation and to Dr. G. Kidder of the Biophysics Department of the Harvard Medical School for their help in some of the spectrophotometric studies, and to Mrs. Jane Ballantine Klubes for her technical assistance.

REFERENCES

1. BRODIE, A. F., in S. P. COLOWICK AND N. O. KAPLAN (Editors), *Methods in enzymology, Vol. 5*, Academic Press, Inc., New York, 1962, p. 51.
2. BRODIE, A. F., AND GRAY, C. T., *Science*, **125**, 534 (1957).
3. PINCHOT, G. B., *J. Biol. Chem.*, **205**, 65 (1953).
4. BRODIE, A. F., AND GRAY, C. T., *Biochim. et Biophys. Acta*, **19**, 384 (1956).
5. SLATER, E. C., AND TISSIÈRES, A., *Nature*, **176**, 736 (1955).
6. BRODIE, A. F., *J. Biol. Chem.*, **234**, 398 (1959).
7. ISHIKAWA, S., AND LEHNINGER, A. L., *J. Biol. Chem.*, **237**, 2401 (1962).
8. KASHKET, E. R., AND BRODIE, A. F., *Biochim. et Biophys. Acta*, **78**, 52 (1963).
9. BRODIE, A. F., AND RUSSELL, P. J., JR., in E. C. SLATER (Editor), *Proceedings of the Fifth International Congress of Biochemistry, Moscow, Vol. 5*, Pergamon Press, London, 1963, p. 89.
10. CHANCE, B., AND WILLIAMS, C. R., in F. F. NORD (Editor), *Advances in enzymology, Vol. 17*, Interscience Publishers, Inc., New York, 1956, p. 65.
11. BRODIE, A. F., DAVIS, B. R., AND FIESER, L. F., *J. Am. Chem. Soc.*, **80**, 6454 (1958).
12. GALE, P. H., ARISON, B. H., TRENNER, N. R., PAGE, A. C., JR., FOLKERS, K., AND BRODIE, A. F., *Biochemistry*, **2**, 200 (1963).
13. CRANE, F. L., in G. E. W. WOLSTENHOLME AND C. M. O'CONNOR (Editors), *Ciba Foundation symposium on quinones in electron transport*, J. and A. Churchill, Ltd., London, 1960, p. 36.
14. GREEN, D. E., in G. E. W. WOLSTENHOLME AND C. M. O'CONNOR (Editors), *Ciba Foundation symposium on quinones in electron transport*, J. and A. Churchill, Ltd., London, 1960, p. 130.
15. ASANO, A., AND BRODIE, A. F., *Biochem. and Biophys. Research Communs.*, **13**, 423 (1963).
16. BRODIE, A. F., AND GRAY, C. T., *J. Biol. Chem.*, **219**, 853 (1956).
17. ASANO, A., AND BRODIE, A. F., *Biochem. and Biophys. Research Communs.*, **13**, 416 (1963).
18. FISKE, C. H., AND SUBBAROW, Y., *J. Biol. Chem.*, **66**, 375 (1925).
19. STADTMAN, E. R., NOVELLI, G. D., AND LIPMANN, F., *J. Biol. Chem.*, **191**, 365 (1951).
20. LOWRY, O. H., ROSEBROUGH, N. J., FARR, A. L., AND RANDALL, R. J., *J. Biol. Chem.*, **193**, 265 (1951).
21. CHANCE, B., *Science*, **120**, 767 (1954).
22. ESTABROOK, R. W., in J. B. FALK, R. LEMBERG, AND R. K. MORTON (Editors), *Haematin enzymes*, Pergamon Press, London, 1961, p. 436.
23. CHANCE, B., *J. Biol. Chem.*, **202**, 383 (1953).
24. ADELSON, J. W., ASANO, A., AND BRODIE, A. F., *Proc. Natl. Acad. Sci. U. S.*, **51**, 402 (1964).
25. CHANCE, B., AND WILLIAMS, G. R., *J. Biol. Chem.*, **217**, 395 (1955).
26. CHANCE, B., AND HAGIHARA, B., in E. C. SLATER (Editor), *Proceedings of the Fifth International Congress of Biochemistry, Moscow, Vol. 5*, Pergamon Press, London, 1963, p. 3.
27. KASHKET, E. R., AND BRODIE, A. F., *Biochim. et Biophys. Acta*, **40**, 550 (1960).
28. CHANCE, B., *J. Biol. Chem.*, **202**, 407 (1953).
29. KAMEN, M. D., BARTSH, R. G., HORIO, T., AND DE KLERK, H., in S. P. COLOWICK AND N. O. KAPLAN (Editors), *Methods in enzymology, Vol. 6*, Academic Press, Inc., New York, 1963, p. 391.
30. TISSIÈRES, A., AND BURRIS, R. H., *Biochim. et Biophys. Acta*, **20**, 436 (1956).
31. HORIO, T., HIGASHI, T., SASAGAWA, M., KUSAI, K., NAKAI, M., AND OKUNUKI, K., *Biochem. J.*, **77**, 194 (1960).
32. DEEB, S. S., AND HAGER, L. P., *J. Biol. Chem.*, **239**, 1024 (1964).
33. HAGIHARA, B., HORIO, T., YAMASHITA, J., NOZAKI, M., AND OKUNUKI, K., *Nature*, **178**, 629 (1956).
34. APPLEBY, C. M., AND MORTON, R. K., *Biochem. J.*, **73**, 539 (1959).
35. WEBER, M. M., AND SWARTZ, M. N., *Arch. Biochem. Biophys.*, **86**, 233 (1960).
36. GREEN, D. E., AND WHARTON, D. C., *Biochem. Z.*, **338**, 335 (1963).
37. KING, T. E., NICKEL, K. S., AND JENSEN, D. R., *J. Biol. Chem.*, **239**, 1989 (1964).
38. CHANCE, B., *J. Biol. Chem.*, **197**, 557 (1952).
39. ESTABROOK, R. W., AND MACKLER, B., *J. Biol. Chem.*, **229**, 1091 (1957).
40. CHANCE, B., AND WILLIAMS, G. R., *J. Biol. Chem.*, **217**, 429 (1955).
41. HANSEN, M., AND SMITH, A. L., *Biochim. et Biophys. Acta*, **82**, 214 (1964).
42. CHANCE, B., *Nature*, **169**, 215 (1952).
43. ERNSTER, L., LJUNGGREN, M., AND DANIELSON, L., *Biochem. and Biophys. Research Communs.*, **2**, 88 (1960).
44. PACKER, L., ESTABROOK, R. W., SINGER, T. P., AND KIMURA, T., *J. Biol. Chem.*, **235**, 535 (1960).
45. ERNSTER, L., DALLNER, G., AND AZZONE, G. F., *J. Biol. Chem.*, **238**, 1124 (1963).
46. BRODIE, A. F., AND BALLANTINE, J., *J. Biol. Chem.*, **235**, 226 (1960).
47. CHANCE, B., AND REDFEARN, E. R., *Biochem. J.*, **80**, 632 (1961).

48. LIGHTBOWN, J. W., AND JACKSON, F. L., *Biochem. J.*, **63**, 130 (1956).
49. ERNSTER, L., in T. W. GOODWIN AND O. LINDBERG (Editors), *Biological structure and function, Vol. 2*, Academic Press, Inc., London, 1961, p. 139.
50. ROSE, I. A., AND OCHOA, S., *J. Biol. Chem.*, **220**, 307 (1956).
51. HOVENKAMP, H. G., *Biochim. et Biophys. Acta*, **34**, 485 (1959).
52. KEARNEY, E. B., *J. Biol. Chem.*, **235**, 865 (1960).
53. RIESKE, J. S., MACLENNAN, D. H., AND COLEMAN, R., *Biochem. and Biophys. Research Communs.*, **15**, 338 (1964).
54. KIELLEY, W. W., AND BRONK, J. R., *J. Biol. Chem.*, **230**, 521 (1958).
55. McMURRAY, W. C., MALEY, G. F., AND LARDY, H. A., *J. Biol. Chem.*, **230**, 219 (1958).
56. PENEFSKY, H. S., PULLMAN, M. E., DATTA, A., AND RACKER, E., *J. Biol. Chem.*, **235**, 3330 (1960).
57. LEHNINGER, A. L., WADKINS, C. L., COOPER, C., DEVLIN, T. M., AND GAMBLE, J. L., JR., *Science*, **128**, 450 (1958).
58. LINNANE, A. W., AND ZIEGLER, D. M., *Biochim. et Biophys. Acta*, **29**, 630 (1958).
59. CHANCE, B., AND SACKTOR, B., *Arch. Biochem. Biophys.*, **76**, 509 (1958).
60. ESTABROOK, R. W., AND SACKTOR, B., *J. Biol. Chem.*, **233**, 1014 (1958).
61. SACKTOR, B., PACKER, L., AND ESTABROOK, R. W., *Arch. Biochem. Biophys.*, **80**, 68 (1959).
62. KLINGENBERG, M., AND SLENCSKA, W., *Biochem. Z.*, **331**, 334 (1959).
63. ZEBE, E., DELBRÜCK, A., AND BÜCHER, T., *Biochem. Z.*, **331**, 254 (1959).
64. VAN DEN BERGH, S. G., AND SLATER, E. C., *Biochem. J.*, **82**, 362 (1962).
65. RINGLER, R. L., AND SINGER, T. P., *J. Biol. Chem.*, **234**, 2211 (1959).
66. KIMURA, T., AND SINGER, T. P., *Nature*, **184**, 791 (1959).
67. ROTHCHILD, H. A., CORI, O., AND GUZMAN BARRON, E. S., *J. Biol. Chem.*, **208**, 41 (1954).
68. COHN, D. V., *J. Biol. Chem.*, **221**, 413 (1956).
69. KIMURA, T., AND TOBARI, J., *Biochim. et Biophys. Acta*, **73**, 399 (1963).
70. KLINGENBERG, M., AND BÜCHER, T., *Annual review of biochemistry, Vol. 29*, Annual Reviews, Inc., Palo Alto, Calif., 1960, p. 669.
71. ANDERSON, L., AND PLAUT, G. W. E., in H. A. LARDY (Editor), *Respiratory enzymes*, Burgess Publishing Company, Minneapolis, 1949, p. 80.
72. CLARK, W. M., *Oxidation-reduction potentials of organic systems*, The Williams and Wilkins Company, Baltimore, 1960.
73. BRODIE, A. F., AND BALLANTINE, J., *J. Biol. Chem.*, **235**, 232 (1960).
74. BRODIE, A. F., *Federation Proc.*, **20**, 995 (1961).
75. WEBER, M. M., BRODIE, A. F., AND MERSELIS, J. E., *Science*, **128**, 896 (1958).
76. WEBER, M. M., AND ROSSO, G., *Proc. Natl. Acad. Sci. U. S.*, **50**, 710 (1963).
77. TSOU, C. L., *Biochem. J.*, **49**, 512 (1951).

Editor's Comments
on Papers 9, 10, and 11

TERMINAL OXIDASES

The enzyme finally reducing an externally supplied oxidant during respiration is a terminal oxidase. The selections presented here describe oxidases that reduce oxygen, and reflect the fact that respiring procaryotes frequently utilize two or more oxidases.

The technique of the relief of carbon monoxide inhibition of respiration by photodissociation, a phenomenon discovered by J. Scott Haldane[1] in 1896 and further developed by Warburg, is used to identify hemoproteins with oxygen-reducing activity. Chance, Smith, and Castor greatly enhanced the usefulness of this procedure by the work described in Paper 9. Although such measurements alone are insufficient to define significant oxidase function, combination of these results with the findings from kinetic experiments clarified the oxidase activity of cytochromes a_1, d (a_2), and o. "*Rhodospirillum* heme protein" (RHP of Paper 5), contrary to expectations of an oxidase role brought about by the ability to bind CO, was shown by kinetic procedures to be without such activity.[2]

The unusual chemical properties of the heme prosthetic group of cytochrome a_2 from *Aerobacter aerogenes* are described by Barrett in Paper 10. This thorough study used the techniques developed over more than a half-century of investigation of pyrrole compounds, especially by Rudolph Lemberg and his associates in Sydney. Cytochrome a_2 was shown to contain an iron-chlorin prosthetic group and is now considered a member of a group of hemo-proteins known as the cytochromes *d*.

Cytochrome *o* was purified and characterized by Webster and Hackett, as described in Paper 11. This oxidase is widely distributed among procaryotes but has not been convincingly demonstrated in eucaryotes. Webster has obtained evidence that H_2O_2 is a product of O_2 reduction by purified cytochrome *o*.[3]

Yamanaka and Okunuki have described an oxidase isolated from a denitrifying *Pseudomonas* and capable of transferring reducing equivalents to either oxygen or nitrite ion.[4] The enzyme possesses two different heme prosthetic groups of types *d* and *c* and has been termed cytochrome d_1c by Lemberg and Barrett.[5] Cytochrome d_1c, unlike branched-chain respiratory systems involving only oxygen, combines multiple oxidase functions within a single macromolecular complex.

Even though containing the same heme prosthetic group, some hemoproteins form complexes with CO while others do not. Lemberg and Barrett have suggested that such a difference is due to modification in which the "prosthetic group is linked to the haem iron coordinately in a linkage which differs from that in haemochromes and the more typical cytochromes."[6] RHP of Paper 5 is accordingly a cytochrome *c'* or *cc'*; "cytochrome a_3 is in fact an *a'* cytochrome and cytochrome *o* a *b'* cytochrome."[6]

REFERENCES

1. Haldane, J. S., and J. L. Smith. *J. Physiol.,* **20**, 497–520, 1896.
2. Chance, B., T. Horio, M. Kamen, and S. Taniguchi. *Biochim. Biophys. Acta,* **112**, 1–7, 1966.
3. Webster, D. *J. Biol. Chem.,* **250**, 4955–4958, 1975.
4. Yamanaka, T., and K. Okunuki. *Biochim. Biophys. Acta.,* **67**, 379–393, 1963.
5. Lemberg, R., and J. Barrett. *Cytochromes.* Academic Press, New York, 1963, pp. 240ff.
6. Ibid, p. 10.

9

Reprinted from *Biochim. Biophys. Acta* **12**:289–298 (1953)

NEW METHODS FOR THE STUDY OF THE
CARBON MONOXIDE COMPOUNDS OF RESPIRATORY ENZYMES*

by

BRITTON CHANCE, LUCILE SMITH AND LAROY CASTOR*

Johnson Research Foundation, University of Pennsylvania,
Philadelphia, Pennsylvania (U.S.A.)

In the past few years it has been possible to improve considerably and to extend the range of three basic methods for the study of respiratory enzymes, especially their carbon monoxide compounds. Visual spectroscopy—used first by MacMunn in 1885[1] to discover the histohemins, by Keilin in 1925[2] to identify and to study the cytochromes in detail, and by Warburg and his co-workers to identify the CO compound of the respiratory enzyme in *Acetobacter pasteurianum*[3]—until recently has had no successful competitor for the study of the absorption bands of the respiratory enzymes in suspensions of intact cells or in muscle tissue. But improved photoelectric surfaces and electronic techniques have in our hands and more recently in the hands of others[4] brought sharply into focus the absorption spectra that could at best be only dimly perceived by earlier photoelectric techniques such as were used by Warburg and Christian to show the presence of flavoprotein in *Bacterium delbrückii*[5] and by Haas to measure the speed of reduction of cytochrome c in *Torula utilis*[6]. It is now possible to observe the reduction of respiratory enzymes in the range 320 to 660 mμ in many types of respiring cell suspensions. In bakers' yeast, for example, the reaction kinetics and spectra of the pyridine nucleotides, flavoproteins and cytochromes of types a, a_3, b and c can be separately studied by rapid and sensitive spectroscopic methods[7,8]. In some cases the sensitivity exceeds that achieved by highly skilful visual observers since we can regularly record the 590 mμ band of cytochrome a_1 in cultures of *Azotobacter chroococcum*. More recently these spectroscopic methods have been improved so that they are suitable for measuring the changes in optical density caused by the formation of the carbon monoxide compounds[9] of the respiratory enzymes[10] or cytochrome oxidases[11] of the cell suspensions.

About ten years ago Bücher and Negelein developed an "optical method" for the study of the kinetics of photodissociation of the CO compounds of the soluble pigments myoglobin and hemoglobin[12]. By introducing new electronic techniques, we now have developed a more sensitive method for use with turbid cell suspensions, first, for demonstrating that the photodissociation of the cytochrome a_3–CO compound actually occurs[13], secondly, for obtaining "photodissociation spectra" of the CO compounds of respiratory enzymes[13], and thirdly, for obtaining accurate values for the molecular extinction of the α-bands of the CO compounds of the respiratory enzymes by direct meas-

---

* This research was supported in part by the National Institutes of Health, United States Public Health Service, by the Office of Naval Research, and by the National Science Foundation.
** Lalor Foundation predoctoral fellow.

urements of the kinetics of photodissociation and recombination of the CO compounds[14]. The latter method is much more direct than the manometric method[15,16] which responds too slowly to permit a direct measurement of the kinetics of photodissociation. We find the molecular extinction coefficient of the a-band of cytochrome a_3–CO to be $\varepsilon = 12$ cm^{-1} $\times$ mM^{-1} for bakers' yeast cells and for heart muscle homogenates[14].

The classical manometric method for determining the relative photochemical action spectrum for the reversal of carbon monoxide inhibition of respiration that was developed twenty-five years ago[17] has been until now the only method so far available. Although this manometric method has given excellent spectra, there seem to be large changes in the heights of the major absorption bands and in the details of the subsidiary bands when the temperature is lowered[18,19]. Also, MELNICK'S action spectrum for yeast[20] does not agree in detail with that of KUBOWITZ AND HAAS[18] nor does his 450 mμ peak for heart muscle preparation agree with any of the other data on cytochrome a_3[13,19]. Thus a new method that permits monochromatic illumination of the sample over a wide range of wavelengths is highly desirable. We can report here preliminary experiments with an apparatus for measuring photochemical action spectra in a drop of cell suspension[21] with the aid of the platinum microelectrode[22,23]. We have not yet perfected the fourth and logical development of these techniques—the plotting of the photochemical action spectra from data on the direct measurement of the photodissociation kinetics for a number of wavelengths of monochromatic photodissociating light, but such an apparatus appears feasible.

We have surveyed the respiratory pigments of various materials with these sensitive methods[24] and have recently focussed our attention upon a rather different "CO-binding pigment" found in *Staphylococcus albus* and in other bacteria. Our absorption spectrum (difference spectrum) for this CO compound shows peaks at 416 mμ[9], 535 and 570 mμ[25], and the photodissociation spectrum shows close agreement with the absorption spectrum; the peak of the Soret band lies at 415 mμ[13]. We here present quantitative data on the kinetics of photodissociation of this CO-binding pigment and find that it is considerably less light-sensitive at 589 mμ than the enzyme of yeast or muscle, but that it has a distinctive band at 546 mμ. Our preliminary value for the molecular extinction of the CO-binding pigment at this wavelength is $\varepsilon = 5$ cm^{-1} $\times$ mM^{-1}. We have also determined the relative photochemical action spectrum for this pigment and find that the action spectrum in the Soret region has a peak at 418 mμ, in agreement with our absorption and photodissociation difference spectra and distinctly different from the 430 mμ peak for yeast and muscle[21]. Our results suggest that this "CO-binding pigment" is a new respiratory enzyme that has a prosthetic group closely allied to that of the protohemin enzymes and distinctly different from the dichroic hemin enzymes, and should therefore be classed as a completely new type of respiratory enzyme.

*Absorption difference spectra**

One of the more useful methods for obtaining difference spectra is illustrated by Fig. 1. This method utilizes the light chopping and demodulating system developed by CHANCE for a double-beam spectrophotometer[8] and an automatic gain control circuit (agc) developed by R.C.A.[26], together with a number of ingenious improvements devised by Dr. C. C. YANG[27]. The apparatus consists of a source of high intensity monochromatic light that is split into two paths by a vibrating mirror (60 cps) and illuminates

---

* *Footnote see page 292.*

two suspensions of respiring cells of equal concentration. Cuvette A is taken to be the reference cell and the photocurrent obtained upon illuminating that cuvette is maintained at a predetermined level by an automatic gain control circuit that receives its signal from the contacts of the first demodulator and adjusts the dynode voltage of the photomultiplier to the appropriate value for constant photocurrent regardless of the intensity of the light illuminating the cuvette, the transmission through the sample, or the sensitivity of the photosurface. This constitutes the "100% transmission" signal. When cuvette B is illuminated, a signal representing the actual transmission is received from the first demodulator and is measured by a second demodulator. In order to record optical densities, the percent transmission is converted into logarithms by a segmented logarithmic characteristic consisting of ten diodes[28, 29]. The optical density values are then plotted by a servo recorder (Leeds and Northrup Speedomax). In order to have a linear wavelength scale on the chart, an appropriately loaded potentiometer operates in the feedback circuit of the chart drive servomechanism[30].

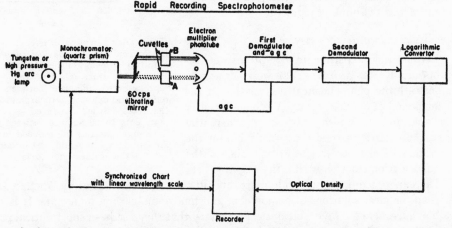

Fig. 1. A schematic diagram of the operation of a spectrophotometer suitable for recording the spectra of the respiratory pigments of cell suspensions and tissue homogenates. agc represents "automatic gain control" (MD-25).

The apparatus has a noise level of $\sim 1 \cdot 10^{-4}$ in optical density and operates with a spectral interval of 2 mμ or less when the cuvettes are filled with a turbid suspension of respiring cells. The spectrum is plotted at the rate of a few millimicrons per second.

In studies with turbid cell suspensions, it is important to gather both the transmitted and the scattered light from the cell suspension in order to obtain adequate sensitivity. This we accomplish by placing the phototube near the cell suspension and thereby avoid the lens and prism as were used earlier by WARBURG AND CHRISTIAN[6].

In actual use, a "base-line" is plotted with cuvettes A and B filled with equal concentrations of oxidized cells. Then the substrate is added to the cell suspension in cuvette B so that the oxygen is consumed and the absorption bands of the reduced cytochromes are recorded. Next the substrate is added to cuvette A and a second base-line is drawn. CO is finally bubbled through cuvette B to form the CO-reduced compound and the spectrum of the CO compound is plotted. (For further details see reference 9.)

Thus this apparatus is especially useful for plotting difference spectra, for example, the spectrum representing the difference between the reduced and oxidized forms of the respiratory pigments of *S. albus* illustrated by the trace labelled "reduced" in Fig. 2.

And the trace labelled "reduced + CO" represents the difference between the CO compounds and the reduced forms of the respiratory pigments. In this case one observes a distinct peak at 416 mμ and a trough at 432 mμ, as contrasted to the peak and trough of the corresponding spectrum for the yeast cells which lie at 430 and 445 mμ respectively.

Similar studies can be carried out for *S. albus* in the visible region of the spectrum and peaks at 535 and 570 mμ are reported by SMITH[25].

Fig. 2 when compared with Fig. 3B of reference 9 shows that cultures of *S. albus* may be treated so as to increase considerably their relative content of this CO-binding pigment.

Photodissociation difference spectra

Because their experimental conditions were inappropriate, KEILIN AND HARTREE were not able to demonstrate the photochemical dissociation of the CO compound of cytochrome a_3. We have recently been able to accomplish this by a differential spectrophotometric method that is suitable for the observation of changes in absorption due to the photodissociation reaction within the respiring cell.

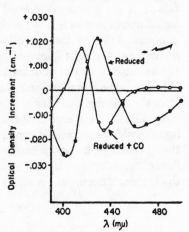

Fig. 2. The absorption difference spectra for a culture of *Staphylococcus albus* obtained by means of the apparatus of Fig. 1. The trace labelled "reduced" represents the differences between the reduced and oxidized cytochromes and the trace labeled "reduced + CO" represents the difference between the CO compound and the reduced form. Similar data can readily be obtained in the visible region (0-37).

This experiment is considerably more difficult than that carried out by BÜCHER AND NEGELEIN on clear solutions of hemoglobin and myoglobin carbon monoxide. It is not possible to use here the favorable optical geometry that they used—a short optical path for the photodissociating light and a long path for the measuring of light. With turbid cell suspensions, we require a fairly large surface area of the suspension near the measuring photosurface (see p. 291, 2nd paragraph under Fig. 1). Thus we have used a square cuvette in which the photodissociating and the measuring paths are both equal to one cm.

Another novel feature of the method that we use is the ability to vary the measuring wavelength and thereby to obtain a "photodissociation difference spectrum"* of the CO compound. Since the turbid suspensions scatter photodissociating light of very high intensity in the direction of the measuring phototube, our method has three features that avoid interference with the spectrophotometric measurement by the photodissociating light.

---

* In order to distinguish between the three types of spectra of the CO compounds that are discussed in this paper, it is useful to define the three terms:

Absorption difference spectrum. This is a spectrum representing the change of light absorption caused by a chemical change of the pigment, for example, from oxidized to reduced (a reduced-oxidized spectrum), or from reduced to the CO compound (a CO-reduced spectrum).

Photodissociation difference spectrum. This is a spectrum representing the change of light absorption caused by a photochemical reaction, for example, the photochemical dissociation of a CO compound of a reduced cytochrome in which case a CO-reduced spectrum is obtained.

Photochemical action spectrum. This is an absolute (not difference) spectrum. The ordinates are inversely proportional to the quantum intensity required at each wavelength to produce a given rate of photochemical decomposition of the CO compound.

First, the photodissociation is accomplished by illuminating the cell suspension with yellow light, for example, the 589 mμ line of the Na arc or the 578 mμ of the Hg arc, other portions of the spectrum of these line sources being readily eliminated by appropriate filters having the characteristics shown in Fig. 3. The observation of the photodissociation of CO compounds is made in the region of the Soret band (410-480 mμ) and the photocell is rendered insensitive to the yellow light not only by the nature of its surface (Cs–Sb) but also by the blue colour filter combination shown by the solid curve of Fig. 3.

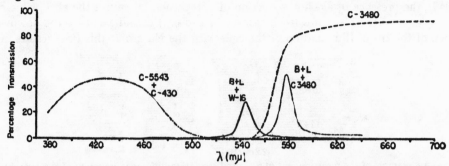

Fig. 3. Transmission curves for optical filters used to isolate photodissociating light (above 520 mμ) from spectrophotometric wavelengths (410–480 mμ). C represents Corning glass filters, W represents Wratten filter, and B + L represents Bausch and Lomb interference filters (MD-27).

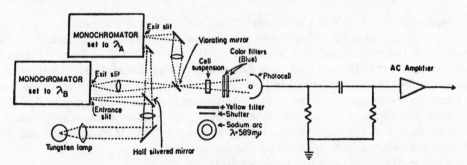

Fig. 4. A schematic diagram of a double-beam spectrophotometer suitable for measuring the kinetics of the photochemical decomposition of the CO compounds of the respiratory enzymes within intact cells. The characteristics of the optical filters are given in Fig. 3. The wavelengths λ_A and λ_B are set in the region 410–480 mμ (MD-28).

Secondly, as Fig. 4 shows, the differential double-beam spectrophotometer employs two wavelengths of light, one a reference wavelength, for example 480 mμ where no appreciable optical density changes due to photodissociation are to be expected, and the other an adjustable wavelength (in the region 410–480 mμ). The photoelectric circuit measures the differences of the light transmission changes at the two wavelengths, and this difference is not affected by leakage of yellow light through the colour filters.

Thirdly, to discriminate further against light leakage, the two beams of monochromatic light are chopped by a vibrating mirror at 60 cps so that first one and then the other is incident upon the sample and the photocell. Thus the output current from the photocell consists of a square 60 cps wave, the amplitude of which represents the difference of light transmission at the two wavelengths of light[8]. Since the arc lamps for causing photodissociation are operated on well-filtered direct current, there is no alternating component of the yellow light that leaks through the filters.

By means of these three design factors, the filtered light from a 100 watt Na or Hg lamp a few inches from the sample cell causes no deflection of the trace of the spectrophotometer. The only detectable effect of the light leakage is an increase in the shot noise output of the photoelectric circuit.

A typical record of the photodissociation and recombination of the CO compound in bakers' yeast cells is shown in Fig. 5. Starting with the steady-state oxidized yeast cells in the presence of alcohol, reduction of cytochrome a_3 causes the abrupt increase of optical density at 445 mμ (with respect to 480 mμ) as indicated by the downward sweep of the trace. Illumination of the cells with the Na arc at this time results in no

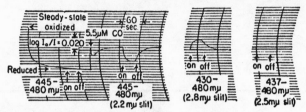

Fig. 5. An example of the measurement of a photodissociation difference spectrum of the cytochrome a_3–CO compound of bakers' yeast cells with the apparatus of Fig. 4. The points "on" and "off" represent the moments at which the photodissociating light is turned on and off. Illuminating light is 589 mμ. (25° C) (Expt. 145e).

deflection of the trace. When reduction is complete and the cells are substantially anaerobic, a solution of CO is added to give a final concentration of 5.5 μM, causing the formation of the cytochrome a_3–CO compound. Illumination of the cells now causes the dissociation of the CO compound while darkness allows its reformation, the latter change corresponding to a decrease of optical density and to a trough in the difference spectrum. If now the wavelength is shifted to 430 mμ, illumination causes the opposite sign of optical density change to occur, corresponding to a peak in the difference spectrum. And if a wavelength of 437 mμ is used no change at all occurs; this is an isosbestic point between the reduced and CO-reduced spectra providing a good control against possible artifacts.

These deflections, plotted as a function of wavelength, form a 'difference spectrum'' that represents the differences between the absorption of the CO compound and the reduced form of cytochrome a_3. The peak of this difference spectrum would be expected to lie very close to that of the absolute photochemical absorption spectrum of the respiratory enzyme at 430 mμ[17] because, as KEILIN AND HARTREE already have shown[11], the respiratory enzyme has many of the properties of cytochrome a_3. The result obtained with direct methods affords a conclusive proof of the identity of the respiratory enzyme of *T. utilis* and cytochrome a_3 of heart muscle preparations.

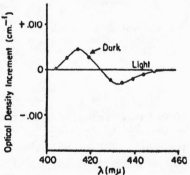

Fig. 6. A photodissociation difference spectrum for the "CO-binding pigment" of *Staphylococcus albus* obtained with the apparatus of Fig. 4 (948 c).

S. albus shows a rather different pigment with a peak at 415 mμ and a trough at 433 mμ as shown in Fig. 6 [18].

In order to demonstrate that our method for measuring the photodissociation spectrum gives a result that agrees accurately with the actual absorption spectrum, we compare in Fig. 7 the spectrum obtained by subtracting the ferromyoglobin–CO spectrum from that of ferromyoglobin (BEZNAK[31]) with a photodissociation spectrum obtained with this apparatus. The agreement of the data shows that the photodissociation method gives nearly as accurate results as the direct measurement of the absorption spectra

It should be noted that exact coincidence of the peaks of the absorption photodissociation difference spectra with those of the relative photochemical action spectra is not to be expected. Fig. 7 (Curve A) clearly shows that for protohemin pigments the peak of the difference spectrum lies 2.5 mμ below that of the absolute spectrum and, in the case of the dichroic hemin enzyme lactoperoxidase, the displacement is 1.5 mμ[13]. Thus the displacement is small, but significant.

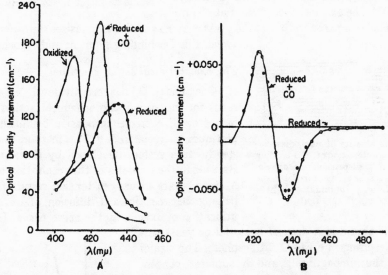

Fig 7. (A), the oxidized, reduced, and reduced-CO spectra for myoglobin (from BEZNAK[31]) and (B), (open circles), the difference spectrum of the CO compound. Solid circles of (B) show experimental data on the photodissociation spectrum of myoglobin-CO obtained by the method of Fig. 4. In order to facilitate the comparison, the ordinates of the photodissociation curve were multiplied by a constant factor to cause the two sets of data to match at the peak of the curve (1 μM Mgb, pH = 7.0, 2.9 μM CO) (Expt. 143a).

Calculation of the molecular extinction coefficients

By measuring the kinetics of photodissociation and recombination of the CO compound on a faster time scale as in Fig. 8, the molecular extinction coefficient may be calculated in a manner similar to that used by BÜCHER AND KASPERS[33] provided the intensity of the photodissociating light is known. But instead of a bolometer we use myoglobin–CO as a standard and thereby avoid the need for an accurate measurement of the light intensity as well as the distribution of intensities in the cuvette. To simulate light scattering when myoglobin is used, *Escherichia coli* are added to give the same scattering effects as the yeast cells (see reference 14 for details). On this basis, we have computed the values of the molecular extinction coefficients for the CO compounds in heart muscle homogenates, bakers' yeast cells, *A. pasteurianum*, and *Bacillus subtilis*[14], and find ε_{589} = 12 cm^{-1} × mM^{-1} for the cytochromes of type a_3. (Reference 14 gives detailed data on the experimental controls and also the method of calculating the results.)

In our previous studies the sensitivity of the apparatus was insufficient to give any quantitative idea of the molecular extinction coefficients of the "CO-binding pigment" of *S. albus*. We now have increased the sensitivity, and satisfactory kinetic data may be obtained as in Fig. 8. A preliminary value can be given for the molecular extinction coefficient of the band at 546 mμ, ε = 5 cm^{-1} × mM^{-1}, about half that of the value for myoglobin–CO at 580 mμ (10.6 cm^{-1} × mM^{-1})[32]. The extinction coefficient at 589 mμ

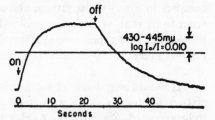

Fig. 8. The kinetics of photodissociation and recombination of the cytochrome a_3–CO compound in bakers' yeast cells as measured by the method of Fig. 4 (Expt. measured by the method of Fig. 4. Illuminating light is 589 mμ (Expt. 144).

is very small compared to that of the yeast enzyme and this emphasizes the difference between this CO-binding pigment and cytochrome a_3.

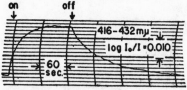

Fig. 9. The kinetics of photodissociation and recombination of "CO-binding pigment" in a suspension of *Staphylococcus albus* cells as measured by the method of Fig. 4. Illuminating light is 578 mμ (Expt. 144).

The photochemical action spectrum

One of us (L. C.) has recently developed an apparatus for measuring photochemical action spectra in a drop of bacterial suspension by means of the platinum microelectrode[21]. This method utilizes the steady-state system developed by CONNELLY AND BRINK[23] in their studies of the respiration of nerve. A steady-state in oxygen tension results from the balance between inward diffusion of oxygen and utilization of oxygen by the nerve tissue. The same conditions obtain in a drop of bacterial or yeast suspension respiring in a CO–O_2 atmosphere. The size of the drop, the number of cells, and the substrate concentration are adjusted so that the steady-state oxygen concentration for maximal effectiveness of the photochemical reaction is obtained. Illumination of the drop will displace this steady-state and the change of oxygen concentration is sensitively recorded by the platinum microelectrode.

Our results for *S. albus* show a Soret band at 418 mμ definitely displaced from the 430 mμ peak measured for yeast cells with the same apparatus. A preliminary action spectrum for the respiratory enzyme in *S. albus* in the Soret region is shown in Fig. 10.

In the visible region of the spectrum, the peaks of the CO compound are found to lie at 535 and 566 mμ in fairly good agreement with the peaks of the absorption difference spectrum that lie at 535 and 570 mμ[25]. These values are similar to those for hemoproteins

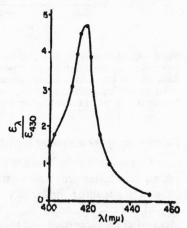

Fig. 10. A relative photochemical action spectrum of the CO-binding pigment in *Staphylococcus albus*. Similar data are readily obtained in the visible region of the spectrum (25°) (0–38).

that have protohemin as their prosthetic group and lead us to suggest that this new respiratory enzyme has a protohemin prosthetic group instead of a dichroic hemin and that it should be classified as a completely new type of respiratory enzyme.

SUMMARY

Several highly refined physical methods have been described for the study of the CO compounds of the respiratory pigments of living cell suspensions. These methods reveal significant differences in the respiratory enzymes of different bacterial cells and our results suggest that *Staphylococcus albus* contains a new respiratory enzyme that has a prosthetic group closely related to the protohemin enzymes and that this respiratory pigment should be classified as a completely new type of respiratory enzyme.

RÉSUMÉ

Plusieurs méthodes physiques très fines pour l'étude des composés oxycarbonés des pigments respiratoires de cellules vivantes en suspension ont été décrites. Ces méthodes révèlent des différences significatives entre les enzymes respiratoires de différentes bactéries et nos résultats suggèrent que *Staphylococcus albus* renferme un nouvel enzyme respiratoire dont le groupement prosthétique est très voisin des enzymes protohémines. Ce pigment respiratoire doit être rangé dans un groupe complètement nouveau des enzymes respiratoires.

ZUSAMMENFASSUNG

Mehrere höchst verfeinerte physikalische Methoden für die Untersuchung der Atmungspigmente von Suspensionen lebender Zellen werden beschrieben. Diese Methoden erlauben bedeutsame Unterschiede zwischen Atmungsfermenten verschiedener Bakterien aufzufinden. Unsere Versuche machen es wahrscheinlich dass *Staphylococcus albus* ein Pigment enthält dessen prosthetische Gruppe mit den Protohäminfermenten nahe verwandt ist, aber als ein ganz neuer Typ von Atmungsferment angesehen werden muss und entsprechend eine Klasse für sich bildet.

REFERENCES

[1] C. A. MacMunn, *Phil. Trans. Royal Soc. London*, 177, (1885) 267.
[2] D. Keilin, *Proc. Roy. Soc. London, Series B*, 98 (1925) 312.
[3] O. Warburg and E. Negelein, *Biochem. Z.*, 262 (1933) 237.
[4] H. Lundegårdh, *Arkiv. Kemi*, 5 (1952) 97.
[5] O. Warburg and W. Christian, *Biochem, Z.*, 266 (1933) 399.
[6] E. Haas, *Naturwissenschaften*, 22 (1934) 207.
[7] B. Chance, *Nature*, 169 (1952) 215.
[8] B. Chance, *Rev. Sci. Instruments*, 22 (1951) 619.
[9] B. Chance, *J. Biol. Chem.*, 202 (1953) 383.
[10] O. Warburg, *Schwermetalle als Wirkungsgruppen von Fermenten*, Chapter 8, Freiburg (1949).
[11] D. Keilin and E. F. Hartree, *Proc. Roy. Soc. London, Series B*, 127 (1939) 167.
[12] T. Bücher and E. Negelein, *Biochem. Z.*, 311 (1942) 163.
[13] B. Chance, *J. Biol. Chem.*, 202 (1953) 397.
[14] B. Chance, *J. Biol. Chem.*, 202 (1953) 407.
[15] O. Warburg and E. Negelein, *Biochem. Z.*, 202 (1928) 202.
[16] O. Warburg and E. Negelein, *Biochem. Z.*, 214 (1929) 64.
[17] O. Warburg and E. Negelein, *Biochem. Z.*, 193 (1928) 339.
[18] F. Kubowitz and E. Haas, *Biochem. Z.*, 255 (1952) 247.
[19] D. Keilin and E. F. Hartree, *Nature*, 171 (1953) 413.
[20] J. L. Melnick, *J. Biol. Chem.*, 141 (1941) 269.
[21] L. N. Castor and B. Chance, to be published.
[22] P. W. Davies and F. Brink, *Rev. Sci. Instruments*, 13 (1942) 524.

[23] C. M. CONNELLY AND F. BRINK, *Rev. Sci. Instruments*, August, 1953.
[24] L. SMITH, to be published.
[25] L. SMITH, *Federation Proc.* 12 (1953) 270.
[26] Radio Corporation of America, personal communication on a normalizing amplifier (1949).
[27] C. C. YANG, *Proc. Institute of Radio Engineers*, 40 (1952) 220.
[28] B. CHANCE, V. HUGHES, E. MacNICHOL, D. SAYRE AND F. C. WILLIAMS, *Waveforms*, Chapter 8, New York (1949).
[29] B. CHANCE, F. C. WILLIAMS, C. C. YANG, J. BUSSER AND J. HIGGINS, *Rev. Sci. Instruments*, 22 (1948) 683.
[30] I. GREENWOOD, J. HOLDAM AND D. MacRAE, Electronic Instruments, p. 94, New York (1948).
[31] M. BEZNAK, *Acta Chem. Scand.*, 2 (1948) 333.
[32] H. THEORELL, *Biochem. Z.*, 268 (1934) 55.
[33] T. BÜCHER AND J. KASPERS, *Biochim. Biophys. Acta*, 1 (1947) 21.

10

Copyright © 1956 by The Biochemical Society

Reprinted from *Biochem. J.* **64**:626–639 (1956)

The Prosthetic Group of Cytochrome a_2

By J. BARRETT*

Institute of Medical Research, Royal North Shore Hospital of Sydney, Australia

(*Received 20 February* 1956)

Cells of *Escherichia coli* and *Shigella dysenteria* which had been grown under aerobic conditions were shown by Yaoi & Tamiya (1928) to possess an absorption band which differed from those of previously described cytochromes in that it lay well within the red region of the spectrum. Keilin (1933) attributed this band to a component of the cytochrome system in these bacteria. Negelein & Gerischer (1934) and Fujita & Kodama (1934) independently published spectroscopic evidence that cytochrome a_2, as it had been designated, was autoxidizable and could combine with carbon monoxide and cyanide. Unlike other cytochromes that had been observed the oxidized form showed a

band in the visible region of the spectrum, at 645 mμ. Fujita & Kodama (1934) also showed that this cytochrome was widely distributed amongst other bacteria, e.g. *Azotobacter chroococcum, Proteus vulgaris, Acetobacter pasteurianum, Eberthella typhosa* and *Salmonella paratyphi*. The spectroscopic evidence of the properties of cytochrome a_2 led to the assumption that in these organisms it had the function of a cytochrome oxidase. This view remained current until the recent work of Tissières (1952), Moss (1952) and Chance (1953) threw doubt on it.

No attempt seems to have been made to establish the nature of the prosthetic group of cytochrome a_2; though Negelein & Gerischer (1934) suggested that it might be related to the ferrophaeophorbides, and

* Working under a grant from the National Health and Medical Research Council of Australia.

Lemberg & Wyndham (1937) considered that there were spectroscopic resemblances to biliviolin–iron complexes. From a study of the difference spectrum of the CO-compound of cytochrome a_2, Chance concluded that the spectrum of its prosthetic group would lack a distinctive Soret band, and considered this as evidence in favour of the assumption of Lemberg & Wyndham.

The probable importance of cytochrome a_2 as an electron carrier and especially its possible role as a terminal oxidase suggested the present attempt to isolate and characterize its prosthetic group.

Aerobacter aerogenes was used as the source of cytochrome a_2, but other organisms have also been examined. Both the haemin and the iron-free pigment, a new chlorin, have been partially purified, the latter to a much greater degree. Comparison of spectra, a study of the side chains and conversion into a porphyrin have led to the conclusion that chlorin a_2 is a dihydroporphyrin derived from either protoporphyrin or a similar porphyrin. A preliminary note covering an early part of this work has been published (Barrett & Lemberg, 1954).

METHODS

Bacteria. A strain of *Aerobacter aerogenes* supplied by Dr F. Moss of Sydney University was used at first, but was later replaced by a more vigorously growing strain isolated from soil in the grounds of this Institute. Both strains constantly gave rise to a mucoid variant which gave extremely viscid cultures on aeration. Consequently the organism was frequently plated out and cultures were made from dew-drop-type colonies. *Aero. aerogenes* was grown in a medium of the following composition: $(NH_4)_2HPO_4$, 64 g.; KH_2PO_4, 16 g.; NaCl, 10 g.; $MgSO_4,7H_2O$, 4 g.; sodium citrate, 18 g.; $FeSO_4,7H_2O$, 0·2 g.; peptone, 32 g.; sucrose, 200 g.; tap water to 15 l.; pH 6·8. Gas mixture $(O_2 + CO_2, 95:5)$ was bubbled through a sintered-glass disk (1 in., grade 4), and provided optimum aeration and gentle stirring of the medium without excessive frothing. Cultures were incubated at 37° for 18 hr. in the early part of this work, but were later left for 72 hr. to give higher yields of cytochrome a_2 per unit weight of cell material. A cell mass equivalent to 15–20 g. in dry weight was normally obtained from 15 l. of culture.

Escherichia coli and *Proteus vulgaris*, *Bacillus subtilis*, *B. mycoides* and *Pseudomonas aeruginosa* were grown at 37° in a similar medium, glucose replacing sucrose and the peptone concentration being increased to 1 %. Aeration was carried out as described above. Cells were harvested after 18 hr. *Azotobacter vinelandii* was grown at 25° in 10 l. amounts, in 16 l. bottles, in the medium of Burk & Lineweaver (1930). Vigorous aeration of the culture was maintained with compressed air. Cells were harvested at 72 hr. *Torulopsis utilis* was grown in a sucrose–mineral salt medium in 10 l. amounts. Cultures were vigorously aerated with $O_2 + CO_2$, and cells were harvested after incubation for 72 hr. at 25°.

Solvents. Peroxide-free ether was used. Acetone, A.R., was used as supplied for extraction of the cells, but for other steps in the preparative work it was stood over CaO overnight, filtered and distilled. All other organic solvents used,

except kerosene, were distilled once if supplied as A.R. but twice if of lower purity.

Silica-gel columns. Silica gel (British Drug Houses Ltd., 100 mesh) was washed twice with 95 % ethanol, twice with water, then dried at 22°. The silica gel (9 g.) was taken into a round-bottom flask and the air was replaced by nitrogen, the flask being continuously shaken. A methanol–water mixture (70:30, 4 ml.) was added and the contents of the flask were shaken under nitrogen. This procedure leaves the particles of silica gel still dispersed, which is essential for smoothly working columns. To the silica gel was added 60 ml. of light petroleum (b.p. 68°). A column 1·5 cm. × 20 cm. was used for the haemins from 20 g. dry weight of cells.

Hydrochloric acid concentrations. Because the term HCl number is widely used throughout the literature of porphyrin chemistry, the form % (w/v) of HCl is used instead of normality.

Paper chromatography. For analytical purposes the method of Chu, Green & Chu (1951) with slight modifications was used. The methyl esters of the porphyrins and chlorins were run on separate sheets in kerosene–chloroform (4·0:2·6) and kerosene–propanol (6:1). Trichloroethylene alone was also used. A 10 cm. migration of the solvent front was used throughout.

For preparative purposes sheets of Whatman no. 1 paper of 19–50 cm. width were used. The paper was washed in 95 % ethanol, followed by 95 % acetone, and dried in air. After development in one of the kerosene systems and marking of the bands that fluoresced under u.v. light, the paper was cut into horizontal strips and these were washed in light petroleum (b.p. below 40°), followed by drying *in vacuo* at 25°. The chlorin or porphyrin was then concentrated by placing one end of the strip in a few ml. of acetone in a test tube. The sharp band of pigment which developed at the top of the strip was cut off and the pigment eluted with acetone. When trichloroethylene was used washing with light petroleum was not necessary.

Spectrophotometry. Absorption spectra were measured with a Hilger Uvispek spectrophotometer. The wavelength scale was set with reference to the hydrogen lines at 656·3 and 486·1 mμ. with the hydrogen-lamp source as supplied with the instrument.

EXPERIMENTAL AND RESULTS

Preparation of haemin a_2

Nomenclature. Throughout this paper the nomenclature of Lemberg & Legge (1949) has been used.

Extraction of haemins from cells of Aero. aerogenes. The cells were dispersed in a Waring Blendor with sufficient water, acetone and HCl to give, for each 10 g. dry weight, 200 ml. of suspension containing 60 ml. of water, 140 ml. of acetone and 0·7 g. of HCl. Extraction was complete in 10–20 sec. Lower concentrations of acetone gave incomplete extraction of the haemins. The use of methanol instead of acetone, or prior extraction of the cells with neutral acetone or methanol, gave rise to low yields of haemin a_2.

The cell residue was separated from the acid–acetone solution by centrifuging. An equal volume of ether was added to the supernatant immediately on separation, and the ethereal solution of haemins obtained washed with 1 % HCl until free from acetone. The ether solution contained much fat, and great care was necessary to avoid the formation of emulsions. At the completion of this stage the combined haemin solutions were stood at $-16°$.

Spectroscopic observation of the brown ethereal solution of haemins showed a diffuse but strong band at 603 mμ., in addition to the bands of protohaemin at 635, 540 and 508 mμ. The intensity of this band relative to the 635 mμ. band of protohaemin was found to be of the same order as the intensity of the 630 mμ. band of reduced cytochrome a_2 relative to the 560 mμ. band of reduced cytochrome b_1. Fig. 1 shows the absorption spectrum of the haemins from cells with a cytochrome a_2 band of medium strength compared with the absorption spectrum of protohaemin. Ether solutions to be measured were washed with 5% HCl to ensure complete formation of the haemin. Extinctions at 635 and 603 mμ. were measured to follow the separation of haemin a_2 from protohaemin. The average batch of cells gave haemin extracts with a value of 1·2 for the ratio $E_{603\,m\mu.}/E_{635\,m\mu.}$. Exceptionally a ratio of 1·3 has been obtained. Cells with weak cytochrome a_2 band gave a ratio of 1·0.

Precipitation of phospholipids. The ether solution of haemins from 100 g. dry weight of cells contains approx. 14 g. of lipids, mainly phospholipids, the greater part of which was removed by acetone precipitation. The ether solution was first chilled at $-16°$, filtered to remove ice crystals, and the volume reduced to one-fiftieth by distillation *in vacuo*, nitrogen being passed through the capillary. Acetone was added in small amounts, the precipitated phospholipid being centrifuged off after each addition. When no more precipitation occurred the volume was reduced *in vacuo*, and any precipitate removed. The solution was cooled to $-16°$. To avoid adsorption of the haemins on the precipitating lipids the temperature was lowered by stages, the phospholipid being filtered off as it precipitated. Finally, all solvent was removed *in vacuo*, thus ensuring removal of residual water, and the oily residue was dissolved in dry acetone and stood at $-16°$.

Chromatography on silica gel. The acetone was removed *in vacuo* from the solution of haemins and the oily residue (approx. 1 g.) taken into a small volume of benzene. The protohaemin that precipitated was removed by centrifuging. By chilling at 5° overnight a second, smaller precipitate could be obtained. The haemins in benzene were applied to a silica-gel column (see Methods). Light petroleum (b.p. 68°) quickly eluted a yellow zone of lipids (fatty acids, phospholipid and a deep-yellow neutral lipid). This solvent was followed by light petroleum (b.p. 68°) which had been equilibrated with an equal volume of a mixture of methanol and water (70:30), then by wet benzene to which was added gradually increasing amounts of methanol. At a concentration of 0·5–1·0% of methanol, separation of a green zone of haemin began to develop at the head of the column, and the haemin was eluted. The methanol content of the benzene was further increased until all the haemin material had been removed from the column. All solvents were run through the column under nitrogen.

The green fraction coming off the columns showed a weak band at 603 mμ. and a strong band at 660 mμ. Washing of the fraction with 1% HCl caused a disappearance of the 660 mμ. band and a considerable increase in the intensity of the 603 mμ. band. The early benzene fractions accounted for 60% of the total absorption at 603 mμ. of the material applied to the column. The ratio $E_{603\,m\mu.}/E_{635\,m\mu.}$ was 2·88. The later benzene fractions of less-pure haemin a_2 were

combined and put through a similar column, yielding haemin a_2 of the same $E_{603\,m\mu.}/E_{635\,m\mu.}$ ratio.

Preliminary work has shown that the crude haemins in light petroleum, without prior precipitation of phospholipids, may be applied to these improved silica columns, and developed in the same manner, except that wet ether is used in place of benzene. Haemin a_2, with a value of 3·18 for $E_{603\,m\mu.}/E_{635\,m\mu.}$, has been obtained readily in this way. Fig. 2 shows a spectral curve for the haemin in ether which had been washed with 5% HCl.

Countercurrent distribution and paper chromatography of haemins a_2. The green haemin obtained from the improved column was still oily on removal of solvent. Therefore,

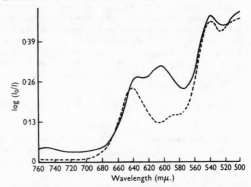

Fig. 1. Absorption spectrum of bacterial haemins, $E_{603\,m\mu.}/E_{635\,m\mu.} = 1·13$, (—) and protohaemin (- - -). Solutions in ether washed with 5% (w/v) HCl.

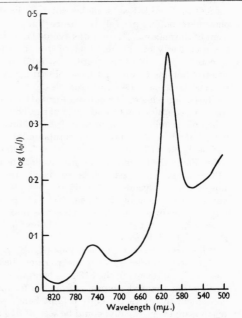

Fig. 2. Absorption spectrum of haemin a_2, $E_{603\,m\mu.}/E_{635\,m\mu.} = 3·18$. Solvent, ether washed with 5% HCl.

attempts were made to remove further lipid by liquid–liquid extraction. The best solvent system was methanol–1% HCl–light petroleum (b.p. 68°) (70:30:100). A six-stage distribution was carried out according to the method of Bush & Densen (1948), six methanol and six light-petroleum fractions being obtained. A small amount of yellow fat moved rapidly with the light petroleum phase, the haemin staying in the first two tubes of the methanol phase. When benzene was used instead of light petroleum some of the haemin migrated with the fat. Haemin a_2, though still oily in appearance, could now be precipitated from acetone by means of light petroleum or benzene.

Attempts were made to obtain separation of haemin a_2 from an accompanying trace of protohaemin by means of paper chromatography. Of many solvent systems tried only benzene–butanol (10:1), with the ascending method of chromatography, gave a marked difference of the R_F value for haemin a_2 (R_F 0·6) and protohaemin (0·1). Haemin a_2 gave a slightly elongated spot, but no separation from the protohaemin impurity was obtained. The failure to obtain separation is attributed to presence of residual lipid.

Spectroscopic properties of haematin a_2 compounds

Haemin a_2 ($E_{603\,m\mu.}/E_{635\,m\mu.} = 2·86$) for these experiments was prepared by silica-gel chromatography, followed by precipitation at $-70°$ of some of the protohaemin and lipid impurity from an acetone solution of the haemin.

The experiments were carried out in a Thunberg tube modified for spectrophotometry. Before the addition of $Na_2S_2O_4$ to obtain the reduced compounds, the tube was evacuated. Sufficient $Na_2S_2O_4$ was added as a molar solution in 0·2 M phosphate buffer, pH 7·6, to ensure full development of the maxima. Excess was avoided as this led to rapid decay of the maxima of the haematin a_2 compounds. Maxima were measured in the spectrophotometer and with the Hartridge reversion spectroscope, in separate samples.

The pyridine haemochrome was formed by adding $Na_2S_2O_4$, contained in the side-arm of the Thunberg tube, to haemin a_2 in a mixture of pyridine and 0·2 N-NaOH (1:2). The ferric compound gave a diffuse band with its maximum at 603–605 mμ.; reduction to the haemochrome gave a sharp peak at 613–615 mμ. This peak decayed fairly rapidly. Lower concentrations of NaOH (to 0·001 N), and various proportions of pyridine to NaOH were tried, but the conditions as stated gave the maximum development of the 613–615 mμ. band and the slowest rate of decay.

When crude haemin preparations ($E_{603\,m\mu.}/E_{635\,m\mu.} = 1·26$) were converted into the pyridine haemochrome, the intensity of the 613 mμ. band was much weaker than that to be expected from the haemin a_2 content of the extracts. Only a faint band, which disappeared very rapidly, could be seen at 613 mμ., though strong bands due to protohaemochrome (at 557 and 525 mμ.) were present and persisted.

Haemin a_2 in 0·001–0·2 N-NaOH or in 0·2 M phosphate buffer, pH 7·6, gave a wide absorption band with its maximum at 664 mμ. (alkaline haematin). Reduction gave a diffuse band at 618 mμ. (haem) as long as the solution remained alkaline.

The CO-haem compound was formed by adding $Na_2S_2O_4$ to the haemin in 0·2 M-NaOH or 0·2 M phosphate buffer, pH 7·6, the solution being saturated with coal gas beforehand. A strong band with its maxima at 618–620 mμ. appeared. Reduction to the haem before gassing did not give as stable a preparation.

The cyanide complex was formed by adding an excess of KCN to haemin a_2 in 0·2 N-NaOH. The 664 mμ. peak of the alkaline haematin disappeared and was replaced by a broad band of absorption with its centre at 603–605 mμ. On reduction with $Na_2S_2O_4$ a strong band with its maximum at 618 mμ. was obtained. This ferrous cyanide compound was the most stable of the ferrous haem a_2 compounds.

Table 1 gives the position of the principal maxima of haematin a_2 compounds.

Chlorin from haemin a_2

Removal of iron from the haemins. The ferrous acetate method of Warburg & Negelein (1932) was used with modifications. First, it was found possible to remove the iron without heating the haemin solution, thus avoiding destruction of the chlorin. Secondly, after much experience it was apparent that the amount of HCl added to the haemin–ferrous acetate mixture was critical, even a small excess causing some destruction of the chlorin.

The iron may be removed from the haemins at any stage after taking them into ether from the acid aqueous–acetone extracts. For preparative purposes precipitation of the phospholipid was first carried out.

The combined haemins were taken into acetic acid to give a solution with $E_{1\,cm.}^{508\,m\mu.} = 2·0$. Carbon dioxide was bubbled through this solution at 20°. To each 8 ml. was added 1 ml. of a ferrous acetate solution prepared by heating under CO_2 2 mg. of Ferrum reductum (British Drug Houses Ltd.) per ml. of acetic acid. The hot ferrous acetate solution did not raise the temperature of the haemin solution

Table 1. *Haematin a_2 compounds*

	Wavelength (mμ.) of the maximum of absorption
Acid haematin (haemin)	603
Alkaline haematin	662–664
Haem	618
CO-haem	618–620
Pyridine haemochrome	613
Cyanide haemochrome	618

above 30°. After 30 sec., 0·1 ml. of conc. HCl was added. The emergence of the main band (630 mμ.) of chlorin a_2 hydrochloride and that of protoporphyrin hydrochloride was followed with a hand spectroscope. After 2–5 min. the acetic acid solution was tipped into ether over dilute sodium acetate. Acetic acid was largely neutralized with $NaHCO_3$, followed by thorough washing with water.

Spectroscopic examination of this ether solution showed, in addition to the bands of protoporphyrin at 633, 576, 537 and 503 mμ., a band at 653 mμ. (the principal band of chlorin a_2).

The ratios $E_{653 m\mu.}/E_{633 m\mu.}$ and $E_{653 m\mu.}/E_{503 m\mu.}$ have been used to follow the separation of chlorin a_2 from protoporphyrin and related porphyrins. Values for these ratios obtained after removal of the iron from haemin preparations of different $E_{603 m\mu.}/E_{635 m\mu.}$ ratios are given in Table 2. This shows that as the haemin a_2 content of these preparations increased there was an increase in the proportion of chlorin a_2 to protoporphyrin.

Chromatography on silica gel. Silica-gel columns (see Methods) of similar dimensions to those used for the haemins readily gave good yields of chlorin a_2 of purity greater than obtainable by any other means, including the classical method of fractionation between ether and HCl. After precipitation of phospholipid with acetone (see haemins) the chlorin was taken into benzene, and the precipitated porphyrin removed by centrifuging. The greenish brown supernatant was applied to a silica column. The sequence of solvents and procedure was as described for the haemins. Benzene which had been equilibrated with water, and to which was then added 1 % of methanol, eluted 40 % of the chlorin a_2 applied to the column. The value of $E_{653 m\mu.}/E_{503 m\mu.}$ for this fraction varied from 2·94 to 2·57. The subsequent fractions obtained by increasing the methanol content of the benzene accounted for 50–55 % of the chlorin applied to the column. These fractions were recombined and run through a second column; a chlorin a_2 fraction with ratio $E_{635 m\mu.}/E_{503 m\mu.}$ of 2·82 was given. Rechromatographing the best fraction did not significantly raise the $E_{653 m\mu.}/E_{503 m\mu.}$ ratio, though a small amount of lipid could be removed.

Further purification of chlorin a_2. The best chlorin fractions from these columns were oily after removal of the solvent. Countercurrent distribution was therefore carried out as described for the haemins, except that ten stages were used. Some fat ran with the light-petroleum phase. Most of the chlorin was in the methanol fractions 1 and 2, and these two fractions were combined and taken into ether. The ratio $E_{653 m\mu.}/E_{503 m\mu.}$ was 3·0. The chlorin could now be completely extracted from ether with 10 % HCl. The chlorin was returned to ether by partial neutralization of the acid extracts with $NaHCO_3$, and this solution exhaustively extracted with 1, 3 and 5 % HCl. A small amount of porphyrin and a trace of chlorin were extracted by 1 % HCl, and the 3 and 5 % fractions contained equal amounts of chlorin a_2. The ratio $E_{653 m\mu.}/E_{503 m\mu.}$ for the 5 % fraction in ether was 3·3. In ether the chlorin showed bands at I 653, II 598, III 573, IV 534 and V 503 mμ. The decreasing order of intensity was I, V, II, IV, III.

Table 2. *Correlation of spectrophotometric ratios for bacterial haemins and for the chlorin–porphyrin mixture obtained on removal of iron from the haemins, with the molar ratio of protoporphyrin to chlorin a_2*

Haemins in ether–HCl $\dfrac{E_{603 m\mu.}}{E_{635 m\mu.}}$	Chlorin a_2–porphyrin mixture in ether $\dfrac{E_{653 m\mu.}}{E_{633 m\mu.}}$	$\dfrac{E_{653 m\mu.}}{E_{503 m\mu.}}$	Molar ratio of protoporphyrin to chlorin a_2*
0·85	0·81	0·34	10·4
1·00	—	—	7·1
1·05	1·23	0·49	6·4
1·09	—	—	5·9
1·14	1·33	0·53	5·3
1·26	—	—	3·6
1·28	1·82	0·81	3·3

* These values have been calculated from the extinctions at 653 and 576 mμ. (see text).

Table 3. *R_F values obtained on paper chromatography of the methyl ester of chlorin a_2 and related chlorins and porphyrins*

	Solvent system		
	Kerosene–propanol	Kerosene–chloroform	Trichloroethylene
Chlorin a_2*	0·55	0·32	0·77
Mesochlorin	0·88	0·89	0·96
Pyrrochlorin	0·96	0·97	0·96
Rhodochlorin	0·90	0·91	0·96
Dioxyprotoporphyrin†	0·34	0·00	0·00
Dioxymonovinylmonohydroxyethyl-deuteroporphyrin‡	0·26	0·00	0·00
Protoporphyrin	0·75	0·80	0·96
Mesoporphyrin	0·82	0·82	0·96
Haematoporphyrin	0·30	0·05	0·05
Monovinylmonohydroxyethyl-deuteroporphyrin	0·40	0·28	0·00
'626 mμ.' porphyrin impurity	0·40	0·28	0·00
Pyrroporphyrin	0·92	0·92	0·96
Rhodoporphyrin	0·77	0·82	0·96

* $E_{653 m\mu.}/E_{553 \mu m.} = 3·3$. † Prepared according to Fischer & Bock (1938).
‡ Prepared similarly from monovinylmonohydroxyethyldeuteroporphyrin.

Chromatography of the methyl esters of chlorin a_2 and porphyrin impurities. The methyl ester was prepared by esterification of chlorin a_2 with diazomethane. The spectra of chlorin a_2 and of its ester were identical.

Paper chromatography. Table 3 gives the R_F values obtained in three solvent systems for the methyl esters of chlorin a_2 and certain related substances and porphyrin impurities. Under u.v. light chlorin a_2 spots in all three systems displayed a brick-red fluorescence, whereas spots due to the porphyrin impurities were bright red.

Various preparations containing chlorin a_2 were chromatographed on a preparative scale. The best fraction from any system did not give a greater value than 2·5 for $E_{653\,m\mu.}/E_{503\,m\mu.}$. This low ratio was found to be due to admixture of a porphyrin of R_F 0·4 in the kerosene–propanol system. The absorption maxima of this porphyrin in ether were at 626, 576, 533 and 502 mμ.

Alumina chromatography. A mixture of chlorin a_2 and porphyrin, after precipitation of phospholipid and in some experiments further removal of lipid by chromatography on silica-gel columns, was esterified with diazomethane and an ether solution of the methyl esters applied to a column of alumina (British Drug Houses Ltd.) set up in ether. On eluting with ether, protoporphyrin moved rapidly down the column, followed slowly by a small amount of a porphyrin with absorption maxima at 626, 576, 534 and 502 mμ. On paper chromatography this porphyrin gave an R_F of 0·4 in the kerosene–propanol system and an R_F of 0·28 in the kerosene–chloroform system.

Chloroform and methanol eluted a small amount of haematoporphyrin (identified by its spectra and by paper chromatography) and a chlorin with a principal maximum of absorption at 648 mμ. The dark-green layer at the head of the column was then separated from the rest of the column and chlorin a_2 eluted from this with 70 % aqueous acetone containing 1 % (w/v) of HCl. In ether the value for $E_{653\,m\mu.}/E_{503\,m\mu.}$ for this fraction ranged from 2·0 to 2·5 in different experiments. The recovery of chlorin a_2 was of the order of 50 %.

Other aluminas (Merck, Savory and Moore) and absorbents, e.g. magnesium oxide, magnesium carbonate, calcium oxide and calcium carbonate, were tried without success.

The '626 mμ.' porphyrin was also obtained from material precipitated with benzene and from certain fractions obtained on silica-gel chromatography of the benzene-soluble material. The amount from any preparation was always very small. It was not possible to crystallize this porphyrin, though protoporphyrin eluted from these columns crystallized readily.

Absorption spectra of chlorin a_2

A curve of the absorption in the visible region of the spectrum of an ether solution of chlorin a_2 is shown in Fig. 3. Chlorin a_2 preparations with a value of 3·3 for $E_{653\,m\mu.}/E_{503\,m\mu.}$ show practically no absorption in the 580–570 mμ. region. Very fatty fractions showed a shift of the two principal maxima of 1–2 mμ. towards longer wavelengths.

A number of the purest preparations of chlorin a_2 in ether solution were examined in the 420–200 mμ. region. These showed a Soret band with its maximum at 405 mμ., and two other main regions of absorp-

tion at 280–270 mμ. and 240–220 mμ. The purest fraction gave the ratios

$$E_{653\,m\mu.} : E_{503\,m\mu.} : E_{405\,m\mu.} : E_{280} : E_{230\,m\mu.}$$
$$= 3\cdot3 : 1 : 12 : 3\cdot0 : 5\cdot0.$$

Some of the absorption in the u.v. region appears to be due to lipid impurity. A number of lipid fractions which had been separated by chromatography and countercurrent distribution from chlorin a_2 showed broad bands in the 280–200 mμ. region.

Chlorin a_2 in dilute HCl showed a strong band at 630 mμ. Higher concentrations exhibited a shading of the band towards the red region of the spectrum. In 20 % HCl the maximum was at 647 mμ. Chlorin a_2 in 10 % HCl gave a value of 0·71 for $E_{647\,m\mu.}/E_{630\,m\mu.}$ initially, but this ratio had risen to 1·1 after 24 hr. Fig. 4 shows spectral curves for chlorin a_2 in 8 % and 16·5 % HCl. The concentration of the chlorin is the same in both, and measurements were made immediately after preparation of the solutions. Dilution of the 16·5 % HCl

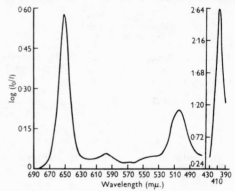

Fig. 3. Absorption spectrum of chlorin a_2, $E_{653\,m\mu.}/E_{503\,m\mu.} = 2\cdot63$. Solvent, ether.

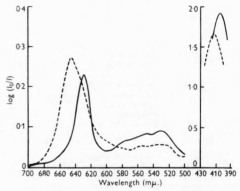

Fig. 4. Absorption spectra of equal concentrations of chlorin a_2 in 8 % HCl (—) and in 16·5 % HCl (- - -).

solution with water to give an 8 % HCl concentration gave a spectral curve identical with that of chlorin a_2 in 8 % HCl.

Metal complexes of chlorin a_2

Haemin. Iron was introduced into chlorin a_2 by the ferrous acetate method (Fischer & Orth, 1940). Quantitative conversion of chlorin a_2 into haemin a_2 could not be obtained. Prolonged heating of the chlorin with ferrous acetate and NaCl in acetic acid caused destruction of the chlorin and of the haemin formed. With short periods of heating or at low temperatures the iron was not introduced into the chlorin.

The haemin was converted into the acid haematin and into the pyridine haemochrome. The positions of the maxima of these compounds were the same as for those formed from the original haemin a_2.

Copper and zinc complex. The Cu–chlorin and Zn–chlorin complexes were formed by the methods of Fischer (Fischer & Orth, 1940). The positions of the maxima of absorption for the Cu complex were I 613, II 562, III 526 and IV 401 mμ.; those of the Zn complex I 615, II 564, III 529 and IV 408 mμ. The decreasing order of intensity was IV, I, II, III in both cases.

Evidence for the nature of the side chains of haemin a_2 and chlorin a_2

Effect of hydroxylamine on haemin a_2 and chlorin a_2. To a solution of the haemin in pyridine, excess of a mixture of equivalent amounts of hydroxylamine hydrochloride and Na_2SO_3 was added, and the mixture was stood for 2 hr. at 22° or gently refluxed for 5 min. After cooling, an equal volume of 0·1 N-NaOH was added to the pyridine solution, followed by a small amount of $Na_2S_2O_4$. No shift of the principal maxima of absorption of the pyridine haemochrome was observed. Chlorin a_2 was similarly heated with hydroxylamine in pyridine, followed by cooling and filtering. No shift of the absorption maxima of chlorin a_2 was found.

The presence of formyl or carbonyl groups in haem a_2 is thus excluded.

Table 4. *Effect of diazoacetic ester (DAE) on the position of the maxima of absorption in the red region of the spectrum*

Compound	Before DAE treatment	After DAE treatment
	Wavelength (mμ.) of the maximum of absorption	
Chlorin a_2	652	646
Phaeophorbide a	667	660
Dioxyprotoporphyrin	668	662
Protoporphyrin	633	626
Monovinylmonohydroxy-ethyldeuteroporphyrin	626	624
'626 mμ.' porphyrin from chlorin a_2	626	626
'626 mμ.' porphyrin from protoporphyrin	626	626

Effect of diazoacetic ester on the absorption spectrum of chlorin a_2. An excess of diazoacetic ester was added to chlorin a_2 in a small tube. The tube was flushed with nitrogen, stoppered and left in the dark for 48 hr. Heating at 70° for 18 hr. as carried out by Fischer (see Fischer & Orth, 1940) gave similar results, but this caused considerable destruction of the chlorin. Ether was added to the tube and the chlorin extracted with 20 % HCl, taken back into ether and the positions of the maxima were determined. Protoporphyrin (two vinyl groups), phaeophorbide a (one vinyl group) and dioxyprotoporphyrin (two vinyl groups) were similarly treated. All these compounds showed the same degree of shift of the principal maxima of absorption after reacting with diazoacetic ester (Table 4). The presence of at least one vinyl group in chlorin a_2 is thus demonstrated.

Paper chromatography of the free chlorin. Chlorin a_2 was chromatographed according to the method of Nicholas & Rimington (1949), in lutidine–water, in an attempt to determine the number of free carboxylic acid side chains. Chlorin a_2 ($E_{653\,m\mu.}/E_{503\,m\mu.} = 3\cdot1$) ran with R_F 0·87 (pyrrochlorin and pyrroporphyrin, R_F 0·95; protoporphyrin and rhodochlorin, R_F 0·8; coproporphyrin, R_F 0·50). The R_F value obtained for chlorin a_2 indicates that it probably has two carboxylic acid side chains (see Discussion).

Effect of acid and alkali on chlorin a_2. Because of the possibility of an esterified carboxylic acid side chain, chlorin a_2 was left to stand in 20 % HCl or in NaOH overnight. No change in the R_F values was found. Esterification of a carboxylic acid side chain can thus be ruled out. Some destruction of the chlorin occurred in the alkali. Similar results were obtained with 1 % methanolic potassium hydroxide. Heating of the chlorin in all these solvents resulted in its total disappearance.

Conversion of chlorin a_2 into porphyrins

As the spectrum of chlorin a_2 did not correspond to that of any known chlorin, further information was sought as to the nature of its side chains by attempting conversion into the porphyrin. Two methods were investigated, both of which had been used extensively by Fischer (see Fischer & Orth, 1940) during his studies on the structure of chlorophyll.

Catalytic hydrogenation and reoxidation. Chlorin a_2, in approx. 100 μg. amounts estimated spectrophotometrically (see below), was hydrogenated at 22° and atmospheric pressure, with palladium black as catalyst. The catalyst was removed from the solvent by centrifuging and the supernatant shaken in air for several hours. In some experiments the solution was left to stand, as a shallow layer, in the dark for several days. The products of the reaction were taken into ether and the spectra determined. Protoporphyrin, phaeophorbide a and dioxyprotoporphyrin were similarly treated.

When the reaction was carried out in acetone, chlorin a_2 gave a small yield of a porphyrin and a still smaller yield of a chlorin. The porphyrin was extracted with 3 % HCl and returned to ether. The spectrum of this porphyrin was of the aetiotype (the four maxima of absorption increasing in strength from the first in the red to the fourth in the blue) and the maxima were at 623, 568, 526 and 496 mμ. On paper chromatography in the kerosene–propanol system the methyl ester of the porphyrin ran with R_F 0·8 with slight streaking (mesoporphyrin, R_F 0·77; pyrroporphyrin, R_F 0·88; protoporphyrin, R_F 0·7). The chlorin had a principal maximum of absorption at 646 mµ. and ran with R_F 0·43 (chlorin a_2, R_F 0·60) in the same system. Similar products were obtained when ethanol was used as a solvent, the amount of 646 mµ. chlorin being greater. No porphyrin and only a trace of the 646 mµ. chlorin was obtained when acetic acid was used, no chlorin a_2 remaining.

Protoporphyrin was converted into mesoporphyrin and phaeophorbide a to phaeoporphyrin a_5 in all solvents.

In acetone or ethanol, hydrogenation converted dioxyprotoporphyrin into the leuco compound; oxidation of this yielded mesoporphyrin. When dioxyprotoporphyrin was hydrogenated in acetic acid the chlorin-like acid spectrum rapidly changed directly to that of mesoporphyrin hydrochloride. In all solvents protoporphyrin and dioxyprotoporphyrin yielded small amounts of a chlorin which in ether had a principal maximum of absorption at 646 mµ.

Conversion of chlorin a_2 into porphyrin with hydriodic acid.
Treatment of chlorin a_2 with HI according to the method of Fischer (see Fischer & Orth, 1940), which involved heating, caused total loss of the chlorin, no porphyrin being obtained. By carrying out the reaction at 18–20°, however, in the presence of a great excess of HI, porphyrins could be obtained from chlorin a_2 without excessive loss of material. To approx. 200 µg. of the chlorin in 0·5 ml. of acetic acid in an atmosphere of CO_2, 0·1 ml. of HI (sp.gr. 1·94) was added, the tube stoppered and placed in the dark for 72 hr. Initially a strong band could be seen at 630–650 mµ. but this slowly disappeared, being replaced by a band at 560 mµ. After 72 hr. there was no further increase in strength of this band. The porphyrin was taken into ether over dilute sodium acetate, and partially neutralized with $NaHCO_3$, the free iodine was removed by washing with 1 % (w/v) sodium thiosulphate and the ether washed thoroughly with water. By this method an ether solution with absorption maxima at 646, 626, 575, 534, 502 and 402 mµ. was obtained (from chlorin a_2 of $E_{653 \text{m}\mu.}/E_{503 \text{m}\mu.} = 2·95$). The maximum at 646 mµ. was caused by the presence of a chlorin of *meso*-type derived by reduction of the vinyl group of chlorin a_2. The other absorption bands indicated that a porphyrin of aetio-type spectrum had been formed.

A major portion of the ether solution was methylated with diazomethane. Paper chromatography, in kerosene-propanol, of the porphyrin esters gave a major spot of R_F 0·41, a secondary spot of R_F 0·26 and a faint spot of R_F 0·75 (haematoporphyrin ester, R_F 0·26; protoporphyrin ester,

R_F 0·75). This mixture of porphyrin esters was chromatographed on an alumina column. Elution with ether gave a rapid-moving (*a*) and a slow-moving (*b*) fraction. A third fraction (*c*) could be eluted with methanol. These all showed aetio-type spectra. The amount of porphyrin in each fraction was estimated by measuring the absorption at 501–503 mµ. Fraction (*b*) contained 60 %, fractions (*a*) and (*c*) 20 % each, of the porphyrin eluted from the column. On paper chromatography in the kerosene–propanol system the major fraction (*b*) gave a strong spot at R_F 0·40 and also a trace of haematoporphyrin ester (R_F 0·2) and a trace of protoporphyrin ester (R_F 0·7). Fraction (*a*) gave a spot with R_F 0·7 and a secondary spot of R_F 0·27, and fraction (*c*) gave a spot of R_F 0·27 with a secondary spot of R_F 0·41. Fraction (*b*) was chromatographed on alumina. The porphyrin ester eluted with ether from this column, when run on paper chromatograms in kerosene–propanol moved with R_F 0·41, in kerosene–chloroform with R_F 0·28. No spots due to protoporphyrin or haematoporphyrin were seen. Fig. 5 shows an absorption curve obtained for this porphyrin. This porphyrin was still oily and could not be crystallized.

The sample that had not been treated with diazomethane was extracted with 0·1, 0·3, 1·0, 2·0, 5 and 10 % HCl successively. The fractions were returned to ether and the absorption at the Soret maximum was read.

The porphyrins were then converted into the ester form and run on paper in the kerosene–propanol system. Table 5 summarizes the data obtained from this fractionation.

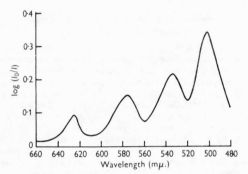

Fig. 5. Absorption spectrum of the principal porphyrin obtained on treating chlorin a_2 with hydriodic acid. Solvent, ether.

Table 5. *Hydrochloric acid fractionation of porphyrins obtained on treating chlorin a_2 with hydriodic acid*

HCl concn.	Wavelength of the Soret maximum (in ether)	Percentage of the total porphyrin based on the extinction of the Soret band	R_F values and relative intensities ($>$, $=$) of spots obtained on paper chromatography in kerosene–propanol of the methyl esters*
0·1	397	15	0·28 > 0·40
0·3	399	18	0·28 = 0·40
1·0	403	37	0·40 > 0·28
2·0	405	7	0·40 > 0·28
5 and 10†	—	—	
Residue	405	22	0·76 = 0·40 = 0·28

Total 97

* Protoporphyrin, 0·76; monovinylmonohydroxyethyldeuteroporphyrin, 0·40; haematoporphyrin, 0·28 (methyl esters).
† These fractions were too small for analysis.

Comparison of the action of HI *on chlorin* a_2 *and other compounds.* At 18–20° it was necessary to use a molar ratio of HI to chlorin a_2 of 140:1. Dioxyprotoporphyrin at this level of HI was converted into protoporphyrin in a few seconds, and phaeophorbide a required a few hours for complete conversion into phaeoporphyrin a_5. When the molar ratio was reduced to 4:1, 18 hr. was required for completion of the reaction for both dioxyprotoporphyrin and phaeophorbide a. Chlorin a_2 at this low molar ratio gave no detectable porphyrin even when left for several days, but some formation of the 646 mμ. chlorin occurred.

Because of the similarity of the principal porphyrin obtained from the action of HI on chlorin a_2 to protoporphyrin and haematoporphyrin, a study of the action of HI on protoporphyrin at low temperatures was made at a molar ratio of HI to porphyrin of 140:1. After 48 hr. at 18–20° a porphyrin with an aetiotype spectrum and maxima at 626, 574, 533, 502 mμ. (R_F 0·40 in kerosene–propanol, R_F 0·28 in kerosene–chloroform) was obtained together with unaltered protoporphyrin and some haematoporphyrin. This study will be reported in full elsewhere.

The spectra obtained for the '626 mμ.' porphyrin from chlorin a_2 and the behaviour on chromatography of the methyl ester suggested that this porphyrin was either monovinylmonohydroxyethyl- or monoethylmonohydroxyethyl-deuteroporphyrin. Dr Granick kindly supplied a sample of monovinylmonohydroxyethyldeuteroporphyrin, obtained from a mutant of *Chlorella*. The maxima of this porphyrin in ether were identical in position with those of the chlorin a_2–porphyrin and of the '626 mμ.' porphyrin derived from protoporphyrin. On paper chromatography of the ester in kerosene–propanol an R_F of 0·40 was obtained, in kerosene–chloroform R_F was 0·28.

Diazoacetic ester (DAE) experiments. The '626 mμ.' porphyrin from chlorin a_2, monovinylmonohydroxyethyl-deuteroporphyrin and the '626 mμ.' porphyrin from protoporphyrin were treated with diazoacetic ester for 24 hr. at 70° under nitrogen. In ether the product from monovinylmonohydroxyethyldeuteroporphyrin showed a small shift of the absorption band in the red end of the spectrum towards shorter wavelengths (Table 4). The other two porphyrins showed no detectable shift.

The diazoacetic ester complexes of chlorin a_2 and dioxyprotoporphyrin and phaeophorbide a were treated with hydriodic acid at molar ratio 140:1. Chlorin a_2 gave a porphyrin with maxima at 626, 574, 533, 501 mμ.; phaeophorbide a yielded a porphyrin with a spectrum corresponding to the DAE compound of phaeoporphyrin a_5, and dioxyprotoporphyrin gave the DAE compound of protoporphyrin.

Attempted oxidation of the copper complex. Fischer & Herrle (1937) were able to convert a number of chlorins into the corresponding vinyl porphyrin by oxidation of the copper complex. The copper complex of chlorin a_2 was shaken in acetic acid for several hours at 40°. In some experiments oxygen was bubbled through the solution. No formation of porphyrin had occurred after several hours. The copper complexes of dioxyprotoporphyrin and phaeophorbide a, similarly treated, also remained unchanged.

Concentration of haemin a_2 and protohaemin in the bacteria

Since it has not been possible to obtain crystalline material, the specific extinction of chlorin a_2 cannot be determined. However, an approximation may be made by utilizing the data published by Stern and his co-workers (Stern & Wenderlein, 1935, 1936; Stern & Deželić, 1937; Stern & Molvig, 1937; Stern & Pruckner, 1937), who determined the molar extinction coefficients (ϵ) of 29 chlorins and related pigments. For the principal maximum of absorption of these, ϵ ranges from 45 000 to 63 000. Of these compounds pyrrochlorin appears to be the most closely related to chlorin a_2 (see Discussion). Pyrrochlorin has a value of 45 000 for $\epsilon_{652\,m\mu}$, and this has been assumed for the principal maximum of absorption of chlorin a_2. Further, it has been assumed (see Discussion) that crystalline chlorin a_2 would be protochlorin, and the value of 566 has therefore been used for the molecular weight throughout the following calculations.

In the region of maximum II (580–570 mμ.) of the spectrum of protoporphyrin and related porphyrins in neutral solvents, chlorin a_2 preparations of $E_{653\,m\mu}/E_{503\,m\mu} = 3·3$ exhibit very little absorption ($E_{653\,m\mu}/E_{576\,m\mu} = 50$). In the initial crude preparations all absorption at 576 mμ. is taken as being due to protoporphyrin, $\epsilon_{576\,m\mu} = 6450$. The absorption of protoporphyrin at 653 mμ. is 0·04 times that at 576 mμ.; thus $E_{653\,m\mu} - 0·04E_{576\,m\mu}$ will give the absorption at 653 mμ. due to chlorin a_2. If E is measured in a 1 cm. layer, the concentration of chlorin a_2 will be 12·6 ($E_{653\,m\mu} - 0·04E_{576\,m\mu}$) μg./ml., and that of protoporphyrin (87·4$E_{576\,m\mu}$) μg./ml. Quantitative determination of the bacterial haemins was carried out by taking the haemins extracted from the bacteria into acetic acid, without prior separation from lipids, and removing the iron from the haemins as previously described. Measurements were made in ether at 653, 633, 576 and 503 mμ.

On the basis of the molecular weight assumed for chlorin a_2, *Aero. aerogenes* contained 1·4–4·3 mg. of haemin a_2 and 16–24 mg. of protohaemin/100 g. dry weight of cells. The amounts of the haemins obtained depended on the degree of aeration and length of incubation of the culture. Table 2 shows the relation between the ratio $E_{603\,m\mu}/E_{635\,m\mu}$ and the molar ratio of protoporphyrin to chlorin a_2 obtained on removal of iron from the haemins, as well as other spectrophotometric ratios (see above) which depend on this ratio. It thus appears possible to estimate roughly the haem a_2/protohaem ratio from the $E_{603\,m\mu}/E_{635\,m\mu}$ ratio of the acid haematins.

Haemin a_2 and chlorin a_2 from other organisms

Az. vinelandii cells harvested at 48 hr. showed a band due to cytochrome a_2 as well as the α-bands of cytochromes a_1, b_1 and c. The cells were extracted as described for *Aero. aerogenes*. The haematins in ether washed with 5 % HCl gave a value of 0·96 for $E_{603\,m\mu}/E_{635\,m\mu}$. This is equivalent to a protohaem/haem a_2 ratio of approx. 8. Haemin a_2 was separated from the mixture of haemins by chromatography on silica gel. From this chlorin a_2 was obtained, identified by its spectrum in neutral and acid solvents and by paper chromatography of the methyl ester.

Esch. coli and *P. vulgaris* cells harvested at 18 hr. showed a band due to cytochrome a_2. On fractionation of the haemins, haemin a_2, and from this chlorin a_2, were obtained. In *Bact. subtilis, Bact. mycoides* and *Ps. pyocyaneus*, the cytochrome a_2 band was very weak, but small amounts of haemin a_2 could be obtained on fractionation of the haemins. No cytochrome a_2 could be seen in *Torulopsis utilis* cells. No band could be detected at 603 mμ. on examination of the acid haematins, nor was any chlorin a_2 found on removal of iron from the haemins.

Anaerobic cultures. Aero. aerogenes, Esch. coli and *P. vulgaris* when grown anaerobically showed no cytochromes. A trace of protohaemin but no haemin a_2 was extracted from these bacteria (30 g. dry weight of cells). A trace of coproporphyrin was found on extracting the culture with ether at pH 3·2.

Free chlorin and porphyrin present in bacterial cells. Small amounts of *a* chlorin, maxima of absorption at 668 and 500 mμ., and protoporphyrin were found in the 5 % HCl washings of the ether solution of crude haemins. If the haemins were not extracted with HCl, the chlorin was found to run with the yellow-lipid fraction on silica-gel chromatography of the haemins. Extraction of the cells with neutral acetone yielded small amounts of the chlorin and porphyrin, and none could be found in the HCl washings of the haemins subsequently extracted from the cells with acid–acetone.

The amount of this free chlorin and porphyrin was always small, but was greater in cells from cultures that had been incubated for several days or from cultures where aeration had been too vigorous, resulting in poor yields of cytochrome a_2.

Haemin a in Aero. aerogenes. The presence of haem *a* in this organism was demonstrated by partitioning crude haemin preparations between ether and pyridine–HCl buffer (see Rawlinson & Hale, 1949). Haemin *a* remained in the ether phase and haemin a_2 went into the aqueous phase together with protohaemin. Haemin *a* was identified by its conversion into the pyridine haemochrome and into the porphyrin.

DISCUSSION

A green haemin which has been shown to be the iron complex of a hitherto undescribed chlorin has been isolated from various bacteria, all of which contained cytochrome a_2. The yield of this haemin was related to the intensity of the 630 mμ. band of the reduced cytochrome, and the haemin was never present in extracts from cells which did not show the band of cytochrome a_2. Further, apart from protohaemin from cytochrome b_1, and a small amount of haem *a* from cells which showed a strong cytochrome a_1 band, no other haemins were found. The green haemin could only be extracted from the bacterial cells by solvents containing acid, and this is evidence for the assumption that the haemin is linked to a protein *in situ*. It is concluded that this haemin is the prosthetic group of cytochrome a_2 and it is designated haemin a_2.

The position of the principal maximum of absorption of the pyridine haemochrome lies 17 mμ. towards the blue end of the spectrum as compared with the absorption band of reduced cytochrome a_2 (630 mμ.), that of the ferrous cyanide compound of haemin a_2 18 mμ. as compared with the position of the absorption band of the reduced cyanide compound of cytochrome a_2 (636 mμ.). The shift found for the pyridine haemochrome is similar in magnitude to that found for pyridine haemochrome *a* (587 mμ.) relative to the α band of reduced cytochrome *a* (604 mμ.), but is greater than that for pyridine protohaemochrome (557 and 527 mμ.) relative to the bands of cytochrome *b* (566 and 528 mμ.), and pyridine mesohaemochrome (547 and 528 mμ.) relative to reduced cytochrome *c* (550 and 521 mμ.). It is well established (see Lemberg & Legge, 1949) that the position of the absorption bands of the compound formed by a haem with a protein varies considerably according to the particular protein used. The small shift found for the latter two cases does not therefore invalidate the assumption that the degree of shift observed for pyridine haemochrome a_2, and for the cyanide compound of haemin a_2, can be ascribed to the replacement of the apoprotein of cytochrome a_2 by a different nitrogenous base rather than to a degradation of the prosthetic group.

Though it has been possible to obtain considerable purification of haemin a_2, protohaemin and lipid impurities are still present in the best preparations. Of several methods of purification, chromatography on a silica gel, which has been treated with aqueous methanol to modify its adsorptive properties, has provided the purest haemin.

By chromatography of the free chlorin on silica-gel columns followed by countercurrent distribution between organic solvents and hydrochloric acid fractionation it has been possible to obtain chlorin a_2 with only a trace of remaining porphyrin impurity. Despite these methods and even after precipitation from benzene the chlorin is still oily in nature. Like the haemin, chlorin a_2 is lipophilic and tends to fractionate according to the partition properties of certain accompanying free lipids. By spectrophotometric analysis and further fractionation of the eluted material it has been shown that chlorin a_2 in the presence of lipids can associate with porphyrins to form a complex which behaves as a single entity on paper chromatography of the methyl esters. Thus it cannot be assumed that a spot of given R_F value represents pure chlorin a_2 where lipids are present.

Since reintroduction of iron into the chlorin obtained from haemin a_2 restores the spectrum of the haemin and of its compounds, it may be taken that no alteration to the nucleus or to the side chains has occurred during removal of the iron.

Of the spectra of the chlorins and related pigments given by Fischer & Orth (1940) only those of meso-chlorin (2:4-diethyl-1:3:5:8-tetramethylchlorin-6:7-dipropionic acid) and pyrrochlorin (4-ethyl-1:3:5:8-tetramethyl-2-vinylchlorin-7-propionic acid), Fig. 6, approach that of chlorin a_2 in respect of the position of the absorption bands (Table 6). The porphyrin obtained by catalytic hydrogenation and reoxidation of chlorin a_2 closely resembles mesoporphyrin; neither the slight difference from mesoporphyrin in the position of the maxima, nor in the R_F value of the ester, would appear to prove a difference.

Pyrrochlorin ester runs with a much higher R_F value than chlorin a_2 on paper chromatography, and pyrroporphyrin ester gave a significantly higher R_F value than did the methyl ester of the porphyrin obtained from chlorin a_2 by catalytic hydrogenation. Thus it is certain that chlorin a_2 is not pyrrochlorin.

The porphyrins obtained by catalytic hydrogenation and by hydriodic acid treatment of chlorin a_2 are evidence also that this chlorin is not a rhodo-chlorin (CO_2H at position 6 of the tetrapyrrole ring). Further, rhodochlorin ester runs with a much higher R_F value than does chlorin a_2 on paper chromatography.

The absorption band of the haemin of meso-chlorin is at 600 mμ. (haemin a_2, 603 mμ.), and that of the copper complex of mesochlorin at 613 mμ. (copper complex of chlorin a_2, 613 mμ.). This is further evidence that chlorin a_2 is closely related to mesochlorin.

The question arises whether chlorin a_2 is a true chlorin, with two extra hydrogens on one of the pyrrole rings, or a 'dihydroxychlorin', with two hydroxyl groups in this position. The 'dihydroxy-chlorins' prepared by Fischer (see Fischer & Orth, 1940) have a principal maximum of absorption which is removed by approximately 10 mμ. further into the red end of the spectrum, as compared with

that of the corresponding true chlorins. It is unlikely that chlorin a_2 is a compound of this type since the position of the principal maximum of absorption of chlorin a_2 is only 9 mμ. further towards the red than that of mesochlorin, and this shift can be accounted for by the presence in chlorin a_2 of a vinyl group (see below). Further, the behaviour of the methyl ester of chlorin a_2 on paper

Fig. 6. Possible structural formulae for chlorin a_2 and those for certain related chlorins and porphyrins.

	Substituents at positions		
	2	4	6
Chlorin series*			
Mesochlorin	E	E	P
Pyrrochlorin	V	E	H
Rhodochlorin	V	E	CB
Chlorin a_2	V / HE / V / E / V	HE / V / E / V / V	P†
Porphyrin series			
Protoporphyrin	V	V	
Mesoporphyrin	E	E	
Haematoporphyrin	HE	HE	
Monovinylmonohydroxy-ethyldeuteroporphyrin	V or HE	HE or V	P
'626 mμ.' porphyrin derived from chlorin a_2	E or HE	HE or E	

Abbreviations: M, methyl; E, ethyl; V, vinyl; HE, hydroxyethyl; H, hydrogen; CB, carboxylic acid; P, propionic acid.
* These contain two extra hydrogens, conventionally placed at positions 7 and 8 of the tetrapyrrole ring.
† Or relatively non-polar carboxylic acid.

Table 6. *Position of the maxima of absorption of certain chlorins*

Wavelength (mμ.) of the maxima of absorption

Compound	I	II	III	IV	Solvent
Chlorin a_2	653	598	534	503	Dioxan
Pyrrochlorin*	652	597	523	491	Dioxan
Mesochlorin*	644	591	522	490	Pyridine–ether
Mesopyrrochlorin*	642	589	518	487	Dioxan

* From Fischer & Orth (1940).

chromatography, and the difficulty with which this chlorin reacts with hydriodic acid, argue against the presence of hydroxyl groups at the β-positions of the pyrrole rings.

Substituents at the methine bridges of the tetrapyrrole ring may be ruled out from a consideration of the porphyrins obtained by catalytic hydrogenation and by hydriodic acid treatment of chlorin a_2. Neither of the methods used would remove a side chain, except a hydroxyl group, from this position. The presence of a hydroxyl group is unlikely, as both dioxyprotoporphyrin (see Fischer & Bock, 1938) and dioxymonovinylmonohydroxyethyldeuteroporphyrin have their principal maxima of absorption well within the red region of the spectrum at 669 and 661 mμ. respectively.

It has been shown that chlorin a_2 does not possess a carbonyl or formyl group, but that at least one vinyl group is present. The residual lipid impurities, which from their ultraviolet spectrum appear to be highly unsaturated, have prevented a determination of the number of vinyl groups by quantitative hydrogenation. Fischer (see Fischer & Orth, 1940) prepared the diazoacetic ester complex of a number of chlorophyll derivatives containing a vinyl group. The shift to the blue of the principal maximum of absorption of the diazoacetic ester compound ranges from 3 to 8 mμ. These values are for chlorins with single vinyl groups, no divinylchlorins having yet been synthesized.

A comparison of the position of the principal maximum of absorption of various vinylchlorins and chlorin-like compounds with that of their meso form, i.e. ethyl instead of vinyl group, shows a shift of 10–13 mμ. to the blue on saturation of the vinyl group. On catalytic hydrogenation of highly purified chlorin a_2 a new chlorin with its principal maximum of absorption at 645–646 mμ. has been obtained as one of the products. The shift to the blue is only 8 mμ. Since this chlorin could have arisen only from chlorin a_2 it can be assumed that it is a meso form of chlorin a_2. The combined evidence of the spectral shift obtained on formation of the diazoacetic ester compound and on hydrogenating chlorin a_2 favours the assumption that only one vinyl group is present in chlorin a_2.

The spectrum and chromatographic behaviour of the principal porphyrin obtained on treatment of chlorin a_2 with hydriodic acid is very similar to, if not identical with, that of monovinylmonohydroxyethyldeuteroporphyrin isolated by Dr Granick from a mutant of *Chlorella*. The failure to demonstrate the presence of a vinyl group in the former porphyrin suggests, however, that it is ethylhydroxyethyldeuteroporphyrin. A similar porphyrin was obtained by the action of hydriodic acid on protoporphyrin under the same conditions. It is evident that formation of a hydroxyethylporphyrin precedes the formation of haematoporphyrin under the specific conditions of these experiments, and this suggests that the hydroxyethyl group is not present in chlorin a_2 itself.

To summarize, it can be concluded that chlorin a_2 is a true chlorin corresponding to protoporphyrin or a porphyrin with only one vinyl group such as monovinylmonoethyldeuteroporphyrin or, less likely, monovinylmonohydroxyethyldeuteroporphyrin. Either isomerism or even replacement of some alkyl groups by others is not excluded.

The R_F value obtained for free chlorin a_2 on paper chromatography in the lutidine–water system is midway between that for a monocarboxylic and that for a dicarboxylic chlorin. It is not known whether in this system lipid impurities could modify R_F values to such an extent. Treatment of chlorin a_2 with acid and alkali did not alter the R_F values obtained on paper chromatography or result in the further separation of lipid. This is evidence against the presence of an esterified side chain. It is possible that one of the side chains of chlorin a_2 is a relatively non-polar carboxylic acid.

The ability of the methyl ester of chlorin a_2 to run on paper chromatograms in kerosene–propanol, kerosene–chloroform and trichloroethylene solvent systems contrasts with its strong adsorption on alumina or magnesium oxide columns, from which the chlorin can be removed only by acid–acetone. The methyl ester of dioxyprotoporphyrin (with two hydroxyl groups on the methine bridges), monovinylmonohydroxyethyldeuteroporphyrin (with one hydroxyethyl side chain) and haematoporphyrin (with two hydroxyethyl side chains), all of which have lower R_F values than chlorin a_2 methyl ester on paper chromatography in these systems, may be readily eluted from alumina with ether or chloroform. The presence of hydroxyl groups in the chlorin would not, therefore, alone account for its behaviour on alumina columns. Mesochlorin was found to run on these columns, so that the reduction of one of the rings of the tetrapyrrole nucleus would not seem sufficient to explain the strong adsorption. It is possible that the adsorption is due to a lipid side chain or to a free lipid with which chlorin a_2 has formed a complex. Indeed the fraction eluted with acid–acetone is fatty, and some lipid can be separated from the chlorin on subsequent partition between ether and hydrochloric acid.

When partition of the haemins between ester and pyridine–hydrochloric acid buffer was carried out, haemin a_2 accompanied protohaemin into the aqueous phase, which contrasts with the behaviour of haemin a. Further, when, in the present work, the method of Kiese & Kurz (1954), by which haemin a may be separated from protohaemin, was applied to the haemins from *Aero. aerogenes*, no separation of haemin a_2 from protohaemin was effected. These partition properties of haemin a_2 suggest that it is unlikely that this haem possesses a long-chain alkyl group such as has been demonstrated to be present in haem a (Warburg & Gewitz, 1953), but the presence of a side chain which may give rise to the formation of complexes between haem a_2, or chlorin a_2, and certain lipids, is not excluded.

The principal porphyrin obtained after hydriodic acid treatment of chlorin a_2 closely resembles a porphyrin which has been found in very small amounts in some preparations of chlorin a_2. The possible identity of those two porphyrins raises the question whether the latter porphyrin is an artifact produced by hydroxylation of one of the vinyl groups of protoporphyrin or whether it arises through removal from chlorin a_2 of the two extra hydrogens. An attractive hypothesis is that the presence of unsaturated lipids is responsible for the dehydrogenation, a fatty acid peroxide being the active agent.

For the purpose of determining approximately the amount of haem a_2 in bacterial cells it has been assumed that the molar extinction of chlorin a_2 would be similar to that of other true chlorins. The molar ratio of chlorin a_2 to protoporphyrin obtained on removal of iron from crude haemin preparations was found to vary with the intensity of the 630 mμ. band of reduced cytochrome a_2 relative to that of the α band of reduced cytochrome b_1 of the bacterial cells. On the basis of the ratios obtained, cells with the strongest cytochrome a_2 band have a ratio of cytochrome a_2 to cytochrome b_1 of 1:4, and those with a weak cytochrome a_2 band a ratio of 1:10. The best synthesis of cytochrome a_2 has been found to occur under conditions of moderate aeration. This has also been found by Moss (in preparation), who has been able to measure accurately the oxygen tension of the medium during growth of the bacteria.

Because of the structural similarity of meso-chlorin to chlorin a_2 it should be possible to use the extinction coefficients of the haemin of meso-chlorin for estimations of haemin a_2 with the haemin spectra directly. This would avoid the difficulties associated with removal of iron from the haemins.

SUMMARY

1. A green haemin has been obtained from *Aerobacter aerogenes* and several other bacteria, all of which contained cytochrome a_2. The yield of this haemin was related to the intensity of the 630 mμ. band of cytochrome a_2.

2. This haemin was partially purified, but its lipophilic nature and the similarity of its side chains to those of protohaemin made complete separation from lipids or protohaemin difficult.

3. The spectroscopic properties of this haemin and of its ferrous, carbon monoxide, cyanide and pyridine compounds have been examined. These are consistent with the view that this haemin is the unaltered prosthetic group of cytochrome a_2.

4. Removal of iron from haemin a_2 yielded a new chlorin. This was highly purified, but still remained oily in nature.

5. The chlorin in ether has a principal maximum of absorption at 653 mμ., and three lesser maxima at 598, 573 and 503 mμ. The Soret band is at 405 mμ. In 8 % hydrochloric acid the chlorin has its principal maximum at 630 mμ., but this is shifted to 647 mμ. in 16 % hydrochloric acid.

6. Paper chromatography of chlorin a_2 methyl ester was carried out in various solvent systems and its behaviour compared with other chlorin-like pigments and with certain porphyrins.

7. Chlorin a_2 was shown to possess at least one vinyl side chain. The presence of a formyl or carbonyl group could not be demonstrated.

8. The chlorin has been converted into a porphyrin by (*a*) catalytic hydrogenation and reoxidation, (*b*) the action of hydriodic acid. The principal porphyrin obtained by the action of hydriodic acid was similar to, but not identical with, monovinyl-monohydroxyethyldeuteroporphyrin. The porphyrin obtained by catalytic hydrogenation was similar to, if not identical with, mesoporphyrin.

9. The experimental evidence is discussed, and it is concluded that chlorin a_2 is a chlorin corresponding to protoporphyrin or to a closely related vinyl-porphyrin possessing a hydroxyethyl or ethyl side chain.

10. A molar extinction for chlorin a_2 based on its similarity to certain other chlorins was assumed. From this value the molar ratio of haemin a_2 to protohaemin has been calculated for the haemins extracted from bacteria of different cytochrome a_2 and b_1 content.

I wish to thank Dr R. Lemberg, F.R.S., for suggesting this problem to me, and for his continued encouragement and advice. I should like to thank my colleagues Dr D. B. Morell, Mrs Judith M. Rigby and Mr W. H. Lockwood for helpful discussions during the course of this work.

REFERENCES

Barrett, J. & Lemberg, R. (1954). *Nature, Lond.*, **173**, 213.
Burk, D. & Lineweaver, H. (1930). *J. Bact.* **19**, 389.
Bush, M. T. & Densen, P. M. (1948). *Analyt. Chem.* **20**, 121.
Chance, B. (1953). *J. biol. Chem.* **202**, 383.
Chu, T. C., Green, A. G. & Chu, E. J. (1951). *J. biol. Chem.* **190**, 643.
Fischer, H. & Bock, H. (1938). *Hoppe-Seyl. Z.* **255**, 1.
Fischer, H. & Herrle, K. (1937). *Liebigs Ann.* **527**, 138.
Fischer, H. & Orth, H. (1940). *Die Chemie des Pyrrols*, vol. 2, part 2. 1st ed. Leipzig: Akademische Verlagsgesellschaft m.b.H.

Fujita, A. & Kodama, T. (1934). *Biochem. Z.* **273**, 186.

Keilin, D. (1933). *Nature, Lond.*, **132**, 783.

Kiese, M. & Kurz, H. (1954). *Biochem. Z.* **325**, 299.

Lemberg, R. & Legge, J. W. (1949). *Hematin Compounds and Bile Pigments*, 1st ed. New York: Interscience Publishers, Inc.

Lemberg, R. & Wyndham, R. A. (1937). *J. Roy. Soc. N.S.W.* **70**, 343.

Moss, F. (1952). *Aust. J. exp. Biol. med. Sci.* **30**, 531.

Negelein, E. & Gerischer, W. (1934). *Biochem. Z.* **268**, 1.

Nicholas, R. E. H. & Rimington, C. (1949). *Scand. J. clin. Lab. Invest.* **4**, 12.

Rawlinson, W. A. & Hale, J. H. (1949). *Biochem. J.* **45**, 247.

Stern, A. & Deželić, M. (1937). *Z. phys. Chem.* A, **179**, 275.

Stern, A. & Molvig, H. (1937). *Z. phys. Chem.* A, **178**, 161.

Stern, A. & Pruckner, F. (1937). *Z. phys. Chem.* A, **180**, 321.

Stern, A. & Wenderlein, H. (1935). *Z. phys. Chem.* **174**, 321.

Stern, A. & Wenderlein, H. (1936). *Z. phys. Chem.* **177**, 165.

Tissières, A. (1952). *Biochem. J.* **50**, 279.

Warburg, O. & Gewitz, H. S. (1953). *Hoppe-Seyl. Z.* **292**, 174.

Warburg, O. & Negelein, E. (1932). *Biochem. Z.* **244**, 9.

Yaoi, H. & Tamiya, H. (1928). Quoted by Keilin (1933).

Reprinted from *J. Biol. Chem.* **241**:3308–3315 (1966)

The Purification and Properties of Cytochrome *o* from *Vitreoscilla**

(Received for publication, January 24, 1966)

D. A. WEBSTER‡ AND D. P. HACKETT§

From the Department of Biochemistry, University of California, Berkeley, California 94720

SUMMARY

By freezing and thawing a suspension of *Vitreoscilla* cells in the presence of 1% sodium deoxycholate, followed by a protamine sulfate step, an ammonium sulfate step, Sephadex G-100 chromatography, and TEAE-cellulose chromatography, two CO-binding pigments have been purified. One (Fraction I) has two α bands and two Soret bands in liquid nitrogen difference spectra and thus appears to possess two heme groups. A molecular weight of 27,000 was determined by chromatography on Sephadex G-75. Protoheme was shown to be the prosthetic group of this pigment, and the E'_0 was found to be +0.10 volt. It is only very slowly autoxidizable. The other pigment (Fraction II) is very autoxidizable and has an E'_0 of −0.09 volt. The prosthetic group of this protein is also protoheme, and it has a molecular weight of 22,500. The properties of both pigments are discussed in relation to their possible roles as the terminal oxidase.

In a survey of the respiratory chain of colorless algae, no evidence was found for the presence of *a*-type cytochromes in the "colorless" blue-green algae; however, all three *Cyanophyta* studied possess what appears to be the same type of CO-binding pigment (1). The absorption bands for the CO compound of this pigment are at approximately 416, 535, and 570 mμ. That this pigment was indeed functioning as the terminal oxidase was demonstrated by performing an action spectrum for the relief of CO-inhibited respiration on *Vitreoscilla* one of the *Cyanophyta* used in the survey (1, 2).

Both the CO difference spectra and the action spectrum observed in these *Cyanophyta* are similar to those which have been observed in certain bacteria by Chance (3, 4), Castor and Chance (5), and Chance, Smith, and Castor (6). The pigment responsible for these spectra has been termed cytochrome *o* (7). This cytochrome appears to have a wide distribution in the bacteria, both as one of several terminal oxidases, as in *Escher-*

* This work was supported by Grant GB 1751 from the National Science Foundation. During the tenure of this work the senior author was a graduate fellow of the National Science Foundation.

‡ Present address, Massachusetts General Hospital, Boston, Massachusetts 02114.

§ Deceased, January 21, 1965.

ichia coli, or as the only terminal oxidase, as in *Acetobacter suboxydans* (8). It has been found in hydrogen-oxidizing bacteria (9), in a fruiting myxobacterium (10), in *Hemophilus parainfluenzae* (11), and in the nitrogen-fixing *Rhizobium* (12).

Bartsch and Kamen (13) have purified a highly autoxidizable, CO-binding heme protein, which they have called RHP,[1] from the facultative photoheterotroph, *Rhodospirillum rubrum*. This pigment, which appears to be localized in the chromatophores (14), has a CO difference spectrum which resembles that of cytochrome *o*. The question of the identity of cytochrome *o* and RHP has been considered by Kamen and co-workers, who at first thought them to be the same pigment (13, 15). In support of this, Horio and Yamashita (16) performed an action spectrum for the relief of the CO-inhibited respiration of dark grown cells of *R. rubrum* and found it to be of the same type as had been found for cytochrome *o* (5). Later, however, Kamen began questioning the role of RHP as an oxidase (17). Recently Taniguchi and Kamen have published strong evidence for the nonidentity of the two CO-binding pigments (18).

This report describes the purification and properties of two CO-binding pigments from *Vitreoscilla*. The CO difference spectra of both pigments have absorption bands similar to difference spectra of cytochrome *o* observed *in vivo*. In agreement with recent results (18), the properties of both pigments are different from the properties of RHP.

METHODS

Growth of Cells—*Vitreoscilla* species was grown on a large scale in 15 liters of medium (1) in 20-liter carboys. Dow-Corning Antifoam B (0.2 to 0.3 ml) was added to each carboy before sterilization. A 1-liter culture in log phase was used as the inoculum. Purified, sterile air was continuously forced through the culture. After growing for 2 days at room temperature (approximately 25°), the cells were harvested with the Sharples supercentrifuge and stored at −15° until used in the purification procedure. About 40 g, wet weight, of cells were obtained from each carboy.

Extraction Procedure—Frozen cells, 100 g, were suspended in 0.1 M phosphate, pH 7.5, containing 2.0 g of sodium deoxycholate, to a final volume of 200 ml. This suspension was distributed into several stainless steel beakers and frozen and thawed four times. Dry Ice in methyl Cellosolve was used for the freezing, and tepid

[1] The abbreviations used are: RHP, *Rhodospirillum* heme protein; TEAE, "triethylaminoethyl" (—C_2H_4—N^+—$(C_2H_5)_3$).

water was used to thaw. All further operations were performed at 0–4°. The suspension was centrifuged at 35,000 × g for 30 min, and the supernatant was carefully decanted.

Protamine Sulfate Step—To the crude extract, 17.5 ml of protamine sulfate solution (Calbiochem, 50 mg per ml) were added; the suspension was centrifuged at 39,000 × g for 2 hours; and the supernatant was carefully decanted. (Before doing this step it is best to take several aliquots of the crude extract and perform a titration to determine the optimum amount of protamine sulfate to add.)

Ammonium Sulfate Step—The supernatant after the protamine sulfate step was brought to 45% saturation with ammonium sulfate (25.8 g added for each 100 ml of supernatant) and allowed to stand for several hours before centrifugation at 25,000 × g for 30 min. The precipitate was discarded, and enough ammonium sulfate was added to bring the supernatant to 65% saturation (12.3 g added to each 100 ml of 45% ammonium sulfate supernatant). After standing for several hours or overnight, the suspension was centrifuged at 25,000 × g for 30 min, and the supernatant was discarded.

Chromatography on Sephadex G-100—The 65% ammonium sulfate precipitate was dissolved in a minimum volume (10 to 20 ml) of 0.02 M phosphate, pH 7.5. When the solution was turbid, it was briefly dialyzed to remove excess salt and to dissolve all the protein. This was then carefully applied to a Sephadex G-100 column (4.1 × 43.5 cm, containing approximately 33 g, dry weight, of gel), and 10-ml fractions were collected (the flow rate was approximately 30 ml per hour). The absorbances of the fractions were read at 280 and 400 mμ. The best fractions were pooled and concentrated by adding 47.6 g of ammonium sulfate to each 100 ml (75% saturation), being allowed to stand for several hours, and then being centrifuged at 25,000 × g for 30 min.

Chromatography on TEAE-cellulose—The concentrated G-100 eluate was dissolved in a few milliliters of 0.015 M phosphate, pH 7.16, and dialyzed for 2 days against the same buffer. A column of TEAE-cellulose (1.1 × 50 cm), containing 10 g, dry weight, of TEAE-cellulose (Bio-Rad Cellex-T, 0.55 meq per g, Control No. 2690), which had been washed according to the method of Peterson and Sober (19), was packed and washed successively with 2 M NaCl and then 0.015 M phosphate, pH 7.16. These solutions were also used for regeneration of the column. The dialyzed sample was then applied, and, with the phosphate buffer as the eluant, 4- to 5-ml fractions were collected (flow rate was approximately 40 ml per hour) until the first red band was completely eluted. This pigment will be referred to as "Fraction I." A linear gradient was then started with the use of 200 ml of 0.5 M NaCl (in the phosphate buffer), which was siphoned into 200 ml of phosphate buffer. This gradient removed the red band, which stayed at the top of the column during the elution with the phosphate buffer alone. This second pigment will be referred to as "Fraction II." Both fractions were concentrated with ammonium sulfate and dialyzed to remove excess salt. Electrophoresis on cellulose acetate strips with 0.02 M phosphate buffer, pH 7.15, followed by staining with 0.001% nigrosin (20) revealed the presence of multiple protein components in both fractions. Fraction I could be further purified by rechromatography on TEAE-cellulose, but the recovery was low, and better results were obtained by chromatography on Sephadex G-75 (see "Estimation of Molecular Weight on Sephadex G-75," below). Frac-

tion II could be further purified by rechromatography on TEAE-cellulose with excellent recovery.

Assay—In the early stages of the purification (before the Sephadex G-100 step) much more consistent results were obtained with the use of the reduced CO Soret band as a measure of the amount of cytochrome present. The absorbance of an appropriate dilution was determined at 280 mμ, a few grains of dithionite were added to the cuvette, and CO was bubbled into the cuvette for 1 min. The absorbance at 420 mμ was determined and from this was subtracted the absorbance at 440 mμ. For the more purified material, the ratio $A_{400}:A_{280}$ is a satisfactory criterion of purity.

Spectra—All spectra were determined with the Cary model 14 equipped with the scattered transmission accessory and the high intensity light source (Cary model 1471200). Cuvettes possessing a path length of 1 cm were used except for the low temperature difference spectra; plastic cuvettes possessing a path length of 3 mm were used for the latter with the procedure described in an earlier report (21). Spectra of the α regions were performed with the 0.0- to 0.1-absorbance unit slide wire.

Removal and Identification of Prosthetic Group—The general procedures used for this determination have been described by Falk (22). Starting with a total of 4.10 absorbance units (at 400 mμ) of Fraction I in phosphate buffer and 3.47 absorbance units of Fraction II in phosphate buffer, the heme was extracted by shaking each fraction with twice its volume of cold acid-acetone (1% 6 M HCl in acetone) and allowing both samples to stand for 10 min at 0°. Each sample was then extracted three times with cold ether. The combined ether extracts were washed with 10 ml of 1.0 M NaCl and evaporated to dryness on a steam bath. The residues were dissolved in a few drops of dimethylformamide and brought to 2.0 ml with methanol. The spectra of the pyridine hemochromogens were determined by the method of Falk (22). The heme was further identified by the lutidine-water paper chromatography system of Shichi and Hackett (23). The iron was extracted from the hemes of both samples by the ferrous sulfate method described by Falk (22). The extracted porphyrins were dissolved in 1.0 ml of 2.7 N HCl, and the spectra were recorded. The number of carboxyl groups on the porphyrin was determined by paper chromatography with the lutidine method of Falk *et al.* (24) and the lithium chloride method of With (25). In the latter method, 0.1 M lithium chloride as the developing solvent and an atmosphere of ammonia are used. Dicarboxylic porphyrins stay at the origin in this system, and they move with an R_F of 0.8 to 0.9 in the lutidine system.

Estimation of Molecular Weight on Sephadex G-75—The method used was in principle that of Whitaker (26). All chromatography was performed at 4° on a column (1.1 × 106 cm) containing roughly 8 g, dry weight, of gel. Phosphate buffer, 0.02 M, pH 7.15, was used as the eluant, and the flow rate was 15 ml per hour. All samples were applied to the column in a total volume of 0.45 ml, which contained 1 to 3 mg of protein. Fractions of 1.0 ml were collected. The hold-up volume (V_0) of the column was determined with blue dextran 2000 (Pharmacia), which has an average molecular weight of 2,000,000. The column was calibrated with crystalline horseradish peroxidase (Worthington, mol wt 40,200), soybean trypsin inhibitor (Sigma, crystallized three times, mol wt 21,500), and equine cytochrome c (Sigma type III, mol wt 12,270). Peaks were located by the absorbance of the fractions at 280 mμ or the absorbance of the oxidized Soret band. The elution volume (V_e) of each protein was measured with a graduated cylinder.

Determination of E'_0—A modified version of the method of Velick and Strittmatter (27) was used. The assay solution for the E'_0 determination for Fraction II contained 0.05 M potassium phosphate, pH 7.0; 0.16 M potassium oxalate; and 10^{-4} M $FeCl_3$ in a total volume of 2.0 ml in an anaerobic cuvette fitted with a serum stopper. The cuvette was evacuated with an aspirator and flushed with purified nitrogen five or six times, and the spectrum was recorded with the Cary spectrophotometer. The cytochrome was then titrated by injecting 0.1 M $FeSO_4$ through the rubber stopper with a calibrated 100-μl microsyringe; the spectrum was recorded after each addition. The cuvette was then opened, a little dithionite was added, and the spectrum was again recorded. The control cuvette, used as a blank, received the same additions as the experimental cuvette. The E'_0 for Fraction I was determined in the same way except that 0.01 M $FeSO_4$ was used for the titrations. The $FeSO_4$ solutions had been flushed with nitrogen and maintained in an anaerobic condition by using bottles fitted with serum stoppers.

RESULTS

Purification—The purification procedure described is quite reproducible. The purity and recovery of cytochrome after each step are given in Table I, which presents the data of a fairly typical purification. If for any reason a particular step did not yield pigment of the approximate purity given in Table I, that step required repetition to ensure the effectiveness of subsequent steps. The number of times the cells were frozen and thawed was varied from 2 to 10 times with little difference in the yield of cytochrome extracted.

An elution diagram for the Sephadex G-100 chromatography is given in Fig. 1. This step is the scale-limiting factor of the purification scheme. No more than 1 g of protein could be applied to the column described without overloading and lessening resolution. A larger G-100 column could be used to increase the preparative scale.

A small amount of 400 mμ absorbing material which came off the column at the hold-up volume (Fig. 1) primarily consisted of small membrane fragments, as evidenced by its chromatographic behavior on Sephadex G-100, which suggested high molecular weight material of rather heterogeneous molecular size. Also, CO difference spectra of this material exhibited a Soret band near

TABLE I
Summary of purification results

Purification stage	Total protein[a]	Total units[b]	Yield	$\Delta : A_{280}$	$A_{400} : A_{280}$
	mg		*%*		
Extract...................	7120	232	100	0.033	0.023
Protamine sulfate supernatant...................	4910	208	90	0.042	0.044
45–65% ammonium sulfate precipitate..............	960	147	63	0.15	0.14
Sephadex G-100 eluate....	169	108	47	0.64	0.39
Fraction I................	7	18	7	2.5	1.4
Fraction II...............	21	36	15	1.7	1.0

[a] Based on 1 unit of absorbance at 280 mμ = 1 mg of protein.

[b] Units (Δ) are defined as A_{420} (the reduced CO Soret band maximum) minus A_{440}.

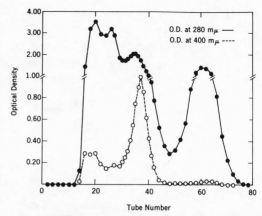

FIG. 1. Elution pattern for chromatography of 45 to 65% ammonium sulfate fraction on Sephadex G-100. Experimental details are given in the text.

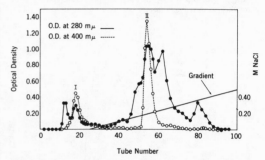

FIG. 2. Elution pattern for chromatography of Sephadex G-100 eluate on TEAE-cellulose. Experimental details are given in the text.

416 mμ, which was closer to the position of the same band in CO difference of whole cells (1) than to the same band in CO difference spectra of the purified heme proteins (Figs. 7 and 8). Most of this high molecular weight material was precipitated by 45% ammonium sulfate, which accounted for the apparent low yield in the ammonium sulfate step.

Fig. 2 shows the elution pattern obtained in the TEAE-cellulose chromatography. Two heme proteins with quite different affinities for the resin were separated by this procedure. After rechromatography, the best preparations of Fraction I had an $A_{400} : A_{280}$ ratio of 2.1, and the best preparation of Fraction II had an $A_{400} : A_{280}$ ratio of 1.9. Neither was pure as judged by cellulose acetate electrophoresis. Both pigments moved strongly anodically at pH 7.0. Thus they both appeared to be acidic proteins. Also, neither pigment bound to carboxymethyl cellulose equilibrated with 0.01 M citrate buffer at pH levels between 6.5 and 5.5.

Spectral Properties—The spectral properties of Fractions I and II are represented in Figs. 3 through 10. Both pigments possessed very small, broad α bands in both absolute (Figs. 3 and 4) and difference spectra (Figs. 5 and 6), and no β bands seemed to

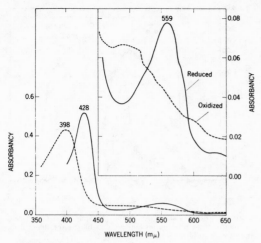

FIG. 3. Absolute spectra of Fraction I. - - -, oxidized form; ——, dithionite-reduced form.

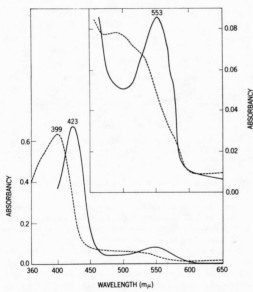

FIG. 4. Absolute spectra of Fraction II. - - -, oxidized form; ——, dithionite-reduced form.

be present. CO difference spectra could not be used to identify the physiological cytochrome *o*, because both purified cytochromes had very similar CO difference spectra (Figs. 7 and 8) and either, or both together, could have been the pigment the CO difference spectrum of which was observed in whole cells (1).

Liquid nitrogen difference spectra revealed the true complexity of the α bands. The α band of Fraction II had three shoulders (Fig. 10); the one at 530 mμ could be called the "vestigial" β

band. The low temperature difference spectrum of Fraction I (Fig. 9) was more informative. Two α bands, two Soret bands, and perhaps two β bands suggested the presence of two hemes.

One of Kamen's major objections against RHP being the terminal oxidase in *R. rubrum* is the fact that the respiration of

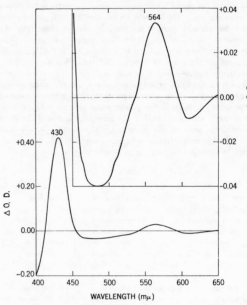

FIG. 5. Difference spectrum of Fraction I (dithionite-reduced — untreated).

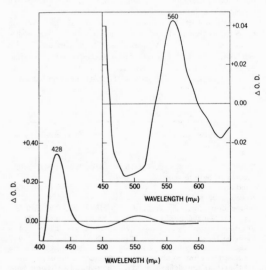

FIG. 6. Difference spectrum of Fraction II (dithionite-reduced — untreated).

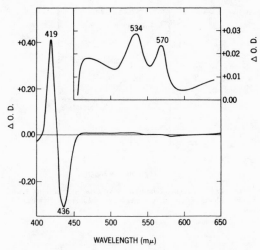

FIG. 7. CO difference spectrum of Fraction I ((dithionite + CO) − (dithionite)).

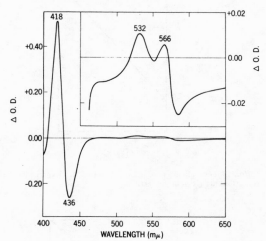

FIG. 8. CO difference spectrum of Fraction II ((dithionite + CO) − (dithionite)).

lutidine-water chromatographic system (23) both unknown hemes and Protoheme IX moved with an R_F of 0.60 to 0.62.

Spectra of the porphyrins, obtained from the unknown hemes, in 2.7 N HCl show absorption maxima at approximately 595 (broad), 554 to 555, and approximately 410 (broad) mμ. A

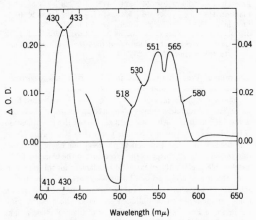

FIG. 9. Difference spectrum of Fraction I at −190° (dithionite-reduced − untreated).

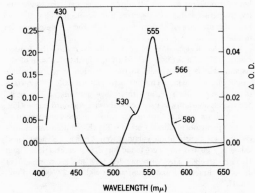

FIG. 10. Difference spectrum of Fraction II at −190° (dithionite reduced − untreated).

R. rubrum is inhibited by cyanide, but RHP does not combine with cyanide (17). The two heme pigments purified from *Vitreoscilla* do combine with cyanide. Absolute spectra of these pigments in 10^{-3} M KCN have absorption maxima at 540 (broad) and 416 mμ. Cyanide difference spectra of both pigments are likewise similar and have maxima at 555 and 421 mμ.

The spectral properties of the two pigments are summarized in Table II.

Identification of Prosthetic Group—The spectral properties of the pyridine hemochromogen of the hemes extracted from Fractions I and II are summarized in Table III, which also contains the corresponding properties of Protoheme IX (22). In the

TABLE II

Spectral properties of Fractions I and II

Bands are in millimicrons.

Fraction	Oxidized bands	Reduced bands	Bands in difference spectra	Bands in 10^{-3} M KCN	Bands in CO difference spectra[a]
I	398	559, 428	564, 430	540, 416	570, 534, 419, 436[b]
II	399	553, 423	560, 428	540, 416	566, 532, 418, 436[b]

[a] CO difference spectrum of *Vitreoscilla in vivo* has bands at 570, 535, and 416 mμ and a trough at 433 mμ.

[b] Trough.

TABLE III

Spectral properties of pyridine hemochromogens of hemes extracted from Fractions I and II

Heme	α	β	γ	α:γ	Heme extracted[a]
Fraction I	556	524	418	0.228	7.4×10^{-3}
Fraction II	556	524	418	0.199	8.6×10^{-3}
Protoheme IX[b]	557	526	418.5	0.180	

[a] In micromoles per absorbance unit (at 400 mμ) of cytochrome.
[b] Data taken from Falk (22).

spectrum of Protophopyrin IX in 2.7 N HCl has absorption maxima at 598, 554, and 408 mμ (22). Both unknowns and Protoporphyrin IX moved with an R_F of 0.74 in the lutidine-water paper chromatographic system, and all stayed at the origin in the LiCl system. All these data supported the identification of the prosthetic group of Fractions I and II as Protoheme IX.

If one assumes that Fraction II possesses one heme per molecule and that the efficiency of the extraction of the heme is 100%, it is possible to calculate an extinction coefficient for this pigment. With the use of the pyridine hemochromogen to estimate the amounts of heme extracted (Table III) a value of 1.15×10^5 liters per mole per cm is obtained for the oxidized Soret band maximum of Fraction II. With the use of the molecular weight value determined on Sephadex G-75, a value of 5.0 ml per mg per cm for the oxidized Soret band maximum for this fraction is calculated. The respective values for Fraction I are 1.36×10^5 liters per mole per cm and 5.0 ml per mg per cm. However, the low temperature difference spectrum of Fraction I (Fig. 9) suggests the presence of two hemes, so that these values may be invalid.

Molecular Weight—According to Whitaker (26) the elution volume (V_e) of a protein divided by the hold-up volume of the column (V_0) is proportional to the logarithm of the molecular weight of the protein. This proportionality is valid for a certain range of molecular size, and this range depends on the resin. Such a relationship was used to establish a standard curve (Fig. 11), which was used in turn to determine the molecular weight of the two pigments obtained from the TEAE-cellulose chromatography, once their elution volumes were known. Experimental values of 1.50 and 1.61 were found for $V_e:V_0$ for Fractions I and II, respectively. This corresponded to a molecular weight of 27,000 for Fraction I and a molecular weight of 22,500 for Fraction II.

It should be noted that there are a few proteins which behave anomalously when chromatographed on Sephadex (26). Thus the values obtained above should be considered tentative until they are confirmed by some other method, such as sedimentation equilibrium. However, this latter method requires knowing accurately the partial specific volume. It would be necessary to measure this parameter for both of these cytochromes because if any detergent used in the extraction procedures was bound to them the density of the molecules may have been altered.

Determination of E'_0—Plots of log $o^2:o^3$ versus log $Fe^2:Fe^3$ for Fractions I and II are given in Figs. 12 and 13, respectively.[2] Since the E'_0 of the ferric-ferrous oxalate couple is 0 (28), the

[2] o^2 and o^3 refer to the concentration of reduced and oxidized cytochrome, respectively. Fe^2 and Fe^3 refer to the concentration of ferrous and ferric ions, respectively. See Reference 23 for the method used to calculate the results.

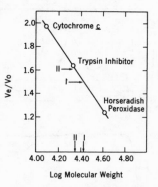

FIG. 11. Estimation of molecular weights of Fractions I and II on Sephadex G-75. Experimental conditions are given in the text.

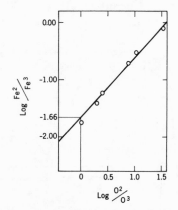

FIG. 12. Determination of E'_0 of Fraction I. Experimental conditions are given in the text.

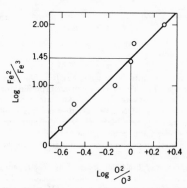

FIG. 13. Determination of E'_0 of Fraction II. Experimental conditions are given in the text.

TABLE IV
Comparison of properties of Fractions I and II

Fraction	Prosthetic group	Molecular weight	E'_0	Autoxidizability
I	Protoheme IX	27,000	+0.10	Very slow
II	Protoheme IX	22,500	-0.09	Very fast

E'_0 for each fraction is simply -0.06 times the logarithm of the $Fe^2 : Fe^3$ ratio at the point where the cytochrome is half reduced. An E'_0 of $+0.10$ volt is found for Fraction I and an E'_0 of -0.09 volt is found for Fraction II.

In agreement with the above results a few grains of ascorbic acid, tipped in from the side arm of an anaerobic cuvette, were found to reduce Fraction I partially but did not reduce Fraction II. Potassium ferrocyanide (5×10^{-3} M) did not reduce either pigment. NADH, which has an E'_0 low enough to be capable of reducing both pigments, also failed to reduce either.

Autoxidizability—Cytochrome c was found to be rapidly and quantitatively reduced by hydrogen in the presence of palladium, 10% on asbestos (K and K Laboratories, Inc.) when tested in an anaerobic cuvette with a side arm to hold the catalyst (*cf.* Reference 29). When Fraction I was tested in this system, only partial reduction resulted. When the cuvette was opened and shaken in air, no reoxidation took place, as judged by the absorbance at 430 mμ, measured with the Cary spectrophotometer. The pigment was slowly reoxidized by oxygen, but about 4 min of bubbling with pure oxygen were required for complete reoxidation.

Fraction II was denatured by the palladium-asbestos catalyst. With the use of an anaerobic cuvette fitted with a serum stopper, this pigment was reduced by titrating it anaerobically with a freshly prepared solution of 0.01 M sodium dithionite, which was added with a microsyringe. On opening the cuvette and shaking with air, this pigment was found to be very rapidly oxidized. From the changes in absorbance at 400 and 430 mμ, the reduced form was estimated to have a half-life of 1 sec or less.

The properties of Fractions I and II are summarized and compared in Table IV.

Stability—Solutions of both proteins could be kept frozen at $-15°$ for months without any change in spectral properties. Both proteins were partially destroyed at pH 3.5 and were totally denatured by heating up to 50° or by treating with acetone at 0°.

Peroxidase Activity—In the o-dianisidine assay of Shichi and Hackett (30), 70 μg of each pigment were found to be completely devoid of peroxidatic activity. This amount of protein is more than 1000 times the amount of horseradish peroxidase normally used in this assay.

DISCUSSION

The basic difficulty in attempting to decide which, if either, of the two purified pigments is the physiological terminal oxidase is that very little is known of the properties of the protein *in vivo*. From the work of Taniguchi and Kamen (18) it is known that cytochrome o has a protoheme prosthetic group; the CO difference spectrum *in vivo* is also known (1). Both Fractions I and II have a protoheme prosthetic group, and the CO difference spectrum of each pigment (Figs. 7 and 8) closely resembles the CO difference spectrum of whole cells.

The more plausible candidate for the role of the terminal oxidase *in vivo* is Fraction II because of its extreme autoxidizabil-

ity. The low E'_0 of this pigment as isolated (-0.09 volt) might seem to be a major objection against its role as a terminal oxidase, but the E'_0 of the protein in the cell, where it is presumably in a lipid environment, may be quite different.

On rechromatography of Fraction II on TEAE-cellulose, a splitting of the single peak into two peaks has been observed sometimes. These two components have been separated and analyzed spectrally. They have identical spectral characteristics as well as the same E'_0, the same molecular weight, and the same prosthetic group. They thus appear to be true isozymes.

Although Fraction I is not very autoxidizable, it cannot be eliminated as a candidate for the physiological cytochrome o. Its properties too could be quite different when it is in the physicochemical milieu of the cell membrane. Purified cytochrome oxidase does not show any appreciable autoxidizability unless cytochrome c is present (31).

It is also possible that neither Fraction I nor Fraction II is the terminal oxidase and that they are both isolation artifacts. The low temperature difference spectra of the purified pigments support the argument that these pigments are physiologically meaningful; the two α bands at 565 and 555 mμ, which are present in these spectra (Figs. 9 and 10), are also visible in low temperature difference spectra of whole cells of *Vitreoscilla* (1); the α band at 551, although not present in the latter spectrum, is present in low temperature difference spectra of *Leucothrix*, one of the other *Cyanophyta* studied (1). Finally, the fact that both purified pigments combine with CO suggests the possibility that the physiological cytochrome o is a complex containing both of these components.

If one of the two purified fractions, or a combination of both of them, is indeed the physiological cytochrome o, then this terminal oxidase is the smallest terminal oxidase yet purified. The molecular weight of cytochrome oxidase is 530,000, while the molecular weight of *Pseudomonas* cytochrome oxidase is approximately 90,000. Cytochrome o is also unlike other terminal oxidases in having protoheme as its prosthetic group.

The reduced and difference spectra of Fractions I and II are characterized by their very broad α bands. At $-190°$ these α bands become complex, and what are apparently the β bands become visible as shoulders. To the authors' knowledge, such spectra have not been previously observed for protoheme proteins.

To elucidate further the roles of the two purified pigments in the respiratory chain of *Vitreoscilla*, physiological experiments were performed. It was hoped that particles isolated from *Vitreoscilla*, which could catalyze the oxidation of NADH (1), could also catalyze the reduction of one or both pigments by NADH anaerobically. This experiment was performed with each pigment alone and with both pigments together, and also in the presence of sodium deoxycholate, but no activity was detected.

REFERENCES

1. WEBSTER, D. A., AND HACKETT, D. P., *Plant Physiol.*, **41**, 599 (1966).
2. WEBSTER, D. A., AND HACKETT, D. P., *Carnegie Inst. Washington, Yearbook*, **63**, 483 (1964).
3. CHANCE, B., *J. Biol. Chem.*, **202**, 383 (1953).
4. CHANCE, B., *J. Biol. Chem.*, **202**, 397 (1953).
5. CASTOR, L. N., AND CHANCE, B., *J. Biol. Chem.*, **217**, 453 (1955).
6. CHANCE, B., SMITH, L., AND CASTOR, L., *Biochim. Biophys. Acta*, **12**, 289 (1953).

7. SMITH, L., in I. C. GUNSALUS AND R. Y. STANIER (Editors), *The bacteria, Vol. II*, Academic Press, Inc., New York, 1961, p. 374.

8. SMITH, L., in I. C. GUNSALUS AND R. Y. STANIER (Editors), *The bacteria, Vol. II*, Academic Press, Inc., New York, 1961, p. 365.

9. PACKER, L., *Arch. Biochem. Biophys.*, **78**, 54 (1958).

10. DWORKIN, M., AND NIEDERPRUEM, D. J., *J. Bacteriol.*, **87**, 316 (1964).

11. WHITE, D. C., AND SMITH, L., *J. Biol. Chem.*, **237**, 1332 (1962).

12. TAZIMURA, K., AND WATANABE, I., *Plant Cell Physiol. (Tokyo)*, **5**, 157 (1964).

13. BARTSCH, R. G., AND KAMEN, M. D., *J. Biol. Chem.*, **230**, 41 (1958).

14. ORLANDO, J. A., LEVINE, L., AND KAMEN, M. D., *Biochim. Biophys. Acta*, **46**, 126 (1961).

15. NEWTON, J. W., AND KAMEN, M. D., in I. C. GUNSALUS AND R. Y. STANIER (Editors), *The Bacteria, Vol. II*, Academic Press, Inc., New York, 1961, p. 397.

16. HORIO, T., AND YAMASHITA, J., in H. GEST, A. SAN PIETRO, AND C. P. VERNON (Editors), *Bacterial photosynthesis*, Antioch Press, Yellow Springs, Ohio, 1963, p. 275.

17. KAMEN, M. D., in H. GEST, A. SAN PIETRO, AND C. P. VERNON (Editors), *Bacterial photosynthesis*, Antioch Press, Yellow Springs, Ohio, 1963, p. 61.

18. TANIGUCHI, S., AND KAMEN, M. D., *Biochim. Biophys. Acta*, **96**, 395 (1965).

19. PETERSON, E. A., AND SOBER, H. A., in *Methods Enzymol.*, **5**, 3 (1962).

20. KOHN, J., *Nature*, **181**, 839 (1958).

21. WEBSTER, D. A., AND HACKETT, D. P., *Plant Physiol.*, **40**, 1091 (1965).

22. FALK, J. E., *Porphyrins and metalloporphyrins*, American Elsevier Publishing Company, New York, 1964.

23. SHICHI, H., AND HACKETT, D. P., *J. Biol. Chem.*, **237**, 2959 (1962).

24. FALK, J. E., DRESEL, E. I. B., BENSON, A., AND KNIGHT, B. C., *Biochem. J.*, **63**, 87 (1956).

25. WITH, T. K., *Scand. J. Clin. Lab. Invest.*, **9**, 395 (1957).

26. WHITAKER, J. R., *Anal. Chem.*, **35**, 1950 (1963).

27. VELICK, S. F., AND STRITTMATTER, P., *J. Biol. Chem.*, **221**, 265 (1956).

28. MICHAELIS, L., AND FRIEDHEIM, E., *J. Biol. Chem.*, **91**, 343 (1931).

29. THEORELL, H., *Biochem. Z.*, **279**, 463 (1935).

30. SHICHI, H., AND HACKETT, D. P., *J. Biol. Chem.*, **237**, 2955 (1962).

31. OKUNUKI, K., in O. HAYAISHI (Editor), *Oxygenases*, Academic Press, Inc., New York, 1962, p. 409.

Editor's Comments
on Papers 12 and 13

12 TISSIÈRES
Role of High-Molecular Weight Components in the Respiratory Activity of Cell-Free Extracts of Aerobacter aerogenes

13 WHITE AND SMITH
Localization of the Enzymes that Catalyze Hydrogen and Electron Transport in Hemophilus parainfluenzae *and the Nature of the Respiratory Chain System*

ORGANIZATION OF THE RESPIRATORY APPARATUS

Respiratory assemblies occupy the plasma membrane in procaryotes. No specialized respiratory organelles have been convincingly demonstrated, and early suggestions that bacteria possessed mitochondria were erroneous.[1] Suggestions that mesosomes were the procaryotic equivalent of mitochondria as sites of respiratory activity were probably due to the concentration of membrane material in those structures. The view that the apparatus of respiration and associated energy conservation is distributed throughout the plasma membrane appears to be a reasonable one.

A. Tissières demonstrated in Paper 12 that subcellular fragments of several million daltons in size were capable of the oxidation of succinate and, when supplemented with soluble factors, of several other compounds of the tricarboxylic acid cycle. These particles were formed as the result of comminution of the cell envelope. Tissières's findings were consistent with those of Weibull, who showed that the entire plasma membrane, isolated from Gram-positive organisms by treatment with lysozyme and subsequent osmotic lysis, contained the bulk of the cytochromes.[2]

The question then arises as to the nature of organization of the components of terminal electron transport within the membrane. C. Jones and E. Redfearn applied to extracts of *Azotobacter vinelandii* fractionation techniques predominantly devised in the laboratory of David Green at Wisconsin, and found that reproducibly different kinds of "subunits" could be separated and isolated.[3] They suggested that two different respiratory sequences, terminating with different cytochrome oxidases, were contained within the two particle fractions: "green" particles were rich in cytochrome a_2 (*d*) and contained cytochromes a_1 and b_1 but respired poorly; "red" particles contained cytochromes o, b_1, and $c_4 + c_5$ as well as much flavoprotein, and oxidized succinate at least fivefold faster than did "green" particles. The physical appearance of the two types of particles were markedly different when examined by electron microscopy. It was subsequently suggested that these two branched and separable respiratory assemblies conserved energy with different efficiencies,[4] although that concept has been challenged (see Editor's Comments on Paper 29). White and Sinclair have reviewed work performed on branched-chain respiratory systems.[5]

At odds with the position adopted by Jones and Redfearn is that taken by David White and Lucile Smith in Paper 23, where it is reported that respiration in *Hemophilus parainfluenzae* is served by components occurring in variable and nonstoichiometric amounts. Such observations suggest a random association of respiratory and other membrane components more consistent with the current view of the cell membrane as a dynamic structure containing constituents capable of rapid and extensive lateral movement.[6] Nonetheless, the possibility remains that certain intramembrane structures are immobile, or move only in association with other components, a hypothesis consistent with the findings of Jones and Redfearn. Continuation of the approach so ably employed by Jones and Redfearn, especially utilizing the sophisticated procedures of Hatefi's group,[7] ought to yield useful results.

REFERENCES

1. Mudd, S. *Ann. Rev. Microbiol.*, **23**, 1–28, 1969 (see especially p. 18).
2. Weibull, C. *J. Bact.* **66**, 696–702, 1953.
3. Jones, C. and E. Redfearn, *Biochim. Biophys. Acta.* **143**, 354–362, 1967.
4. Meyer, D., and C. Jones. *Eur. J. Biochem.*, **36**, 144–151, 1973.
5. White, D., and P. Sinclair. *Adv. in Microbial Physiol.*, **5**, 173–211, 1970.
6. Singer, S. J. *Ann. Rev. Biochem.*, **43**, 805–833, 1974.
7. Hatefi, Y., D. Stiggal, and Y. Golante. In S. Fleischer and L. Packer, eds. *Meth. Enzymol.* **53**(Part D):3–54 1978.

12

Reprinted from Nature (London) **174**:183–184 (1954)

ROLE OF HIGH-MOLECULAR WEIGHT COMPONENTS IN THE RESPIRATORY ACTIVITY OF CELL-FREE EXTRACTS OF *AEROBACTER AEROGENES*

By Dr. A. TISSIÈRES

IT has been shown that clear cell-free extracts from a strain of *Aerobacter aerogenes* catalyse the oxidation of glucose, glucose-6-phosphate, hexose diphosphate, pyruvate and succinate[1]. As the rate of oxidation with these substrates was not appreciably modified by 20-min. centrifugation in a field of 15,000 g, and as the extract was transparent by transmitted light, it was obvious that the enzyme systems concerned were attached to very small elements.

The experiments reported here show that the bulk of the succinic oxidase system, in these cell-free extracts, is bound to one, or possibly two, high-molecular weight components, which have sedimentation constants of approximately 40 and 22 S respectively. The same components are also necessary, in addition to soluble factors, for the oxidation of glucose, pyruvate, citrate, α-ketoglutarate and fumarate.

The strain of *Aerobacter aerogenes* used and the methods of cultivation have been described previously[1]. The bacteria from a 24-hr. culture were washed three times with twenty volumes of distilled water by centrifugation and the well-packed cells were ground by hand in a cold mortar for 2–3 min. with three parts (w/w) of a very fine 'Pyrex' glass powder (passed through a 200-mesh sieve) and extracted with 2·5 parts (w/v) of ice-cold distilled water. A first centrifugation at 4,000 g for 20 min. removed the glass powder, the intact cells and the larger cell debris, and the supernatant was centrifuged again at 18,000 g for 20 min., to give a clear supernatant (Sup. 1). This fraction was again centrifuged for 90 min. at about 110,000 g in a model L Spinco centrifuge, yielding a supernatant (Sup. 2) and a small gelatinous pellet which was resuspended in one-fifth the volume of Sup. 1 of 0·05 M phosphate buffer pH 7·0 to give fraction P. The preparation was kept at 0–4° C. throughout these manipulations.

The various fractions Sup. 1, Sup. 2 and P were examined in the ultracentrifuge. As seen in Figs. 1–4, three major components were found in Sup. 1, with sedimentation constants of about 40, 22 and 9 S respectively. In Sup. 2 (Figs. 5–7) only the third component (9 S) was present, while fraction P contained the two larger components only (40 and 22 S,

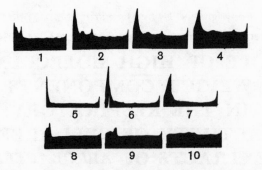

Ultracentrifugal patterns of Sup. 1 (1–4, time interval 600 sec., average speed 38,400 r.p.m. increased after picture 3 to 43,100 r.p.m.); Sup. 2 (5–7, time interval 840 sec., average speed 43,000 r.p.m.); and *P* (8–10, time interval 300 sec. between 8 and 9, and 900 sec. between 9 and 10, average speed 39,600 r.p.m.)

Figs. 8–10). Thus, by centrifugation at about 110,000 *g* for 90 min., it was possible to separate the two larger components from the rest of the extract. Of these two components, that of 40 *S* was the major one; it showed a sharp boundary in the ultracentrifuge, and its molecular weight, based on ultracentrifugal data, is of the order of 1–3 millions. Further experiments are required to determine accurately the molecular weights and to study the homogeneity of both the 40 and 22 *S* components.

Schachman, Pardee and Stanier[2] found that cell-free extracts prepared by different methods and from different species of bacteria all gave essentially similar patterns on examination in the ultracentrifuge. The extracts contained four major components with sedimentation constants of about 40, 20–30, 9 and 5 *S*. An electron micrograph of the purified 40 *S* fraction showed that it was formed of particles which appeared to be spherical with a diameter of about 150 A., and the molecular weight of these elements, calculated either from ultracentrifugal or electron microscopic data, was about one million. Although they did not give any data on the matter, Schachman *et al.*[2] stated that the 40 *S* fraction contained "considerable amounts of ribonuclease, catalase, apyrase, formic dehydrogenase and succinodehydrogenase". Siegel, Singer and Wildman[3], in the course of their study of high-molecular weight components of normal and infected *E. coli* cells, observed very similar ultracentrifugal patterns, and the data presented here are in good agreement with those given by both groups of authors.

The ability of Sup. 1, Sup. 2 and *P* to oxidize various substrates was tested in Barcroft differential

Table 1. OXIDATION OF VARIOUS SUBSTRATES BY .FRACTIONS FROM
CLEAR CELL-FREE EXTRACTS OF *Aerobacter aerogenes.*

Results given as Qo_2 (μl. oxygen uptake/mgm. protein/hr.) corrected
for blanks. Substrate concentration: 0·03 M. Experimental
conditions : see text

	Sup. 1	Sup. 2	P
Glucose (with 0·04 m.mol. diphospho-pyridine nucleotide	49	4	0
Pyruvate (with 0·04 m.mol. diphos-phopyridine nucleotide and 36 units of coenzyme A)	16	1	0
Pyruvate (with 0·04 m.mol. diphos-phopyridine nucleotide. no coenzyme A)	10	1	0
Citrate	5·5	0	0
α-Ketoglutarate	6	0·7	0
Fumarate	8	0	0
Succinate	8	0	42

manometers at 36° C., in the presence of 0·05 M
phosphate buffer pH 7·0 and with potassium
hydroxide in the centre well. 1·5 ml. of either Sup. 1
or Sup. 2 and 0·3 ml. of P were used in each manometric flask in a total volume of 3 ml. The results,
presented in Table 1, show that Sup. 1 contained
the catalysts necessary for the oxidation of glucose,
pyruvate, citrate, α-ketoglutarate, fumarate and
succinate. Sup. 2 alone was inactive in the oxidation
of these substrates, while P contained the bulk of
the succinic oxidase system present in Sup. 1.
Further fractionation of P will show whether the
40 S component alone carries all the enzymes of the
succinic oxidase system. Whatever the answer, however, the experiments reported here show that the
very fine particles—or macromolecules—of fraction P,
of which the largest have a molecular weight of the
order of 1–3 millions, support a complete succinic
oxidase system, and, with the soluble factors found
in Sup. 1, are able to catalyse the oxidation of some
intermediates of the citric acid cycle.

It has been known for some time that clear cell-free
extracts from some bacterial species are able to
catalyse the oxidation of various substrates, including
Krebs-cycle intermediates. Thus Stone and Wilson[4]
presented evidence that in an extract from *Azotobacter* the citric acid cycle was operating. As this
extract was said to be translucent, and in view of
the results of Schachman *et al.*[2] with different species
of bacteria, it is not unlikely that the largest particles
were of the same order of magnitude as those found
in Sup. 1.

It is of great interest that some of the reactions,
which in animal tissues are known to depend upon
the integrity of the mitochondria, can take place in a
bacterial extract in which the largest element would
have a diameter of about 150 A., and therefore a
volume of nearly one-millionth that of a mitochondrion.

However, as the activity of these bacterial extracts

in the oxidation of some of the citric acid cycle intermediates is low compared with that of mitochondria,
it is not inconceivable that when the cells are disrupted a cellular organization, necessary for optimum
activity of the enzyme systems concerned, is dis-
turbed.

I am indebted to Dr. P. Johnson for carrying out
the experiments in the analytical ultracentrifuge and
to Miss J. Moyle for her assistance in running the
preparative Spinco centrifuge.

[1] Tissières, A., *Nature*, **169**, 880 (1952).

[2] Schachman, H. K., Pardee, A. B., and Stanier, R. Y., *Arch. Biochem. Biophys.*, **38** 245 (1952).

[3] Siegel, A. Singer, S. J., and Wildman, S. G., *Arch. Biochem. Biophys.*,
41, 278 (1952).

[4] Stone R. W., and Wilson, P. W., *J. Bact.*, **63**, 605 (1952).

Localization of the Enzymes That Catalyze Hydrogen and Electron Transport in *Hemophilus parainfluenzae* and the Nature of the Respiratory Chain System*

DAVID C. WHITE† AND LUCILE SMITH‡

From the Departments of Biochemistry, University of Kentucky College of Medicine, Lexington, Kentucky 40506, and Dartmouth Medical School, Hanover, New Hampshire

(Received for publication, April 20, 1964)

Hemophilus parainfluenzae possess a respiratory chain system with many characteristics similar to those of the mammalian system (1) and of a number of other bacteria (2): it is composed of typical flavoprotein dehydrogenases and six cytochrome pigments, three of which appear to be oxidases (3–5). These pigments are bound to particles which presumably are derived from the cytoplasmic membrane. Unusual aspects of the respiratory chain of *H. parainfluenzae* are the accumulation, under some conditions of growth, of large amounts of one cytochrome that is not reducible in the presence of substrates (4, 6, 7), and the variability of the proportions of the different pigments observed under different growth conditions and in different phases of growth (5–7). Further studies, reported here, show that bacteria having widely varying proportions of the different cytochromes can have respiration rates that are similar with a number of substrates.

These bacteria are readily permeable to substrates and pyridine nucleotides (8). Thus it is possible to compare the reactions of the membrane-bound system in intact bacteria and in the small membrane fragments derived from it upon rupture of the cells. Such studies show little modification of the reactivity immediately after preparation of the membrane fragments, but upon standing some pigments become dissociated from the membrane. As long as the pigments are associated with the membrane in proper orientation, electron transport can proceed rapidly, and the cytochromes and flavoproteins can be seen to undergo oxidation and reduction during electron transport. In either intact cells or particles, the over-all rate of electron transport is always limited by the reaction of the membrane-bound flavoprotein dehydrogenases with the appropriate substrate. Pyridine nucleotide is reduced by dehydrogenases which are not membrane-bound, and the rates of reduction of diphosphopyridine nucleotide are low.

Taken together, all of the studies on the respiratory chain system of *H. parainfluenzae* show that its properties resemble those of mammalian mitochondria in most aspects. However, there is compelling evidence that in these bacteria the system is not composed of fixed units of pigments with a definite "stoichiometry" of the components.

* Supported by Grants GM 10285 and GM 06270 of the Institute of General Medical Sciences, United States Public Health Service.
† Department of Biochemistry, University of Kentucky College of Medicine, Lexington, Kentucky 40506.
‡ Department of Biochemistry, Dartmouth Medical School, Hanover, New Hampshire.

EXPERIMENTAL PROCEDURE

The bacteria used in most of the experiments are a mutant of the strain of *H. parainfluenzae* (Boss No. 7) previously studied with respect to the cytochrome system (3, 4). The mutant, which appeared spontaneously during transfers of the parental type, has the same cytochrome components as the parental type as shown by measurements of difference spectra (7). However, cytochrome c_1 is synthesized at a lower rate by the mutant, with the result that cytochrome b_1 predominates in the late log phase cells under the growth conditions used. In contrast, when grown under the same condition, the parental type contains a large amount of cytochrome c_1 that is not reducible with substrate and is not membrane-bound (3, 4). The effect of DPN added to intact bacteria in increasing the rate of respiration in the presence of substrate is much more pronounced with the parental type. An advantage of working with the mutant is that the respiration rate shows less variability with the growth phase than does the parent type. The data of Table I, Part A, show that the respiration rates of parent and mutant bacteria are comparable with a number of substrates. The extent of reduction of the predominant cytochrome (c_1 in the parent strain, b_1 in the mutant) is also similar with the different substrates. About 50% of the cytochrome c_1 of the parent strain cannot be reduced by substrates and is reduced only by $Na_2S_2O_4$. The bacteria were grown in 2500-ml Parrot (low form Erlenmeyer) flasks with 400 ml of proteose-peptone medium (3) containing 0.02 M glucose or gluconate (autoclaved separately). After incubation for 14 hours at 37° without agitation, the cells were harvested by centrifugation in the cold, washed once with cold 0.05 M phosphate buffer, pH 7.6, then suspended in buffer to a final concentration of about 100 mg of bacterial protein per ml. The suspension was stored in an ice bath and usually used within 4 hours after harvesting. Contamination of the stock culture was checked (3). These conditions of growth yield bacteria containing high concentrations of the cytochrome pigments (6) as well as flavoprotein dehydrogenases (5).

Suspensions of insoluble respiratory particles were prepared by grinding the bacteria with Alumina A-305 (generously supplied by the Aluminum Company of America) as described (4).

The content of respiratory pigments was estimated from the anaerobic minus aerobic difference spectra (3, 6) in Cary spectrophotometers, models 14CM and 15.

Oxygen uptake was measured polarographically with the Clark electrode (Yellow Springs Instrument Company) in the

TABLE I

Comparison of respiratory rates produced by adding D-lactate, L-lactate, succinate, DPNH, and formate to H. parainfluenzae which formed principally cytochrome b_1 with bacteria which formed primarily cytochrome c_1

Oxygen uptake was measured polarigraphically after addition of approximately 10 mg of bacterial protein and substrates at concentrations of 10 mM, except for DPNH (5 mM), at 30° in 50 mM phosphate buffer, pH 7.6, as reported (9), and is expressed as millimicromoles of O_2 per second per 10 mg of protein. Cytochrome b_1 was estimated as the difference in absorbance between 561 and 575 mμ in anaerobic (in the presence of the substrate) minus aerobic difference spectrum; cytochrome c_1 was estimated similarly at 553 and 575 mμ per 10 mg of protein.

Substrates	Mutant (cytochrome b_1 predominant)			Parental type (cytochrome c_1 predominant)		
	Rate of oxygen uptake	Rate expected if additive	Cytochrome b_1 reduced	Rate of oxygen uptake	Rate expected if additive	Cytochrome c_1 reduced
A. Added singly						
D-Lactate	2.23		0.028	0.67		0.048
L-Lactate	4.60		0.033	3.68		0.053
Succinate	1.48		0.026	2.12		0.064
DPNH	1.77		0.032	2.95		0.064
Formate	43.5		0.034	46.0		0.053
$Na_2S_2O_4$			0.034			0.102
B. Added sequentially						
Succinate + DPNH	2.95	3.25	0.033	5.10	5.07	0.062
Succinate + DPNH + L-lactate	6.75	7.85	0.031	8.90	8.75	0.063
Succinate + DPNH + formate	18.9	46.75	0.030	44.0	51.07	0.054
D- + L-lactate	3.85	6.83	0.031	1.35	4.35	0.054

manner described previously (9). Rates of oxygen uptake are expressed as millimicromoles of oxygen per second per 10 mg of bacterial protein or as millimicromoles of oxygen per second × 0.05/the difference in absorbance at 561 and 580 mμ in the anaerobic minus aerobic difference spectrum.

Ferricyanide reduction was followed spectrophotometrically at 425 mμ (4, 5). Under these conditions of assay, the rate of reduction is zero order (5).

Protein was measured by the biuret method (10) in the presence of 0.06% sodium deoxycholate.

Reagents—Rotenone (K and K Laboratories), thenoyltrifluoroacetone (Fisher Scientific Company), 2,4-dinitrophenol (Amend Drug Company), and carbonyl cyanide *m*-chlorophenylhydrazone (CalBioChem) were added as solutions in 95% ethanol. The inhibitor 2-*n*-heptyl-4-hydroxyquinoline *N*-oxide, the generous gift of Dr. J. W. Lightbown, was dissolved in 0.001 M KOH, and Dicumarol (Mann Research Laboratories) in 0.02 M KOH. The addition of equivalent volumes of ethanol or of KOH to the buffered reaction mixtures has no measurable effect on the rate of oxygen uptake. Quinacrine (3-chloro-7-methoxy-9-(1-methyl-4-diethylaminobutylamino)acridine hydrochloride), from Nutritional Biochemicals Corporation, and sodium secobarbital (sodium 5-allyl-5-(1-methylbutyl)barbiturate), from Eli Lilly and Company, were prepared in aqueous solutions. Crystalline perfluorosuccinate was synthesized by oxidation of cyclic $C_4F_4Cl_2$ (synthesized by Dr. T. R. Walton, Ohio State University) with permanganate (11).

RESULTS

H. parainfluenzae is characterized by an unusual permeability to pyridine nucleotides and substrates. One washing with weak buffer usually removes endogenous respiration, and an additional washing with weak buffer uniformly removes endogenous respiration. Addition of DPNH to intact bacteria results in an immediate rapid oxygen uptake with no measurable lag (3). Somewhat lower rates of respiration are observed in the presence

of substrates involved with pyridine nucleotide-linked enzymes (8). Since these bacteria have no apparent mechanism capable of oxidizing reduced pyridine nucleotide at a rate sufficient to promote growth at a detectable rate that does not involve electron transport to oxygen or nitrate (8), the addition of various substrates to bacteria suspended in phosphate buffer results in the accumulation of reduced pyridine nucleotide once the oxygen in the suspension is utilized. Consequently, the addition of substrates to bacteria suspended in phosphate buffer is followed by an increase in absorbance at 340 mμ, after the oxygen in the suspension is exhausted. This absorbance change is not a light scattering phenomenon as indicated by the sharp maximum at 340 mμ. These results are illustrated in Fig. 1. Various substrates produce reduced pyridine nucleotide at different rates, but the total amount produced is always the same. Adding other metabolites, TPN, or DPN after reduced pyridine nucleotide production is complete (*right-hand arrow* in Fig. 1A) does not result in further increases in reduced pyridine nucleotide. Adding two substrates simultaneously produces a greater rate of reduced pyridine nucleotide production than either added singly but does not effect the total amount produced. Nitrate can cause the reoxidation of reduced cytochromes in this bacterium (3), and the addition of nitrate can cause the disappearance of reduced pyridine nucleotide absorbance. The capacity of the electron transport system to reduce pyridine nucleotide is much greater than the rate at which it is generated. The amount of reduced pyridine nucleotide produced in the presence of substrates is between 100 and 200 mμmoles per g, dry weight.

If stationary phase bacteria are held at 0° for several hours in phosphate buffer, the rates of oxygen utilization with these substrates can be increased by adding DPN. Such an experiment with the use of citrate is illustrated in Fig. 2. Anaerobically these bacteria can produce DPNH from the DPN added to intact cells in the presence of a suitable substrate. The DPNH produced can reach levels 100 times that detected with freshly harvested bacteria in the presence of substrate. The

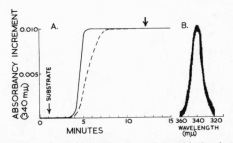

FIG. 1. *A*, change in absorbance at 340 mμ with time in the presence of 10 mM α-ketoglutarate (———) or 10 mM citrate (– – –) to suspensions of intact parental type *H. parainfluenzae*. The sample cuvette was allowed to go anaerobic in the presence of substrate, which was added when indicated by the *left-hand arrow*. Experiments with an identical suspension with the oxygen electrode established that pyridine nucleotide reduction began after anaerobiosis and that there was no endogenous respiratory activity. Addition of other substrates or 1 mM DPN or TPN at the time indicated by the *right-hand arrow* had no effect on the amount of pyridine nucleotide reduced. Data were obtained with the Cary model 14CM spectrophotometer with the scattered transmission accessory and intense visible light source between identical bacterial suspensions containing 14.5 mg of protein per cm of light path in 50 mM phosphate buffer, pH 7.6, at 25°. Under these conditions the dispersion of the spectrophotometer at 340 mμ was ±9 A. *B*, the difference spectrum of the reduced pyridine nucleotide produced 18 minutes after the addition of α-ketoglutarate, plotted to give an indication of the noise level. Similar difference spectra are produced with glucose, malate, citrate, and pyruvate.

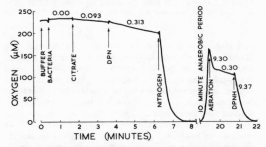

FIG. 2. Tracing of the respiration of intact parental type *H. parainfluenzae* (34.0 mg of protein) grown with 20 mM glucose, added to 3 ml of 50 mM phosphate buffer, pH 7.6, at 30° in the oxygen electrode as described (7, 9). Irregularities result from adding bacteria, substrates, or bubbling nitrogen or air (aeration). The bacteria have no endogenous respiration, and utilize oxygen in the presence of 20 mM citrate and 6 mM DPN. The suspension is then deoxygenated with nitrogen and incubated with bubbling nitrogen for 10 minutes in the presence of 0.05 ml of Dow-Corning Antifoam B. After 10 minutes, the suspension is aerated with air, and the initial rate observed after aeration is equivalent to that of added DPNH (3 mM). Respiratory rates are written above the tracing, expressed as millimicromoles of O₂ per second.

parental type reacts more readily with added DPN. The ability to reduce added DPN can be used to show that DPNH formed anaerobically can be oxidized in the presence of oxygen at the same rate as DPNH added to the bacterial suspension. This result is illustrated in Fig. 2.

Although intact cells can oxidize a large variety of substrates (8), the insoluble particles which bear the electron transport

chain can only respire in the presence of formate, DPNH, D- and L-lactate, and succinate. These are the substances most rapidly oxidized by the intact cells (8). A comparison of the rates of respiration of intact cells with respiratory particles is shown in Table II. The electron transport system is concentrated in the membrane fragments as indicated by the increase in specific activity of the substrate-provoked respiration (Table II) and the demonstration that all the substrate-reducible cytochromes are found in this fraction (4). The membrane-linked primary dehydrogenases of these bacteria can be assayed readily by use of ferricyanide reduction in the presence of cyanide (5). The ferricyanide reduction capacity of the particles with DPNH, lactate, or succinate corresponds to the oxygen uptake per electron transferred. Formate ferricyanide reductase has about one-fourth of the activity predicted from its respiratory activity (5). Very little ferricyanide reductase activity is found in the supernatant, indicating that these primary dehydrogenases are all membrane-bound.

The respiratory capacity of the particles can be reduced differentially by prolonged incubation in phosphate buffer at 0° as seen in Table III. There is considerable decrease in specific activity with D- or L-lactate. Even so, the rates of respiration expressed in terms of the extent of reduction of cytochrome b₁ by a given substrate are quite similar for the intact bacteria and aged particles. When fresh membrane preparations are exposed to ultrasonic energy, there ensues a loss of both ferricyanide and oxygen utilization capacity in the membrane fraction, which is exactly balanced by ferricyanide reductase in the supernatant (5). The concentration of substrate giving half-maximal reaction rates for the different substrates are not very different with whole cells and with the small particles, as seen in Table IV.

TABLE II

Comparison of rates of oxygen utilization and ferricyanide reduction of bacteria, respiratory particles, and supernatant fractions of H. parainfluenzae

Bacteria were harvested after 12 hours of incubation, centrifuged, washed with 50 mM phosphate buffer, pH 7.6, ruptured with alumina, and resuspended in phosphate buffer. Centrifugation at 6,000 × *g* for 10 minutes removed alumina and whole cells; then the particles were collected at 12,000 × *g* for 10 minutes. The supernatant was centrifuged at 105,000 × *g* for 45 minutes, and the small membrane fragments were combined with those in the 12,000 × *g* pellet in phosphate buffer. Oxygen uptake measurements were made as in Table I. Ferricyanide reduction was followed spectrophotometrically at 425 mμ after addition of substrates to cuvettes containing about 5 mg of protein, 0.5 mM ferricyanide, and 5 mM KCN in 50 mM phosphate buffer, pH 7.6, at 30° as described (5). DPN (10 mM) was added with glucose and malate.

Substrate	Oxygen uptake		Ferricyanide reduced	
	Bacteria	Particles	Particles	Supernatant
	mμmoles/sec/10 mg protein			
Formate..............	52.00	58.00	63.0	<0.02
DPNH...............	6.40	14.00	61.5	6.6
D-Lactate.............	1.88	2.54	11.2	<0.02
L-Lactate.............	3.40	6.24	25.0	<0.02
Succinate.............	1.27	3.00	13.6	<0.02
Malate (+DPN).......	0.68	<0.01		
Glucose (+DPN)......	0.62	<0.01		

The relative concentrations of substrate-reducible cytochrome c_1 can be varied over a wide range and still provide the organism with the efficient electron transport system that it needs to survive. The same variability is also possible in the relative concentration of cytochrome b_1. Some of the data on which this conclusion is based are illustrated in Fig. 3. Since the α maximum of reduced cytochrome c_1 is 553 mμ (3) and that of reduced cytochrome b_1 is 561 mμ, the presence of one cytochrome could obscure the presence of the other. Certain information is necessary to evaluate the relative concentration of cytochrome b_1 in the presence of membrane-bound cytochrome c_1. Membrane preparations can be depleted of cytochrome c_1 (4). The membrane-bound and the cytochrome c_1 rendered soluble have essentially identical absorption spectra (4), indicating that functionally active, membrane-bound cytochrome c_1 and soluble cytochrome c_1 have very similar if not identical extinction coefficients. Membrane preparations depleted of cytochrome c_1 have an absorbance at 561 mμ that is proportional to the protein content of the membrane. Intact bacteria of the mutant strain harvested in the late log phase of an appropriate growth condi-

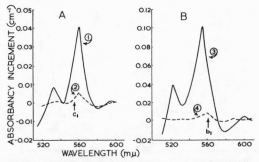

FIG. 3. The difference spectra between membrane fragments of *H. parainfluenzae* allowed to go anaerobic in the presence of DPNH (10 mM) compared to an identical aerobic suspension. Spectra were measured at a protein concentration of 10 mg per ml with membranes prepared by grinding with alumina (4) in 50 mM phosphate buffer, pH 7.6, at 25°. *A*, washed membrane fragments of the mutant which does not form large amounts of cytochrome c_1: *Curve 1* (——), measured with bacteria grown anaerobically with nitrate harvested in the late log phase; *Curve 2* (– – –), measured with bacteria grown with vigorous aeration (7). *B*, *Curve 3* (——), resuspended alumina-ruptured cells of the parental type grown in a deep, unshaken culture flask in medium without glucose were harvested at the initiation of the stationary phase; *Curve 4* (– – –), difference spectrum of these particles washed four times with phosphate buffer, frozen, and thawed twice as described (4). Rates of oxygen uptake were measured at DPNH concentrations that were not rate-limiting and are expressed as millimicromoles of oxygen per second per 10 mg of protein at 30°: *Curve 1*, 3.48; *Curve 2*, 1.00; *Curve 3*, 3.43; *Curve 4*, 0.005. The *arrow* in *Part A* indicates 553 mμ; the *arrow* in *Part B* indicates 561 mμ.

TABLE III

Comparison of respiratory rate of bacteria and aged respiratory particles of H. parainfluenzae

Bacteria were harvested after 24 hours of incubation, centrifuged, washed with 50 mM phosphate buffer, pH 7.6, ruptured with alumina, and resuspended in phosphate buffer. After centrifugation at 6,000 × g for 10 minutes to separate intact bacteria and alumina, particles were collected by centrifugation at 12,000 × g and aged at 0° for 6 hours before use. Oxygen utilization was measured as in Table I and expressed as rate per 10 mg of protein or as rate per 0.05 absorbance unit of cytochrome b_1 reduced after anaerobiosis produced with that substrate.

Substrate	Oxygen utilization per 10 mg of protein		Oxygen utilization per 0.05 absorbance of cytochrome b_1	
	Bacteria	Particles	Bacteria	Particles
	mμmoles/sec		*mμmoles/sec*	
Formate	26.0	16.0	35.0	34.0
DPNH	4.16	3.12	7.9	7.9
D-Lactate	6.31	0.13	6.5	6.1
L-Lactate	7.40	0.25	7.1	7.0
Succinate	4.66	3.48	6.7	6.7

TABLE IV

K_m values for formate, DPNH, D-lactate, L-lactate, and succinate measured with intact bacteria and respiratory particles

K_m values were obtained from a Lineweaver-Burk (12) plot of reciprocal respiratory rate *versus* reciprocal substrate concentration with bacteria and respiratory particles similar to those used for Table II.

Substrate	K_m with intact bacteria	K_m with respiratory particles
	mM	*mM*
Formate	0.04	0.16
DPNH	0.20	0.06
D-Lactate	1.7	0.37
L-Lactate	2.0	0.31
Succinate	0.29	0.10

tion contain no detectable cytochrome c_1 on reduction with $Na_2S_2O_4$. On rupture of the bacteria by grinding with alumina, sonic vibration, or the Hughes press, no detectable cytochrome b_1 is found in the supernatant suspension, and all the cytochrome b_1 found in the intact bacteria can be accounted for by that found in the membrane fraction. Subjecting the membranes to the washing and freeze-thaw procedure (4), which removes cytochrome c_1, does not alter the content of cytochrome b_1. If the washings are lyophilized and treated with acid-acetone, and the resultant protohemin chromatographed and detected by its pyridine-hemochromogen or by the ultrasensitive benzidine spray according to classical methods (13), essentially no protohemin can be detected. Bacteria harvested under these growth conditions contain an insignificant catalase activity (6). Treatment of the membrane by this procedure uniformly yields protohemin with a content that roughly parallels the cytochrome b_1 content (14). Consequently the absorbance at 561 mμ on reduction is a real measure of the relative cytochrome b_1 concentration if the influence of cytochrome c_1 on this spectrum can be established. We have established that soluble cytochrome c_1 has a c-type pyridine-hemochromogen (3) and that hematohemin is liberated only after reduction of the thioester bonds (14). If membranes similar to those used for the experiments illustrated in Fig. 3*A*, which show no spectral evidence for cytochrome c_1, are treated with acid-acetone, then reduction with Ag_2SO_4 followed by isolation of hemin or porphyrin, no significant evidence for amounts of the hemato derivative can be found.

The absorbance of soluble reduced cytochrome c_1 at 553 mμ is proportional to the protein concentration. Examination of the spectra of reduced, soluble, partially purified cytochrome c_1 indicates that at 561 mμ it has 65% of the absorbance that it shows at 553 mμ. The influence of cytochrome b_1 on the absorbance of cytochrome c_1 is a bit more difficult to access. We can set an upper limit on the possible effect of cytochrome b_1 on membrane-bound cytochrome c_1 by use of a preparation of the mutant strain incubated in the stationary growth phase until it develops a respiratory system that has the spectrum illustrated in Fig. 1B of Reference 7. Bacterial membranes can be depleted of all detectable cytochrome c_1 by repeating the washing and freeze-thaw technique (4) 10 times. This treatment reduces the respiratory activity 1000-fold, and no further cytochrome c_1 can be removed. The soluble cytochrome c_1 removed and the absorption of the remaining cytochrome b_1 roughly correspond to the facts that at 561 mμ cytochrome c_1 accounts for 61% of the absorbance, and that at 553 mμ cytochrome b_1 accounts for 45% of the absorption at 553 mμ. In the case of the wild-type strain illustrated in Fig. 3B, the complication of the overlap of reduced cytochrome b_1 and c_1 is readily corrected. Removing all detectable cytochrome c_1 as described (4), a procedure which lowers the rate of oxygen uptake with DPNH 400-fold, indicates that cytochrome b_1 can account for less than 3% of the absorbance at 553 mμ. We have established that this procedure does not remove cytochrome b_1.

With this information in hand, the data of Fig. 3 can be examined. The maximal rates of oxygen utilization measured

TABLE V

Inhibition of respiration of intact H. parainfluenzae in presence of various substrates

Data were calculated from the initial rate of oxygen utilization with substrate alone and the slowest rate achieved within 30 seconds after addition of inhibitor. Inhibitors were added when oxygen tension was greater than 100 μM. Oxygen utilization was measured as in Table I.

Inhibitor	Concentration	Inhibition in the presence of:				
		Formate	DPNH	D-Lactate	L-Lactate	Succinate
	μmoles/3 ml	%	%	%	%	%
Quinacrine	0.12	34	59	97	56	84
Secobarbital	12.0	86	89	98	92	97
Thenoyltrifluoroacetone	30	50	71	96	89	92
Oxalate	60	14	53	95	92	99
Rotenone	0.05	0	0	0	0	25
Malonate	60	0	0	0	0	87
Monoethyloxalacetate	30	0	0	0	0	100
Perfluorosuccinate	60	0	0	0	0	61
Oxamate	60	0	0	0	0	0
2,4-Dinitrophenol	0.1	25	30	50	33	40
CCP	0.01	40	96	60	60	95
Dicumarol	0.09	60	56	96	66	85
2-n-Heptyl-4-hydroxyquinoline N-oxide	0.006	74	73	94	87	98
Azide	60	73	97	97	50	88
Cyanide	5	97	100	100	100	100
Carbon monoxide	40% (v/v)	27	25	20	27	26

in the presence of DPNH concentrations that are not rate-limiting are given in Fig. 3. By comparing the mutant bacteria grown with high aeration (*Curve 2*) and the parental type (*Curve 3*), a respiratory system capable of rapid electron transport can be fashioned by the living bacteria, involving at a *minimum* a 32-fold variability in functional cytochrome c_1 concentration. This assumes that all the absorbance at 553 mμ in *Curve 2* is due exclusively to cytochrome c_1. With correction for the increment that cytochrome b_1 adds to the absorbance at 553 mμ, the *maximal* level of cytochrome c_1 that could be present in this bacterium is 72-fold less than that constructed by the bacterium grown under conditions producing maximal enzymatically reducible cytochrome c_1. This is also an underestimate of the variability of functional cytochrome c_1, since the absence of hematohemin isolated from the membranes similar to those reduced in *Curve 2* indicates that actually little if any cytochrome c_1 is present. *Curve 4* (Fig. 3) clearly indicates that essentially all the absorbance at 553 mμ is due to cytochrome c_1.

In Fig. 3A, variation in the growth condition can lead to a 9-fold change in the content of enzymatically reducible cytochrome b_1 and yet provide for an active electron transport system. This assumes that cytochrome c_1 makes no contribution to the absorbance at 553 mμ. On the assumption that there is no cytochrome c_1 in the bacteria grown with high aeration and that the maximal amount is present in the anaerobically grown bacteria, the range of variability would still be 6-fold.

It has been established that the rate-limiting component in the electron transport system of this bacterium is near the flavoprotein dehydrogenases (5). It has also been established that the greater the concentration of a given membrane-bound primary dehydrogenase, the greater the proportion of cytochromes c_1 or b_1 or both reduced, and the more rapid the rate of oxygen utilization produced in the presence of the particular substrate (Table VII of Reference 5). In the experiments illustrated in Fig. 3, conditions of growth were chosen such that DPNH reduced all the membrane-bound cytochrome reducible by $Na_2S_2O_4$. If growth conditions are chosen in such a way that all five dehydrogenases are present in roughly similar amounts, combinations of substrates can be tested effectively for their effects on the level of cytochrome reduction and the rate of electron transport in both mutant and parental types. Such data are illustrated in Table I, Part B, and show that the respiratory rate in the presence of combinations of substrates is additive with the parental strain except for the mixture of D- and L-lactate and a combination containing formate. The order of addition has no effect on the final rate of respiration. With the mutant, the rates observed with mixtures of substrates were always less than additive, and the discrepancy was particularly marked with mixtures containing formate. The cytochrome b_1 of the mutant could be completely reduced in the presence of formate and L-lactate and was incompletely reduced by the other substrates. In the parental type, the greatest amount of cytochrome c_1 was reduced by DPNH and succinate, and somewhat less was reduced with the other substrates. As reported previously (3, 4, 6), some of the cytochrome c_1 could only be reduced with $Na_2S_2O_4$, and this is the cytochrome c_1 which is not membrane-bound (4). Addition of mixtures of substrates does not produce increases in the proportions of cytochromes b_1 and c_1 reduced with either strain.

The effect of the addition of a number of known respiratory chain inhibitors is shown in Table V. Both inhibited and uninhibited rates were measured when the respiratory chain system was saturated with both substrate and oxygen. This was done by making the measurements at relatively high oxygen concentrations, since inhibition of electron transport can result in an apparent increased K_m value for oxygen (7). In most cases maximal inhibition was observed within 30 seconds after the addition of inhibitor to the cells or particles.

Azide, cyanide, and carbon monoxide, typical inhibitors of cytochrome oxidases, showed the expected inhibitory effect on the respiration of whole cells and insoluble particles. Representative data with whole cells are shown in Table V. The inhibition by carbon monoxide was observed to be partially relieved by illumination with strong white light.

2-n-Heptyl-4-hydroxyquinoline N-oxide, which inhibits the oxidation of cytochrome b in some bacteria (15) and inhibits transfer of electrons from cytochrome b to cytochrome c_1 in the mammalian cytochrome system (16), depressed respiration between 70 and 100% with all substrates tested when present in a concentration of 18 μM.

Respiration in the presence of succinate is strongly inhibited by malonate and by monoethyloxaloacetate, typical inhibitors of succinic dehydrogenase (17, 18), and by perfluorosuccinate. The enzyme of *H. parainfluenzae* is unusually sensitive to inhibition by malonate. However, no inhibition was observed on addition of 0.05 M oxaloacetate.

The respiration of the cells is inhibited to varying extents with the five substrates if tested by a number of substances which inhibit flavoprotein enzymes: quinacrine (19), secobarbital (20), thenoyltrifluoroacetone (21), and oxalate (Table V). The respiration with D-lactate is unusual in that it varies depending upon whether the cells are grown in glucose or in gluconate (or glucuronate). When glucose is the carbon source during growth, the respiration of the cells in the presence of D-lactate can be blocked by all inhibitors of electron transport down the cytochrome chain, and the cytochromes are reduced in the presence of D-lactate under anaerobic conditions. If the bacteria are grown in media supplemented with gluconic or glucuronic acid, the addition of D-lactate produces respiration insensitive to inhibition by 2-n-heptyl-4-hydroxyquinoline N-oxide or inhibitors of cytochrome oxidases, and the cytochromes are not reduced when the cells are anaerobic in the presence of D-lactate. The respiration of cells grown in gluconate is inhibited by secobarbital, thenoyltrifluoroacetone, oxalate, and, to a small degree, by quinacrine. The respiration is dependent upon the concentration of oxygen in solution up to 100%; this resembles the respiration of the hemin-requiring *Hemophilus* species grown with aeration in the presence of limiting concentrations of hemin; under these conditions an autoxidizable flavoprotein mediates the respiration (9).

The data of Table V also show that rotenone and oxamate, which inhibit DPNH dehydrogenase and lactate dehydrogenases, respectively, in mammalian cells (22, 23), were without effect on the DPNH- and lactate-stimulated respiration of intact cells. The uncoupling agents of mammalian systems, 2,4-dinitrophenol, CCP,[1] and Dicumarol, showed inhibitory effects on respiration. The inhibition with CCP always occurs after a lag period in agreement with observations of Avi-Dor (24) on *E. coli*.

[1] The abbreviation used is: CCP, carbonyl cyanide m-chlorophenylhydrazone.

The respiration of the insoluble particles was also inhibited by the above substances.

DISCUSSION

From the data presented in this paper plus our previous observations (3–7), the following picture of hydrogen and electron transfer in *H. parainfluenzae* emerges.

1. The cytochrome system and at least five dehydrogenases can be bound to insoluble cellular membranes, presumably the cytoplasmic membrane. The five dehydrogenases appear to be flavoproteins (see also White (5)). The five flavoproteins, like the cytochromes, are synthesized at different rates, and these vary with the growth conditions and the growth phase. They appear to be arranged in varying numbers around the different cytochrome chains in a three-dimensional array, as previously suggested for two of the dehydrogenases (4, 6), with some overlapping of the flavoproteins and the different cytochrome assemblies. This arrangement would explain the observations in Table I, Part B, and in Table VII of White (5) that (a) respiration with a combination of substrates of these dehydrogenases may or may not be additive, and (b) the extent of reduction of the predominant cytochrome under anaerobic conditions is different with the different substrates and is usually the same as the amount reduced with one substrate when a combination of substrates is added.

The linkages of some of the dehydrogenases (e.g. D- or L-lactate) with the membrane system are more easily broken than others (formate or succinate or DPNH); they are dissociated at different rates as a suspension of the particles ages, even at 0°. The formate dehydrogenase is particularly tightly bound and appears to be less accessible for reaction with added oxidation-reduction substances (ferricyanide) or inhibitors.

2. The numerous other cellular dehydrogenases are not membrane-bound, or are so loosely associated with the membrane that they are easily detached on rupture of the cells (8). Various substrates can reduce what appears to be a single pool of pyridine nucleotide. The pool of pyridine nucleotide that is capable of enzymatic reduction is not in rapid equilibrium with DPN added to intact bacteria unless the cells have been damaged by incubation at 0°. The reduced pyridine nucleotide formed enzymatically can be oxidized by the membrane-bound electron transport system as rapidly as DPNH added to the bacterial suspension. There is no evidence for compartmentation of DPN or DPNH within this bacterium.

3. The rate of oxidation of substrates of pyridine nucleotide-linked enzymes is low compared to the oxidation of DPNH by the DPNH dehydrogenase and the cytochrome chain. The capacity for electron transport in the cytochrome chain is still larger than the rate of oxidation of DPNH by the DPNH dehydrogenases, as shown by the rate of oxidation of formate. Apparently, various metabolic reactions in this bacterium produce DPNH, succinate, formate, D-lactate, and L-lactate, which diffuse to the membrane-bound electron transport system where they are rapidly oxidized.

4. The ease of removal of substrates and pyridine nucleotides from the electron transport system of *H. parainfluenzae* and the rapid penetration of these substances into intact cells make these bacteria suitable for comparison of the reactions of this system in intact bacteria with that on the derived membrane fragments collected on rupture of the cells. Immediately upon rupture, the specific activity of the isolated respiratory chain

particles with the different substrates is increased on a protein basis, and the K_m values for the different substrates are rather similar with intact cells and particles. As the dehydrogenases dissociate from the membranes on standing, the respiratory rates with the appropriate substrates decrease; then the respiratory rates are related to the amount of cytochrome that can be reduced under anaerobic conditions. Experiments reported elsewhere (5) show that the dehydrogenases lost from the membrane are found in the supernatant fluid. Thus only the dehydrogenases that remain associated with the membrane system are active in electron transport. Similar observations have been reported (4) for the cytochrome c_1 of the parental type.

5. The respiratory chain system of *H. parainfluenzae* is sensitive to inhibition by a number of substances which inhibit other respiratory chain systems. For example, the oxidases of the mutant used in these experiments are inhibited by cyanide, azide, and carbon monoxide. 2-*n*-Heptyl-4-hydroxyquinoline *N*-oxide inhibits the bacterial electron transport chain in the region of cytochrome b_1, as in mammalian cells, and the flavoprotein dehydrogenases are inhibited by typical inhibitors of other flavoprotein enzymes. The succinate dehydrogenase of *H. parainfluenzae* is unusually sensitive to inhibition by malonate, as compared with the mammalian enzyme (25), but is insensitive to oxaloacetate. Rotenone, which is strongly inhibitory to the mammalian DPNH dehydrogenase (22), has no effect on the dehydrogenase of *H. parainfluenzae*. The most startling difference in the effect of inhibitors on the bacterial respiration is seen in the strong inhibition by dinitrophenol, Dicumarol, and CCP, which are uncouplers of mammalian oxidative phosphorylation but do not inhibit respiration in such low concentrations.

The data presented above give a picture of the localization of the enzymes for hydrogen and electron transport in this bacterial cell. They also show that in most aspects the bacterial system resembles that in mammalian mitochondria. On rupture of the cells, electron transport proceeds rapidly to the extent that the pigments remain associated with the membrane in the proper orientation. There is one really important difference between the bacterial and mammalian respiratory chain systems. This difference is the great variability of the relative proportions of the different pigments (both cytochromes and flavoproteins) in bacteria grown under different conditions or harvested at different times during the growth cycle. The bacteria have the ability to modify greatly the composition of the electron transport complex. Also, the differences in the relative rates of synthesis of the various cytochromes by the mutant as compared to the parental type make possible the harvesting of bacteria with widely different proportions of the cytochromes. We have established that a membrane-bound respiratory system capable of rapid electron transport can be fashioned by the living bacteria with a 3-fold range in DPNH dehydrogenase, a 27-fold range in formate dehydrogenase, a 500-fold range of D-lactate dehydrogenase, a 1400-fold range of L-lactate dehydrogenase, and an 8-fold range of succinate dehydrogenase activities (5). The cytochrome b_1 concentration can be modified over *at least* a 6- to 10-fold range, and the cytochrome c_1 concentration over *at least* a 32- to 72-fold range that is compatible with the rapid electron transport system which we have shown to be absolutely necessary for growth in this bacteria. The cytochrome oxidase *o* can vary over a 4-fold range, the cytochrome oxidase a_1 can vary over *at least* a 70-fold range, and the cytochrome oxidase a_2 can vary over *at least* a 10-fold range (3). Three, four, or five dehydrogenases or one,

two, or three oxidases may be present in the functionally active electron transport system. In spite of the great variabilities in the quantities of the different cytochromes making up the respiratory chain system, the rates of respiration do not differ greatly (Table I and Fig. 3) (2, 5) unless the content of the flavoprotein dehydrogenases is changed. The rate-limiting step never appears to be in the cytochrome chain. It has been suggested that these observations with these bacteria mean that the pigments are synthesized separately, then incorporated into the membrane-bound system (4, 6, 7). In addition, the data also give additional insight into the structure of the respiratory chain system. There is no evidence that this system in *Hemophilus* is composed of several multienzyme packets, each with a fixed proportion of respiratory pigments. In fact, the type of elementary repeating unit of electron transport formed by the stoichiometric accretion of four multienzyme complexes, each of fixed composition, used as a model for beef mitochondria (26), obviously does not apply to this bacterium. In spite of the lack of consistency of the proportion of the different pigments, the bacterial respiratory chain system is always capable of rapid electron transport.

The two lactate dehydrogenases of *H. parainfluenzae* are not DPN-linked enzymes; in this respect they resemble the enzymes of yeast (27, 28). The L-lactate dehydrogenase of *H. parainfluenzae* can pass reducing equivalents to the cytochrome system, although it is not clear that the enzyme of yeast can do this (29). It has recently been reported that the D-lactate dehydrogenase of yeast does react with the respiratory chain system (30, 31).

The D-lactate dehydrogenase activity of *H. parainfluenzae* is different in cells grown in different media. In cells grown with glucose, the dehydrogenase appears to be a membrane-bound enzyme which can react directly with the cytochrome system. Like the other dehydrogenases, it does not react with oxygen at a detectable rate when dissociated from the membrane (5). In cells grown with gluconate, the enzyme is not linked to the respiratory chain system and reacts with oxygen as a typical flavoprotein oxidase. This observation is reminiscent of the work of Somlo (32), who showed that the activity of yeast L-lactate dehydrogenase is different depending upon whether or not it is membrane-bound.

SUMMARY

Studies of respiration and difference spectra in the presence of a number of substrates and inhibitors show the respiratory chain system of *Hemophilus parainfluenzae* to have many properties similar to that in mammalian tissues. The main differences are the marked inhibition of respiration produced by uncouplers of oxidative phosphorylation and the variability in the proportions of the respiratory pigments that can be induced environmentally. Two forms of *H. parainfluenzae*, one a mutant of the other, show similar respiratory activity even when they contain widely differing proportions of cytochromes. These data, plus previous observations with these bacteria, show that the bacterial respiratory chain system cannot be composed of "elementary particles" with a fixed composition. The data can only be explained in terms of a variable three-dimensional array of pigments.

The membrane-bound respiratory chain system contains the cytochromes and five flavoprotein dehydrogenases, while the pyridine nucleotide-linked dehydrogenases are in the cytoplasm.

The reduced diphosphopyridine nucleotide generated diffuses rapidly to the membrane-bound reduced diphosphopyridine nucleotide dehydrogenase. The over-all rate of respiration is always limited by the activity of the dehydrogenases. Insoluble respiratory particles collected after rupture of the cells contain the respiratory chain system with increased specific activity. On aging, even at 0°, the pigments become dissociated at different rates. Only the pigments which remain membrane-bound participate in rapid electron transport.

Acknowledgments—The authors wish to express appreciation for the skillful assistance of Miss Marjorie Krause and Miss Willa A. Duke.

REFERENCES

1. CHANCE, B., AND WILLIAMS, G. R., in F. F. NORD (Editor)' *Advances in enzymology*, Vol. 17, Interscience Publishers' Inc., New York, 1956, p. 65.
2. SMITH, L., in I. C. GUNSALUS AND R. Y. STANIER (Editors), *The bacteria*, Vol. 2, Academic Press, Inc., New York, 1961, p. 215.
3. WHITE, D. C., AND SMITH, L., *J. Biol. Chem.*, **237**, 1332 (1962).
4. SMITH, L., AND WHITE, D. C., *J. Biol. Chem.*, **237**, 1337 (1962).
5. WHITE, D. C., *J. Biol. Chem.*, **239**, 2055 (1964).
6. WHITE, D. C., *J. Bacteriol.*, **83**, 851 (1962).
7. WHITE, D. C., *J. Biol. Chem.*, **238**, 3757 (1963).
8. WHITE, D. C., *J. Bacteriol.*, in press.
9. WHITE, D. C., *J. Bacteriol.*, **85**, 84 (1963).
10. GORNALL, A. G., BARDAWILL, C. J., AND DAVID, M. M., *J. Biol. Chem.*, **177**, 751 (1949).
11. HENNE, A. L., AND ZIMMERSCHIED, W. J., *J. Am. Chem. Soc.*, **69**, 281 (1947).
12. LINEWEAVER, H., AND BURK, D., *J. Am. Chem. Soc.*, **56**, 648 (1934).
13. FALK, J. E., *Porphyrins and metalloporphyrins*, Elsevier Publishing Company, Amsterdam, New York, 1964, pp. 94–103, 181–212.
14. WHITE, D. C., Ph D. thesis, The Rockefeller Institute, 1962.
15. LIGHTBOWN, J. W., *J. Gen. Microbiol.*, **11**, 477 (1954).
16. LIGHTBOWN, J. W., AND JACKSON, F. W., *Biochem. J.*, **63**, 130 (1956).
17. KREBS, H. A., AND EGGLESTON, L. V., *Biochem. J.*, **34**, 442 (1940).
18. HELLERMAN, L., REISS, O. K., PARMAR, S. S., WEIN, J., AND LASSER, N. L., *J. Biol. Chem.*, **235**, 2468 (1960).
19. HAAS, E., *J. Biol. Chem.*, **155**, 321 (1944).
20. ERNSTER, L., JALLING, O., LÖW, H., AND LINDBERG, O., *Exptl. Cell. Research*, **3** (suppl.), 124 (1955).
21. TAPPEL, A. L., *Biochem. Pharmacol.*, **3**, 289 (1960).
22. ÖBERG, K. E., *Exptl. Cell. Research*, **24**, 163 (1961).
23. PAPACONSTANTINOU, J., AND COLOWICK, S. P., *Federation Proc.*, **18**, 298 (1959).
24. AVI-DOR, Y., *Acta Chem. Scand.*, **17**, 144 (1963).
25. SINGER, T. P., AND KEARNEY, E. B., in P. D. BOYER, H. LARDY, AND K. MYRBÄCK (Editors), *The enzymes*, Vol. 7, Academic Press, Inc., New York, 1963, p. 383.
26. GREEN, D. E., *Sci. American*, **210**, 63 (1964).
27. NYGAARD, A., *Ann. N. Y. Acad. Sci.*, **94**, 774 (1961).
28. APPLEBY, C. A., AND MORTON, R. K., *Biochem. J.*, **71**, 492 (1959).
29. CHANCE, B., in J. E. FALK, R. LEMBERG, AND R. K. MORTON (Editors), *Haematin enzymes*, Pergamon Press, New York, 1961, p. 597.
30. ROY, B. R., *Nature*, **201**, 80 (1964).
31. GREGOLIN, C., AND D'ALBERTON, A., *Biochem. and Biophys. Research Communs.*, **14**, 103 (1964).
32. SOMLO, M., *Biochim. et Biophys. Acta*, **65**, 333 (1962).

Editor's Comments
on Papers 14 and 15

14   McCORD, KEELE, and FRIDOVICH
      An Enzyme-Based Theory of Obligate Anaerobiosis: The Physiological Function of Superoxide Dismutase

15   HERBERT and PINSENT
      Crystalline Bacterial Catalase

CONSEQUENCES OF OXYGEN UTILIZATION

The use of oxygen as terminal electron acceptor for respiration is not without biological hazard, since highly reactive products arise by partial reduction of dioxygen. The following selections consider the mechanisms that have developed to "detoxify" such reagents.

Following the discovery by McCord and Fridovich that superoxide dismutase activity was displayed by a copper-containing erythrocyte protein,[1,2] McCord, Keele, and Fridovich surveyed the superoxide dismutase contents of bacteria and found it absent from obligate anaerobes. They accordingly offered a satisfying hypothesis to explain obligate anaerobiosis in Paper 14.

Destruction of hydrogen peroxide formed as the result of superoxide dismutase or other activity is accomplished by peroxidatic or catalatic activity. Denis Herbert and Jane Pinsent (Jane Gibson) describe in Paper 15 their achievement of the first crystallization of an enzyme from a bacterial source, the hemoprotein catalase.

REFERENCES

1. McCord, J., and I. Fridovich. *J. Biol. Chem.*, **243**, 5753–5760, 1968.
2. McCord, J., and I. Fridovich. *J. Biol. Chem.*, **244**, 6049–6077, 1969.

14

Reprinted from *Proc. Nat. Acad. Sci.* **68**:1024–1027 (1971)

An Enzyme-Based Theory of Obligate Anaerobiosis: The Physiological Function of Superoxide Dismutase

JOE M. McCORD, BERNARD B. KEELE, JR.*, AND IRWIN FRIDOVICH

Department of Biochemistry, Duke University Medical Center, Durham, North Carolina 27706

Communicated by Philip Handler, February 11, 1971

ABSTRACT The distribution of catalase and superoxide dismutase has been examined in various microorganisms. Strict anaerobes exhibited no superoxide dismutase and, generally, no catalase activity. All aerobic organisms containing cytochrome systems were found to contain both superoxide dismutase and catalase. Aerotolerant anaerobes, which survive exposure to air and metabolize oxygen to a limited extent but do not contain cytochrome systems, were found to be devoid of catalase activity but did exhibit superoxide dismutase activity. This distribution is consistent with the proposal that the prime physiological function of superoxide dismutase is protection of oxygen-metabolizing organisms against the potentially detrimental effects of the superoxide free radical, a biologically produced intermediate resulting from the univalent reduction of molecular oxygen.

Pasteur's discovery that certain organisms are not only capable of growing in oxygen-free environments, but in many cases are restricted to such environments, has never been satisfactorily explained. Obligately anaerobic organisms are strongly inhibited or killed by exposure to molecular oxygen (1). The possible role of catalase in protecting aerobic microorganisms from death by hydrogen peroxide poisoning was rather quickly recognized. In 1893 Gottstein discovered that certain bacteria decomposed H_2O_2 with the liberation of a gas (2). In 1907 it was observed that certain anaerobic bacteria contain no detectable catalase, whereas all the aerobes examined exhibited significant catalatic activity (3). This led to proposals that oxygen toxicity was occasioned by its reduction product, hydrogen peroxide (4, 5). Proceeding from this assumption investigators reasoned (4) that: (a) H_2O_2 should accumulate in aerobic cultures of anaerobes, as a result either of bacterial metabolism or of the action of light on the medium, (b) anaerobes should be sensitive to externally added hydrogen peroxide and, (c) anaerobes should grow aerobically when catalase is present in the medium. Technical limitations at the time prevented detection of the low but toxic concentrations of H_2O_2 that anaerobes produce. It was, however, subsequently shown that nearly all anaerobes do produce H_2O_2 (6). The sensitivity of anaerobes to H_2O_2 was readily shown, and a high degree of variation was apparent (4, 7). It could *not* be shown that the presence of catalase would allow aerobic growth of anaerobes (4, 5), although one anaerobe grew better at low oxygen tension with catalase present (4). Thus, although catalase aids the survival of some microorganisms in aerobic media, catalase activity does not provide a sufficient answer. Many organisms capable of aerobic growth do not contain catalase, e.g., the streptococci, pneumococci, and lactic acid bacteria. More recently, *Agromyces ramnosus*, the predominant soil organism, was found to lack catalase, despite its aerobic metabolism (8, 9). Further, some strict anaerobes have catalase activity, yet cannot tolerate exposure to air (10).

The recent discovery and characterization of superoxide dismutase (11, 12) raised the question of its physiological role. The substrate, a reactive and potentially detrimental free-radical form of oxygen, had long been implicated as an intermediate in the reduction of O_2 by a family of metalloflavoenzymes (13–17). Evidence that the superoxide radical is released into free solution from the enzyme surface was not obtained until 1968 (11), but was then quickly confirmed for the xanthine oxidase system by the detection of its electron paramagnetic resonance signal (18). The reaction catalyzed by superoxide dismutase,

$$O_2^- + O_2^- + 2H^+ \longrightarrow O_2 + H_2O_2,$$

proceeds spontaneously at pH 7.7, with a rate constant of approximately $2 \times 10^5 \, M^{-1} \, sec^{-1}$ (19). The ubiquity and constancy of this enzymic activity in a wide variety of tissues and organisms led us to seek its physiological importance. Interest was heightened by the discovery that the superoxide dismutase of *Escherichia coli* is a manganoprotein (20), which bears little resemblance to the copper- and zinc-containing mammalian enzyme (12, 21), but which is nevertheless present in the organism at similar concentration and displays a nearly identical specific activity.

The data presented in this report strongly implicate superoxide dismutase as being vital to the existence of any organism that metabolizes oxygen.

MATERIALS AND METHODS

Frozen or lyophilized cells of certain microorganisms were generously supplied for this study as follows: *Salmonella typhimurium* and an unidentified pseudomonad from Dr. Henry Kamin; *Halobacterium salinarium* from Dr. Jayant Joshi; *Rhizobium japonicum* from Dr. Gerald Elkan; *Mycobacterium* sp. from Dr. Jerome Perry; *Veillonella alcalescens* and *Butyribacterium rettgeri* from Dr. Charles Wittenberger; *Clostridium pasteurianum*, *Clostridium sticklandii*, *Clostridium lentoputrescens*, *Clostridium barkeri*, and *Clostridium* sp. (strain M.E.) from Dr. T. C. Stadtman; *Butyrivibrio fibrisolvens* from Dr. Sam Tove; *Clostridium cellobioparum* and N2C3, an unclassified rumen organism, from Drs. Robert Mah and R. E. Hungate; *Zymobacterium oroticum* from Dr.

---

* Present address: Institute of Dental Research, University of Alabama Medical Center, Birmingham, Ala. 35233.

K. V. Rajagopalan; and *Clostridium acetobutylicum* from Mr. Robert Waterson. *E. coli* cells were obtained as a frozen paste from Miles Laboratories. *Micrococcus radiodurans*, *Saccharomyces cerevisiae* (ATCC 560), *Streptococcus fecalis*, *Streptococcus mutans*, *Streptococcus bovis*, *Streptococcus mitis*, *Streptococcus lactis*, and *Lactobacillus plantarum* were grown by us on either trypticase soy broth or APT broth, available from BBL, Cockeysville, Md., or on Brain–Heart Infusion Broth obtained from Difco. Cultures were obtained as follows: *M. radiodurans* from Dr. Jane Setlow; *S. fecalis* and *L. plantarum* from Dr. John McNeill; and *S. mutans* 6715, *S. lactis* (ATCC 19435), *S. bovis* (ATCC 9809), and *S. mitis* (ATCC 9811) from Dr. James Sandham.

Cells were suspended in 50 mM potassium phosphate buffer, pH 7.8, containing 0.1 mM EDTA, and sonicated in an ice bath by means of a Branson sonifier at a power setting of 100 W to disrupt the cells. After centrifugation, the cell-free extracts were assayed for superoxide dismutase activity as previously described (12). In certain cases, the presence of low molecular weight substances capable of reducing cytochrome *c* necessitated an overnight dialysis of the cell-free extracts to remove these interfering substances. The extracts were assayed for catalase activity by means of a Gilson Oxygraph equipped with a Clark electrode and a thermostatted cell. The assay mixture contained 0.02 M hydrogen peroxide in 50 mM potassium phosphate buffer at pH 7.8, containing 0.1 mM EDTA, at 25°C. Rates of oxygen production were compared to the rate obtained with a standardized solution of bovine liver catalase obtained from Sigma. Alternatively, catalase was assayed spectrophotometrically by the method of Beers and Sizer (22). Protein contents of cell-free extracts were estimated at 280 nm assuming E_{lem} (c = 1%) = 10.0.

RESULTS AND DISCUSSION

The superoxide dismutase and catalase contents of 26 species of microorganisms of three categories are reported in Table 1. The *aerobes* are the microorganisms that can utilize molecular oxygen as the terminal electron acceptor. The *obligate anaerobes* not only lack the cytochrome system necessary for aerobic respiration, but are unable to survive under conditions of aeration. The organisms termed *aerotolerant anaerobes* do not utilize molecular oxygen as the terminal electron acceptor for their energy metabolism, but, with one exception, are capable of reducing oxygen to a limited extent. Many aerotolerant anaerobes grow as well under vigorous aeration as under anaerobic conditions and, at any rate, are not killed by such exposure to oxygen. *Aerotolerant anaerobe* seems to be a more accurate description of most of the organisms in this category than the term *microaerophile*, which has frequently been used to describe this kind of behavior.

The aerobes

The eight organisms in this category (Table 1), chosen at random, represent a broad spectrum of organisms, some Gram-positive, some Gram-negative, one yeast. All of these organisms contain both catalase and superoxide dismutase. The catalase activity of these organisms ranged from 0.7 unit/mg (*R. japonicum*) to 289 units/mg (*M. radiodurans*), a 400-fold variation. The activity of superoxide dismutase of these organisms ranged from 1.4 units/mg (*S. typhimurium*) to 7.0 units/mg (*M. radiodurans*), only a 5-fold variation.

TABLE 1. *Superoxide dismutase and catalase contents of a variety of microorganisms*

	Superoxide dismutase (units/mg)	Catalase (units/mg)
Aerobes:		
Escherichia coli	1.8	6.1
Salmonella typhimurium	1.4	2.4
Halobacterium salinarium	2.1	3.4
Rhizobium japonicum	2.6	0.7
Micrococcus radiodurans	7.0	289
Saccharomyces cerevisiae	3.7	13.5
Mycobacterium sp.	2.9	2.7
Pseudomonas sp.	2.0	22.5
Strict Anaerobes:		
Veillonella alcalescens	0	0
Clostridium pasteurianum, sticklandii, lentoputrescens, cellobioparum, barkeri	0	0
Clostridium acetobutylicum	0	—
Clostridium sp. (strain M.C.)	0	0
Butyrivibrio fibrisolvens	0	0.1
N2C3*	0	<0.1
Aerotolerant Anaerobes:		
Butyribacterium rettgeri	1.6	0
Streptococcus fecalis	0.8	0
Streptococcus mutans	0.5	0
Streptococcus bovis	0.3	0
Streptococcus mitis	0.2	0
Streptococcus lactis	1.4	0
Zymobacterium oroticum	0.6	0
Lactobacillus plantarum	0	0

* N2C3 is an unclassified cellulolytic Gram-negative rod isolated from the rumen of an African zebu steer and has been described by Margherita, S. S., and R. E. Hungate, *J. Bacteriol.*, **86**, 855 (1963).

The strict anaerobes

The ten organisms in this classification represent various clostridial species and three organisms that were isolated originally from the bovine rumen. Aeration is lethal for all these species. Strict anaerobes are nearly always catalase-negative. Two species of the rumen bacteria displayed very low levels of catalase activity. The existence of significant catalase activity in certain strict anaerobes has been observed by others (10). The consistent absence of superoxide dismutase activity among the obligate anaerobes contrasts with the presence of nearly constant levels of this activity in the organisms that possess oxygen-metabolizing capabilities.

The aerotolerant anaerobes

Examination of the third class of organisms in Table 1 casts additional light on the relative importance of catalase and superoxide dismutase. While none of these organisms utilizes oxygen as a primary electron acceptor, most of them consume some oxygen by the action of flavoprotein and metalloprotein oxidases not coupled to ATP synthesis (23). The apparent product of these oxidative processes is usually hydrogen peroxide. Despite their limited abilities to consume oxygen and to produce hydrogen peroxide, the data show that none of these organisms contains a significant amount of catalase activity. With only one exception, though, all aerotolerant anaerobes contained superoxide dismutase activity, at levels averaging 30% of that shown by the aerobes. The ability of these organisms to survive without catalase probably depends upon their low rate of production of H_2O_2 and upon the relative chemical stability of this compound that enables it to diffuse from these cells without causing damage. An accumulation of H_2O_2 in the medium surrounding these cells would be prevented by the catalatic action of substances in the medium or, in a mixed culture, by the catalatic action of other species of cells containing catalase. This explanation has already been proposed (9).

The single aerotolerant organism that contained no superoxide dismutase was *Lactobacillus plantarum*. Importantly, no consumption of oxygen by *L. plantarum* could be detected. The cells studied were grown under aerobic conditions and harvested during log phase. They were resuspended in fresh growth medium and oxygen consumption was measured using a Clark electrode with a Gilson Oxygraph. Under identical conditions, oxygen consumption by a known consumer such as *S. cerevisiae* was easily measurable. If the rate of consumption by *L. plantarum* had been as much as 5% that of *S. cerevisiae*, it would have been detected.

The presence of superoxide dismutase in the aerotolerant anaerobes and its absence among the strict anaerobes suggests that the normal physiological function of this enzyme is, indeed, the dismutation of superoxide radicals. It appears possible that this activity may be the single most important enzymic activity for enabling organisms to survive in the presence of molecular oxygen. Presumably, the great chemical reactivity of superoxide anion precludes the possibility of depending upon diffusion from the cell as a means of disposal of this radical and necessitates the presence, within the cell, of superoxide dismutase. Admittedly, were an organism obligately anaerobic for some other reason, there would be no reason for it to continue to carry the genetic burden of the genes for catalase and superoxide dismutase and this correlation might have some other, as yet unsuspected, explanation.

An organism without superoxide dismutase could survive in an oxygen environment if it does not produce quantities of the superoxide radical sufficient to jeopardize its survival. *L. plantarum* appears to be such an organism. Even an oxygen-metabolizing organism need not possess the enzyme, providing the *direct* products of its limited oxygen-metabolizing pathways be hydrogen peroxide and water rather than the superoxide radical.

The ubiquity of superoxide dismutase among all aerobic organisms and its uniform distribution among the various tissues of mammals implies that the superoxide free radical is a commonly occurring but quite undesirable physiological species. Relatively few biological reactions have been shown to produce the radical *in vivo*. The first enzyme shown to release the radical into free solution was milk xanthine oxidase (11, 18), a metalloflavoprotein containing nonheme iron. Two other nonheme-iron flavoenzymes, rabbit liver aldehyde oxidase and dihydroorotate dehydrogenase from *Zymobacterium oroticum* (17), also produce the radical. (*Z. oroticum* is an aerotolerant anaerobe and contains super-

oxide dismutase.) Of a variety of flavoprotein oxidases and dehydrogenases, several were shown to produce superoxide to very limited extents (24). Clostridial ferredoxin, a nonheme-iron protein, was shown to produce the radical upon air oxidation of its reduced form (25). Pig kidney diamine oxidase, a copper-containing enzyme, has recently been shown to produce the superoxide radical (26). The autoxidation of hemoglobin and myoglobin and all similar one-electron transfers to oxygen are processes that almost certainly produce O_2^- (27–29), and a variety of low molecular weight electron carriers such as reduced flavins and hydroquinones likewise produce the radical upon autoxidation (30). Since improved methods now exist for the detection of the superoxide radical, we expect that additional biological sources of O_2^- will be discovered in the near future.

Superoxide dismutase activity appears to be a concomitant and perhaps necessary condition for the survival of oxygen-metabolizing organisms. Other factors in addition to the lack of superoxide dismutase might render an organism unable to survive in the presence of oxygen, e.g., enzymes that are autoxidized and thereby inactivated by molecular oxygen. Conceivably, membranes containing easily autoxidizable unsaturated lipids could be rendered nonfunctional by contact with molecular oxygen. However, the data presented herein strongly suggest that superoxide dismutase is a factor of primary importance in enabling organisms to survive the challenge presented by the reactive intermediate species resulting from the univalent reduction of molecular oxygen. Further study of this process may lead to a greater understanding of the mechanisms of oxygen toxicity.

This work was supported by grant GM-10287 from the National Institutes of Health, Bethesda, Md.   J. M. M. and B. B. K. were postdoctoral fellows of the National Institutes of Health.

1. Stanier, R. Y., M. Doudoroff, and E. A. Adelberg, *The Microbial World*, 3rd ed. (Prentice-Hall, Inc., Englewood Cliffs, N.J., 1970), p. 75.
2. Gottstein, A., *Virchows Arch.*, **133**, 295 (1893).
3. Rywosch, D., and M. Rywosch, *Zentralbl. Bakteriol. Parasitenk. Infectionskr. Hyg. Abt. Orig.*, **44**, 295 (1907).
4. McLeod, J. W., and J. Gordon, *J. Pathol. Bacteriol.*, **26**, 332 (1923).
5. Callow, A. B., *J. Pathol. Bacteriol.*, **26**, 320 (1923).
6. Gordon, J., R. A. Holman, and J. W. McLeod, *J. Pathol. Bacteriol.*, **66**, 527 (1953).
7. McLeod, J. W., and J. Gordon, *J. Pathol. Bacteriol.*, **26**, 326 (1923).
8. Gledhill, W. E., and L. E. Casida, Jr., *Appl. Microbiol.*, **18**, 340 (1969).
9. Jones, D., J. Watkins, and D. J. Meyer, *Nature*, **226**, 1249 (1970).
10. Prevot, A. R., and H. Thouvenot, *Ann. Inst. Pasteur Paris*, **83**, 443 (1952).
11. McCord, J. M., and I. Fridovich, *J. Biol. Chem.*, **243**, 5753 (1968).
12. McCord, J. M., and I. Fridovich, *J. Biol. Chem.*, **244**, 6049 (1969).
13. Fridovich, I., and P. Handler, *J. Biol. Chem.*, **233**, 1581 (1958).
14. Fridovich, I., and P. Handler, *J. Biol. Chem.*, **236**, 1836 (1961).
15. Greenlee, L., I. Fridovich, and P. Handler, *Biochemistry*, **1**, 779 (1962).
16. Fridovich, I., and P. Handler, *J. Biol. Chem.*, **237**, 916 (1962).
17. Handler, P., K. V. Rajagopalan, and V. Aleman, *Fed. Proc.*, **23**, 30 (1964).

18. Knowles, R. F., J. F. Gibson, F. M. Pick, and R. C. Bray, *Biochem. J.*, **111**, 53 (1969).
19. D. Behar, G. H. Czapski, J. Rabani, L. M. Dorfman, and H. A. Schwarz, *J. Phys. Chem.*, **74**, 3209 (1970).
20. Keele, B. B., Jr., J. M. McCord, and I. Fridovich, *J. Biol. Chem.*, **245**, 6176 (1970).
21. Keele, B. B., Jr., J. M. McCord, and I. Fridovich, *J. Biol. Chem.*, in press.
22. Beers, R. F., and I. W. Sizer, *J. Biol. Chem.*, **195**, 133 (1952).
23. Stanier, R. Y., M. Doudoroff, and E. A. Adelberg, *The Microbial World*, 3rd ed. (Prentice-Hall, Inc., Englewood Cliffs, N.J., 1970), p. 663.
24. Massey, V., S. Strickland, S. G. Mayhew, L. G. Howell, P. C. Engel, R. G. Matthews, M. Schuman, and P. A. Sullivan, *Biochem. Biophys. Res. Commun.*, **36**, 891 (1969).
25. Orme-Johnson, W. H., and H. Beinert, *Biochem. Biophys. Res. Commun.*, **36**, 905 (1969).
26. Rotilio, G., L. Calabrese, A. Finazzi-Agro, and B. Mondovi, *Biochim. Biophys. Acta*, **198**, 618 (1970).
27. George, P., and C. J. Stratmann, *Biochem. J.*, **51**, 163 (1952).
28. George, P., and C. J. Stratmann, *Biochem. J.*, **51**, 418 (1952).
29. George, P., and C. J. Stratmann, *Biochem. J.*, **57**, 568 (1954).
30. McCord, J. M., and I. Fridovich, *J. Biol. Chem.*, **245**, 1374 (1970).

15

Reprinted from *Biochem. J.* **43**:193–202 (1948)

Crystalline Bacterial Catalase*

By D. HERBERT (Leverhulme Research Fellow) AND JANE PINSENT (Leverhulme Research Scholar),
Medical Research Council Unit for Bacterial Chemistry, Lister Institute, London, S.W. 1

(*Received* 13 *January* 1948)

[*Editor's note:* Because of poor reproducibility, the photograph of catalase crystals (Plate 1) originally included in Paper 15 has been deleted.]

In recent years, the trend of enzyme research has shifted from the study of the reactions catalyzed to a study of the chemical nature of the enzymes themselves. This has led in the last fifteen years to the isolation of some forty enzymes in a crystalline or highly purified state, and in many cases to the identification of their prosthetic groups, resulting in a completely new outlook on enzyme chemistry.

Little progress, however, has been made in the study of bacterial enzymes from this standpoint, and up to the present there has not been recorded the isolation of a single bacterial enzyme in a pure state. This is the more regrettable since many interesting enzymes exist in bacteria which have not been found elsewhere, and some bacterial enzymes at least (e.g. lactic dehydrogenase, cytochromes a_1 and a_2) are known to differ greatly from their counterparts in animal tissues. This relative neglect of bacterial enzymes is in part due to purely technical reasons, namely, the difficulties involved in growing the large quantities of bacteria required, and the problem of liberating endo-enzymes from the bacterial cell. The first of these problems is well on its way to solution, but the second is more difficult. Most of the techniques hitherto used for destroying the cell wall and liberating intracellular enzymes (for example, autolysis, vacuum- or acetone-drying followed by extraction, shaking with glass beads (Curran & Evans,

* A preliminary account of part of this work appeared in *Nature, Lond.*, 160, 125 (1947).

1942) or grinding with powdered glass (Kalnitsky, Utter & Workman, 1945), the roller-crushing mill (Booth & Green, 1938), ultrasonic disintegration (Stumpf, Green & Smith, 1946, and others)) either tend to destroy labile enzymes, are difficult to employ on a large scale, or require specialized apparatus.

This paper describes the use of a relatively little-used method of liberating enzymes from bacterial cells, namely, lysis of the bacteria with lysozyme. This substance, which is now easily prepared in crystalline form from egg white, rapidly brings about smooth and complete lysis of susceptible bacteria; no specialized apparatus is required, and the method can be employed on any scale. Penrose & Quastel (1930), Quastel (1937) and Epps & Gale (1942) have used lysozyme to determine the true enzyme content of bacterial cells grown under different conditions, but it has not previously been used as an aid to enzyme purification.

The present paper describes the application of this method to the isolation of catalase from *Micrococcus lysodeikticus*. Catalase was one of the first enzymes to be described in bacteria (Gottstein, 1893) and much work has been done on it since, but no attempts have been made to isolate it in a pure state or determine its chemical nature. Using lysozyme to liberate the enzyme from the bacteria, we have been able to isolate *M. lysodeikticus* catalase as a pure, crystalline protein. As far as we are aware, this is the first bacterial enzyme to have been crystallized.

Bacterial catalase is on the whole very similar to the catalases that have been isolated from mammalian tissues, but there are certain differences. It is a conjugated protein with haematin as the prosthetic group, but unlike liver catalase it contains no verdohaematin. The protein part of the molecule has the same molecular weight as liver catalase protein, but differs in its resistance to organic solvents and low pH. The catalytic activity of the bacterial enzyme is considerably higher than that of blood or liver catalases; this difference also is to be attributed to the protein part of the molecule. Finally, it differs from other catalases in its crystalline form.

METHODS

Bacterial suspensions. The strain of *M. lysodeikticus* used (National Collection of Type Cultures no. 2665) was a descendant of that originally isolated by Fleming (1922). For large-scale production, the bacteria were grown on C.C.Y.-lactate agar (Gladstone & Fildes, 1940) in enamelled trays (photographic developing dishes) measuring 11 × 16 in., with overlapping lids, each containing 500 ml. of agar. Three ml. of inoculum, prepared by suspending the 24 hr. growth from a Roux bottle in 50 ml. of saline, was spread evenly over the surface of each tray with a glass spreader, and the trays incubated at 35°. Growth was almost complete in 24 hr., but the catalase activity of the bacteria continued to increase

up to 40 hr., which was therefore adopted as the standard time for incubation. The bacterial growth was then removed from the agar surface with a scraper. The average yield was c. 1·5 g. bacteria (dry wt.)/tray.

Estimation of catalase activity. The activity of catalase preparations was measured essentially according to Euler & Josephson (1927). Suitably diluted catalase solution (1 ml., containing c. 0·3 μg. of pure enzyme) is added to 49 ml. of 0·015 N-H_2O_2 in 0·015 M-phosphate buffer of pH 6·8, kept at 0° in an ice-water bath. Five ml. are immediately withdrawn, pipetted into 5 ml. of 2 N-H_2SO_4, and titrated with 0·01 N-$KMnO_4$. Further samples are withdrawn and titrated after 3, 6, 9 and 12 min. For each time interval, the first-order velocity constant is calculated as $k = \dfrac{1}{t} \log_{10} \dfrac{a}{a-x}$, where a is the initial $KMnO_4$ titre and $a-x$ the titre after t min.

Under these conditions the reaction is approximately first order but, as with catalase of plant and animal origin, significant destruction of the enzyme by the H_2O_2 occurs, causing falling values of k. Following Sumner (1941), we plot k against t and determine k_0, the value of k at zero time, by extrapolation. The amount of catalase taken should be such that k_0 falls between 0·025 and 0·04 min.$^{-1}$; the value of k_0 is then directly proportional to the amount of enzyme taken.

Catalase solutions always have to be highly diluted for testing; the activity of the undiluted solution is calculated by multiplying the value of k found in the test by the overall dilution factor; e.g. if 1 ml. of a 1/10,000 dilution gives a k value of 0·03 in the test, then k for the undiluted solution is 0·03 × 50 × 10,000 = 15,000. The purity of an enzyme preparation is expressed according to Euler & Josephson (1927) as $Kat.\text{-}f. = \dfrac{k}{\text{g. enzyme in 50 ml.}}$, or under the above test conditions, $Kat.\text{-}f. = \dfrac{k \text{ in test}}{\text{g. enzyme in test}}$.

To obtain reliable results by this method, it is essential that all glassware should be cleaned with H_2SO_4-$K_2Cr_2O_7$, and that the very dilute enzyme solutions necessary for the test should be used immediately after diluting. Even so, we consider the error to be about 5%. All measurements reported in this paper are the means of duplicates.

Dry weights. Well-dialyzed enzyme solutions, or bacterial suspensions thoroughly washed in distilled water, were dried to constant weight at 105° and weighed on a micro-balance. The colorimetric method of Pressman (1943) was used as a rapid, rough method of determining the protein content of enzyme fractions; all measurements reported, however, are based on direct weighings. Dry weights of bacterial suspensions were as a routine measured turbidimetrically using a Hilger photoelectric absorptiometer previously calibrated with suspensions of known dry weight.

Haemin estimations. The method chiefly used was the pyridine-haemochromogen method of Keilin & Hartree (1936) and Rimington (1942). Results were occasionally checked by the cyanhaematin method of King & Gilchrist (1947); the two methods gave identical results.

Crystalline lysozyme. This was initially prepared from egg white by bentonite adsorption according to Alderton, Ward & Fevold (1945). Once a supply of seed crystals had been prepared, subsequent batches were made by direct crystallization from egg white (Alderton & Fevold, 1946); this method was found very simple and reliable.

Absorption spectra were observed with a Hartridge reversion spectroscope (calibrated with a neon lamp), and a Beckman spectrophotometer.

RESULTS

Action of lysozyme on Micrococcus lysodeikticus suspensions

When a dilute suspension (say 1 mg./ml.) ot *M. lysodeikticus* in 0·5 % saline is treated with a small amount of lysozyme, the turbidity rapidly disappears leaving an almost water-clear solution in which no intact bacteria are observable microscopically; the phenomenon has been described in detail by Fleming (1922, 1929) and subsequent workers.

An interesting finding is that the catalase activity of *M. lysodeikticus* suspensions invariably increases after lysis with lysozyme, usually by about tenfold. For example, a typical suspension gave the following results (tested at 30°):

	Bacteria in test (mg.)	*k*	*Kat.-f.*
Before lysis	0·424	0·0382	89
After lysis	0·071	0·0606	854

The same effect is observed if the bacteria are disintegrated by shaking with glass beads. Similar results were observed by Penrose & Quastel (1930), and Krampitz & Werkman (1941) found that intact *M. lysodeikticus* suspensions had no action on oxaloacetic acid, whilst lyzed or acetone-dried bacteria rapidly decarboxylated this substance. The simplest explanation is that diffusion of substrate into the cell is a limiting factor.

Fleming (1929) noted that high salt concentrations inhibit lysis by lysozyme. We find also that in the total absence of salts (bacteria washed with distilled water and treated with dialyzed lysozyme solutions) lysis is almost completely inhibited for prolonged periods. The optimal salt concentration is about 0·5 % for NaCl and 0·02–0·05 M for phosphate buffers; under these conditions, 1 mg. of crystalline lysozyme is more than sufficient to bring about complete lysis of 1 g. of *M. lysodeikticus* in 1 hr. at 30°.

Previous workers on lysozyme have only studied its action on quite dilute bacterial suspensions. When large amounts of bacteria in thick (1–8 % dry weight) suspension are lyzed, interesting new phenomena are observed. When acted on by lysozyme, such suspensions of *M. lysodeikticus*, which are originally canary yellow and completely opaque, rapidly become greenish yellow and semi-transparent though not completely water-clear; the residual turbidity is due to the high concentration of 'ghosts'. As these changes take place the initially mobile suspension becomes highly viscous and slimy. The solution produced by lysis of a 1 % bacterial suspension has

about the consistency of egg white, while an 8 % solution is a semi-solid gel which cannot be pipetted or poured out of a test-tube; a 4 % solution is the strongest that can conveniently be handled. Besides being highly viscous, such solutions have marked elastic properties. They are readily drawn out into threads, and on pouring from a measuring cylinder emerge as an elongated 'blob' which slowly descends while the cylinder is tilted and runs back into the cylinder if the latter is restored to an upright position. When caused to flow along a 2 mm. horizontal capillary under pressure (in an apparatus similar to that used by Scott Blair, Folley, Malpress & Coppen (1941) for testing the flow-elasticity of bovine cervical mucus), they show marked recoil when the pressure is suddenly released.

The chemical nature of this viscous substance or substances is unknown, nor is it known whether they are initially present inside the bacterial cell and released from it by lysis, or formed by the action of lysozyme; it is hoped to investigate these problems in the future. The phenomenon is not peculiar to *M. lysodeikticus*, similar viscous substances being formed when other sensitive bacteria are treated with lysozyme.

Isolation of crystalline catalase from lysed bacteria

The essentials of the purification method we have adopted are as follows. The solution of lyzed bacteria is treated with 0·5 vol. of ethanol at pH 5·6, which precipitates the viscous substances formed on lysis, and then shaken with chloroform, which denatures considerable quantities of inert proteins. The aqueous-ethanolic solution is then treated with solid ammonium sulphate which, with correct proportions of the three components, causes it to separate into two liquid phases, one containing all the catalase while the other contains most of the contaminating proteins. This 'partition' method is, as far as we know, a novel procedure in protein purification, and may well be applicable to other problems.

After repetition of the above process, two fractionations with ammonium sulphate bring the enzyme to 70–80 % purity, when it can be crystallized either by prolonged dialysis or by careful addition of ammonium sulphate.

The following are the details of a typical preparation:

Stage 1. The bacterial growth from 156 trays (78 l. of medium) was harvested, suspended without washing in c. 3 l. of 0·5 % NaCl, and strained through muslin to remove flakes of agar. Turbidimetric estimation showed that the total dry weight of bacteria was 203 g., and 0·5 % NaCl was added to make the final concentration of the suspension 4 % on a dry-weight basis (5085 ml.). Crystalline lysozyme was then added (1 mg./g. bacteria) and the suspension incubated 1 hr. at 30°, when lysis was complete. *Kat.-f.* of lyzed suspension = 910.

Stage 2. The highly viscous lyzed suspension was treated successively with 509 ml. of M-acetate buffer of pH 5·6, and 2800 ml. of ethanol (final ethanol concentration 33·3 % v/v). A bulky yellow gelatinous precipitate was centrifuged off, washed with 2500 ml. of M/15 acetate (pH 5·6) containing 33·3 % ethanol, and the washings added to the original supernatant fluid. This gave 8180 ml. of a pale yellow mobile liquid; *Kat.-f.* = 4020. (All the above operations were carried out at 0°; this is not absolutely essential, but gives better yields.)

Stage 3. The above liquid was treated with 1820 ml. of chloroform, shaken on a fast mechanical shaker for 15 min. and centrifuged, when two liquid layers formed with a thick layer of denatured protein at the interface. The top layer (7610 ml.) was siphoned off; *Kat.-f.* = 5200.

Stage 4. The top layer from the last stage was treated with $\frac{1}{16}$ vol. of M-sodium acetate and 2400 g. of solid $(NH_4)_2SO_4$ added (30 g. to each 100 ml.). This caused the separation on standing of two liquid layers, the lower containing most of the $(NH_4)_2SO_4$ and the upper most of the ethanol, some $(NH_4)_2SO_4$ and water. The smaller top layer (2760 ml.) was pale brown and contained all the catalase, whose characteristic absorption band at 631 mμ. could now be seen with a hand spectroscope; *Kat.-f.* = 15,650. (It is essential for the success of this step that the proportions of aqueous solution, ethanol and chloroform specified in stages 2 and 3 should be adhered to; otherwise two layers may not separate, or the catalase may be precipitated at the interface. The sodium acetate is added to keep the pH at about 5·6 on addition of the $(NH_4)_2SO_4$.)

Stage 5. The top layer from the above stage was shaken for 15 min. with an equal volume of chloroform, allowed to stand, and the top layer (1890 ml.) removed. (Comparatively little inert protein is removed by this step; the main purpose is to reduce the ethanol concentration.) Solid $(NH_4)_2SO_4$ was now added (23 g. to each 100 ml.) when two layers again separated. The top layer was much the smaller, and dark brown; it was removed in a separating funnel and dialyzed against running tap water overnight; final volume 600 ml., *Kat.-f.* = 20,200.

(Stages 4 and 5 bring about a fourfold purification and decrease the volume to $\frac{1}{13}$; this concentration is important for the subsequent $(NH_4)_2SO_4$ fractionation which is less effective if the protein concentration is too low.)

Stage 6. The dialyzed solution from stage 5 was brought to pH 5·6 by the addition of $\frac{1}{16}$ vol. of M-acetate buffer, and roughly fractionated by adding successive portions of solid $(NH_4)_2SO_4$ and centrifuging off the resulting precipitates. Fraction 6a (obtained with 1·96M-$(NH_4)_2SO_4$) which was greyish white and contained little catalase, was rejected.

Fractions 6b, c and d, taken off at 2·27, 2·38 and 2·52M-$(NH_4)_2SO_4$, were brown and contained most of the catalase, little being left in the final supernatant. These three fractions were combined and dissolved in M/20 acetate pH 5·6 to give a volume of 61 ml., *Kat.-f.* = 40,000.

Stage 7. The combined fractions b, c and d were now carefully fractionated by dropwise addition of a 4M-$(NH_4)_2SO_4$ solution adjusted to pH 5·6 with NH_4OH. (It was found impossible to standardize these fractionations completely. The exact $(NH_4)_2SO_4$ concentration at which catalase begins to precipitate is markedly affected by the catalase concentration, the temperature and probably other factors. It is necessary to proceed empirically, adding the $(NH_4)_2SO_4$ drop by drop and with good stirring, taking off fractions at intervals. Fortunately, the colour of the catalase makes it easy to determine its distribution in the precipitates.) Three successive precipitates were taken off, after which little catalase remained in the supernatant fluid. The smaller 1st and 3rd precipitates were visibly paler than the 2nd, and obviously contained colourless protein impurities. The 2nd dark brown precipitate contained the bulk of the catalase and was dissolved in M/20-acetate pH 5·6 to give a volume of 63 ml., *Kat.-f.* = 62,900.

Stage 8 (*crystallization*). The solution resulting from the last stage was crystallized in three different ways. (i) A portion (10 ml.) of the solution was dialyzed against repeated changes of distilled water at 0°. After 5 days (longer than this may be necessary) it had mostly crystallized. (ii) Another 10 ml. portion of the solution was cautiously treated with 4M-$(NH_4)_2SO_4$ until the faintest turbidity appeared. The solution was allowed to stand at room temperature, and by the next day it had almost completely crystallized, leaving a nearly colourless mother liquor. (iii) The rest of the solution (43 ml.) was treated with just enough 4M-$(NH_4)_2SO_4$ to precipitate all the catalase. The precipitate was centrifuged down and redissolved by adding distilled water drop by drop, very slowly and with good stirring, until all but a small portion had dissolved; this was centrifuged off. The supernatant fluid was then saturated with amorphous catalase; it was allowed to stand at room temperature, and most had crystallized within 24 hr. (iii a). A smaller second crop of crystals (iii b) was obtained by adding a few drops of $(NH_4)_2SO_4$ to the mother liquor of the 1st crop. The four batches of crystals were separately dissolved in M/15-phosphate buffer pH 6·8, well dialyzed, and tested; *Kat.-f.* = 90,000–98,000, which is the highest value we have obtained. There is thus a considerable increase in purity on crystallization.

The yields and purities at each stage of the isolation procedure are shown in Table 1.

Table 1. *Purification of bacterial catalase*

Stage	Volume (ml.)	Total protein (g.)	Total catalase (g.)	*Kat.-f.*
1. Lyzed bacteria	5,085	203	1·94	910
2. Ethanol supernatant	8,180	40·2	1·69	4,020
3. Chloroform supernatant	7,610	29·5	1·60	5,200
4. First ethanol-$(NH_4)_2SO_4$ partition	2,760	8·9	1·46	15,650
5. Second ethanol-$(NH_4)_2SO_4$ partition	600	5·4	1·14	20,200
6. First $(NH_4)_2SO_4$ fractionation	61	2·1	0·90	40,000
7. Second $(NH_4)_2SO_4$ fractionation	63	0·735	0·485	62,900
8. Crystals: (i)	—	0·050	0·050 ⎫	93,300
(ii)	—	0·065	0·065 ⎪ 0·376	98,000
(iii a)	—	0·206	0·206 ⎬	99,000
(iii b)	—	0·055	0·055 ⎭	90,000

Properties of the crystalline enzyme

General properties. Solutions of the pure enzyme have a red-brown colour resembling that of methaemoglobin. Strong solutions (1 % or over) are stable for many weeks at 0°, or even at room temperature, if bacterial contamination is avoided, but very dilute solutions such as are used in *Kat.-f.* determinations lose their activity fairly rapidly, and must be tested immediately. In this they resemble liver catalase (Sumner & Dounce, 1937).

Crystalline form. The pure enzyme crystallizes as regular octahedra, which are isotropic when viewed between crossed polaroids; they have the same form, however the enzyme is crystallized (Pl. 3). In this respect bacterial catalase differs from beef-liver catalase, which according to Sumner & Dounce (1937) may crystallize as needles, plates or prisms, according to the conditions of crystallization.

Prosthetic group. Bacterial catalase has a higher activity (*Kat.-f.*) than catalases from other sources (Tables 1 and 3). It is important to discover whether this is to be attributed to differences in the protein

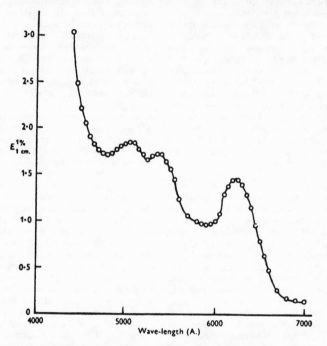

Fig. 1. Absorption spectrum of bacterial catalase. Crystalline enzyme
(*Kat.-f.* = 99,000) in M/15 phosphate pH 6·8.

Bacterial catalase is fairly stable at high pH values (e.g. in 0·1N-ammonia) but much less stable to acid pH. Horse liver and erythrocyte catalase are stable down to pH 3·2 (Agner & Theorell, 1946), but bacterial catalase is instantly denatured and precipitated at pH 4·0, and fairly rapidly at pH 4·6. Hence, treatment with acetate buffer pH 3·8, which Bonnichsen (1947) used effectively for purifying mammalian catalases, cannot be employed for purifying the bacterial enzyme. Dioxan, which Sumner & Dounce (1937, 1939) used to purify liver catalase, denatures bacterial catalase very rapidly at room temperature and still rapidly at 0°; we were able to obtain fairly pure preparations by Sumner's method working at 0°, but only in very low yields.

or the prosthetic group, and the nature of the latter was investigated in some detail.

Strong solutions of bacterial catalase have a characteristic absorption spectrum (Fig. 1), showing three bands centred at 506, 545 and 631 mμ. (in M/15 phosphate pH 6·8), which are close to the values reported for other catalases. The exact positions and intensities of the bands are affected both by the pH and the nature of the buffer anion (cf. Agner, 1942). These data are not always recorded in the literature; it is uncertain, therefore, whether the slight spectroscopic differences observed between different catalases are apparent or real.

On treatment with pyridine and sodium hyposulphite (Na₂S₂O₄) in 0·1N-NaOH bacterial catalase gives a typical haemochromogen spectrum, and it forms characteristic compounds with cyanide and azide. Neither azide-catalase nor cyanide-catalase, nor catalase itself, is reduced by hyposulphite. Azide-catalase forms a characteristic pink compound with hydrogen peroxide, which gradually reverts to the original spectrum as the hydrogen peroxide decomposes. This behaviour is exactly similar to that of liver catalase as described by Keilin & Hartree (1937), and the absorption bands of the compounds have similar positions (Table 2).

at 502, 547 and 644 mμ., identical with those of haemin in this solvent. It contained no detectable trace of the 'blue pigment' (biliverdin) that is produced when liver catalases are treated in a similar way (Sumner & Dounce, 1939). On evaporating off the acetone *in vacuo*, the haemin precipitated, leaving a colourless supernatant fluid. The haemin was centrifuged off, washed with water, and dissolved in 10 ml. of dilute Na_2CO_3. Part of this alkaline haematin solution was reserved for conversion to the cyanide- and pyridine-haemochromogen derivatives; the remainder was immediately coupled with a *c*. 1·5% solution of globin prepared from human-blood haemoglobin by the method of

Table 2. *Absorption bands of catalase and catalase-haematin derivatives*

(Positions of the absorption bands, determined with the Hartridge reversion spectroscope, are given in mμ.)

	Catalase derivatives	
	M. lysodeikticus catalase (this paper)	Horse-liver catalase (Keilin & Hartree, 1937)
Catalase	506, 545, 631·5	506·5, 544, 629·5
Azide-catalase	504, 541, 623	506·5, 544, 624·5
Azide-catalase—H_2O_2	548, 588	547, 588
Cyanide-catalase	555·5, 592	556·5, 595·5
	Haematin derivatives	
	Bacterial catalase haematin	Blood haematin
Haematin (in ether-acetic acid)	505, 545, (584), 638	506, 544·5, (585), 637
Cyanhaematin	547	547
Reduced cyanhaematin	537, 578·5	536·5, 578
Pyridine haemochromogen	525, 557	526, 557
	'Resynthesized haemoglobin' derivatives	
	From globin + bacterial catalase haematin	From globin + blood haematin
Methaemoglobin (alkaline)	542, 575·5, 603·5	541·5, 575·5, 603
Haemoglobin	557	560
Oxyhaemoglobin	540, 577·5	540·5, 577
CO-haemoglobin	536·5, 572	537, 572

The above facts strongly suggest that the prosthetic group of bacterial catalase is haematin, but further evidence is needed. This was obtained by splitting off the prosthetic group with acetone-hydrochloric acid and coupling the isolated pigment to globin, when it formed methaemoglobin which could be converted to reduced haemoglobin, oxyhaemoglobin and carboxyhaemoglobin, identical with the corresponding derivatives formed from globin and pure haemin. This is proof that the prosthetic group of bacterial catalase actually is haematin; the same experiment also showed that it contains no verdohaematin or similar substance giving rise to biliverdin on treatment with acetone-hydrochloric acid. Details are given below:

Bacterial catalase (15 ml. of 1·5%) was run into 300 ml. of pure acetone containing 5 ml. of conc. HCl. The flocculent protein precipitate was filtered off and washed with acetone-HCl, the washings being added to the original filtrate. The washed protein precipitate was pure white. The acetone-hydrochloric acid filtrate was brown, showing diffuse bands

Anson & Mirsky (1929–30). The globin solution (which was free from denatured globin) was added drop by drop to the solution of catalase haematin until visual and spectroscopic observation showed that all of the latter had coupled with the globin; the solution then showed the absorption bands of methaemoglobin. This was reduced with the minimum quantity of Stokes's reagent (1% $FeSO_4$ in 2% tartaric acid) required to convert it to reduced haemoglobin. On shaking vigorously with air this was converted to oxyhaemoglobin, which was further converted to CO-haemoglobin by saturation with CO. The same series of compounds was formed from the same globin solution by coupling with a freshly prepared solution of recrystallized blood haemin; the absorption bands of both series, and of the other catalase haematin derivatives, are shown in Table 2. The spectra of the two series of haemoglobin derivatives were identical within the errors of reading (Table 2).

For comparison, samples of purified horse-liver catalase and crystalline human-blood catalase were treated with acetone-hydrochloric acid in the same way. The blood catalase behaved exactly like the bacterial catalase, giving a brown acetone solution

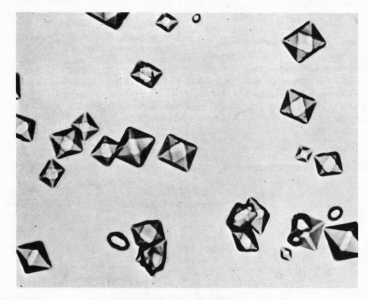

(a) Crystallized from $(NH_4)_2SO_4$; ×500.

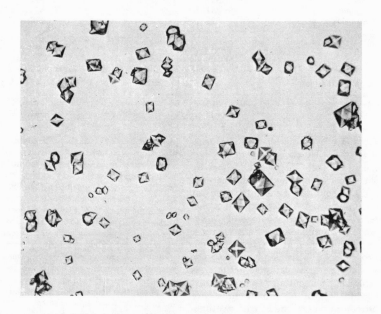

(b) Crystallized by dialysis; ×200.

Crystalline catalase from *Micrococcus lysodeikticus*.

D. HERBERT AND J. PINSENT—CRYSTALLINE BACTERIAL CATALASE

containing, as far as could be ascertained, only haematin. The liver catalase, however, gave a bright blue acetone solution, containing both haematin and biliverdin, as Sumner & Dounce (1939) have described. This could be detected with even a few-drops of a 1·5 % liver catalase solution; bacterial catalase contains none of the substance (probably verdohaematin, see Lemberg & Legge, 1943) that gives biliverdin on treatment with acetone-hydrochloric acid.

Solutions of bacterial catalase and blood catalase are identical in colour to the naked eye, while horse-liver catalase is distinctly greener in colour, and can be seen spectroscopically to have a higher end-absorption in the red. This difference in colour is almost certainly due to the presence of verdo-haematin in the liver catalase. and its absence in the other two catalases.

Catalytic activity, haematin content and molecular weight

Table 3 records the *Kat.-f.* and haematin content of crystalline bacterial catalase preparations compared with those of other catalases, and also the ratio *Kat.-f.*/percentage of haematin. Evidently this ratio should be independent of the purity of the catalase preparation provided that impurities present (*a*) contain no haematin, (*b*) have no effect on the activity of the enzyme. Fig. 2 shows *Kat.-f.* plotted against

the percentage of haematin for bacterial catalase preparations of varying degrees of purity, the lowest

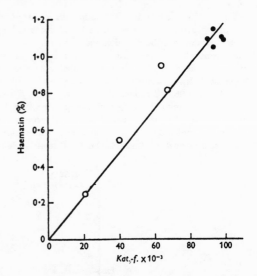

Fig. 2. Relation between haematin content and *Kat.-f.* for bacterial catalase at different stages of purification. Crystalline preparations, ●; amorphous, ○.

only 20 % pure. The points are well fitted (within the limits of error) by a straight line passing through the

Table 3. *Catalytic activity and haematin content of bacterial catalase compared with liver and erythrocyte catalases*

Source	*Kat.-f.*	Haematin (%)	Bile pigment (%)	*Kat.-f.*/% of haematin	Sedimentation constant	References
			Liver catalases			
Ox	30,000–35,000	0·46–0·54	0·49–0·55*	57,000–67,000	11·2 × 10⁻¹³	Sumner & Dounce (1939); Sumner & Gralén (1938)
Horse	25,000–40,000	0·41–0·68	0·37–0·62*	58,000–61,000	—	Sumner, Dounce & Frampton (1940)
	34,000–48,000	0·67–0·92	+	50,000–53,000	—	Keilin & Hartree (1945a)
	50,000	0·89–0·91	+	55,000–56,000	11·3 × 10⁻¹³	Bonnichsen (1947), Agner (1938)
			Erythrocyte catalases			
Ox	48,000	?	Nil	?'	—	Laskowski & Sumner (1941)
Horse	65,000–70,000	1·042	Nil	62,000–67,000	—	Agner & Theorell (1946)
	65,000	1·08	Nil	60,000	—	Bonnichsen (1947)
Human	50,000	0·83	Nil	60,300	—	Bonnichsen (1947)
	63,000	1·15	Nil	54,700	11·26 × 10⁻¹³	Herbert & Pinsent (1948); Cecil & Ogston (1948)
			Bacterial catalase			
M. lysodeikticus	93,300†	1·042	Nil	89,500	—	This paper
	98,000‡	1·103	Nil	89,000	—	This paper
	99,000§	1·096	Nil	90,000	11·0 × 10⁻¹³	This paper; Cecil & Ogston (1948)
	90,000‖	1·096	Nil	82,200	—	This paper

* From 'bile pigment Fe' analyses.
† Crystallized by dialysis, stage 8 (i).
‡ Crystallized by (NH₄)₂SO₄, stage 8 (ii).
§ Crystallized by (NH₄)₂SO₄, stage 8 (iiia).
‖ Crystallized by (NH₄)₂SO₄, stage 8 (iiib).

origin. This shows that our preparations are not contaminated with other iron-porphyrin proteins.

Table 3 shows that the haematin content of our preparations is the same as those recorded by other workers for blood catalases and higher than those reported for liver catalases; the *Kat.-f.*, however, is *c.* 50 % higher than the most active catalases of animal tissues, the average value being *Kat.-f.* = 95,000. Similarly, the ratio *Kat.-f.*/percentage of haematin is higher, being *c.* 88,000. To make certain that this is not due to any error in our analytical methods, we prepared crystalline blood catalase by a new method (Herbert & Pinsent, 1948),

Cecil & Ogston (1948) have examined our crystalline preparations in the ultracentrifuge and found them to consist essentially of a single homogeneous protein with sedimentation constant 11.0×10^{-13} (Table 3). In the best preparation examined in the ultracentrifuge, the catalase accounted for 85 % of the sedimenting material. As the error of this determination is *c.* 5 %, we may conclude that our preparations were essentially homogeneous. The haematin content and the agreement between the chemical and ultracentrifugal calculations of the molecular weight lead us to suspect that the small amount of impurity apparently present is probably denatured catalase. If this is so, then the activity

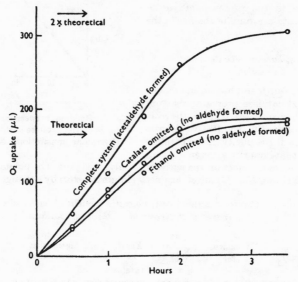

Fig. 3. Coupled oxidation of ethanol. Warburg manometers contained xanthine oxidase 8 mg., hypoxanthine 1 mg., ethanol 0·1 ml., crystalline bacterial catalase 0·8 mg., M/20 phosphate pH 7·2, total vol. 3 ml. Temp. 30°, gas phase air.

and determined its activity and haematin content in parallel with determinations on bacterial catalase. Any systematic errors in our *Kat.-f.* and haematin determinations would apply equally to both enzymes. In fact our values for blood catalase (Table 3) are in good agreement with those of other workers. We concluded, therefore, that bacterial catalase actually has a considerably higher activity, whether measured on a dry weight or on a haematin basis, than the catalases of mammalian tissues. Since the prosthetic groups are the same, the difference must be attributed to the protein component of the enzyme.

Assuming our crystalline preparations to be pure, the mean haematin content of 1·09 % corresponds to a molecular weight of $58,000 \times n$, where n is the number of haematin groups/mol. Assuming $n = 4$, as for catalases of mammalian tissues, this gives a value for the molecular weight of 232,000.

of the completely pure enzyme may be some 10 % higher than the values given above.

Once the molecular weight and *Kat.-f.* of the pure enzyme are known, it is possible to calculate the 'Turnover Number', defined by Warburg & Christian (1933) as the number of molecules of substrate decomposed by one molecule in 1 min. The relation between Turnover no. and *Kat.-f.* is obtained as follows. The initial velocity is obtained from the velocity constant k_0 by the first-order reaction equation $\left(\dfrac{-dS}{dt}\right)_{t=0} = 2.303\, k_0 S_0$. By definition,

$$Kat.\text{-}f. = \frac{k_0}{\text{g. catalase/50 ml.}} = 20\, k_0/EM,\ \text{where } S_0 \text{ and}$$

S are the concentrations of hydrogen peroxide at 0 and t min., and E is the concentration of catalase (all in mol./l.), and M is the molecular weight of catalase.

Hence,

$$\text{Turnover no.} = \frac{1}{E}\left(\frac{-dS}{dt}\right)_{t=0} = Kat.\text{-}f. \times 0\cdot115\,MS_0.$$

For bacterial catalase of mol. wt. $= 232,000$ and $Kat.\text{-}f. = 95,000$, under the test conditions $(0\cdot0075\,\text{M-}H_2O_2$ at $0°)$, this gives a Turnover no. of 19×10^6, the highest recorded for any enzyme.

By similar calculations, the relation between $Kat.\text{-}f.$ and the Q_{O_2} (μl. O_2 evolved/mg. of enzyme/hr.) is given by

$$Q_{O_2} = Kat.\text{-}f. \times 77,500\,S_0.$$

Under the test conditions, bacterial catalase has a Q_{O_2} of 55×10^6. (The activity of catalase is usually measured at low hydrogen peroxide concentrations, when the percentage of total enzyme combined with substrate is small and proportional to the substrate concentration, so that the reaction is first order. Under these conditions k and $Kat.\text{-}f.$ are independent of the initial substrate concentration, but the Turnover no. and Q_{O_2} are directly proportional to the hydrogen peroxide concentration, which should always be stated.)

Coupled oxidation of alcohols

Keilin & Hartree (1936, 1945b) have shown that if catalase and ethanol are added to any enzyme system which produces hydrogen peroxide, the latter is used by the catalase to bring about a 'coupled oxidation' of the ethanol to acetaldehyde. In other words, under these special conditions (continuous slow supply of hydrogen peroxide at a very low concentration), the catalase acts as a peroxidase.

Fig. 3 shows that bacterial catalase behaves exactly like liver catalase in this respect. Xanthine oxidase-hypoxanthine was used as the source of hydrogen peroxide; the coupled oxidation is shown by a doubling of the theoretical oxygen uptake and the formation of acetaldehyde, recognized by its smell and the brown coloration imparted to the potassium hydroxide papers in the manometer cups. Acetaldehyde is only formed when catalase, ethanol, xanthine oxidase and hypoxanthine are all present.

DISCUSSION

The objects of this work were twofold: to investigate the use of lysozyme for the liberation of enzymes from the bacterial cell, and to apply this technique to the isolation of bacterial catalase.

Our present results indicate that the lysozyme technique is an excellent one, though not entirely without drawbacks. It is, of course, only applicable to lysozyme-sensitive micro-organisms. The viscous substances released from the bacteria by lysozyme (or possibly formed by its action) are a decided hindrance in the initial stages of enzyme purification. Nevertheless, the simplicity of the technique, the

fact that it is unlikely to destroy labile enzymes, and its ready applicability on either a large or a small scale, should make it a useful tool in studying the intracellular components of bacteria.

The isolation of the catalase of *M. lysodeikticus* was undertaken partly in the hope that interesting differences might be revealed between the bacterial enzyme and the catalases of mammalian tissues. In fact, the differences observed are less striking than the similarities. The prosthetic group is the same as that of mammalian catalases, the molecular weight is the same, and there are the same number of haematin groups in the molecule. The main difference is that the catalytic activity of the bacterial enzyme is considerably higher than that of mammalian catalases; this difference must be attributed to the protein component of the enzyme.

The protein components of sheep, ox, horse and human catalases have all been shown to be different by immunological methods (Tria, 1939; Campbell & Fourt, 1939; Bonnichsen, 1947), and there is little doubt that the protein of bacterial catalase is different again. All these proteins, however, when combined with haematin, have the common property of catalyzing specifically the decomposition of hydrogen peroxide. It seems reasonable to suppose that this common property is related to some common structural element of the molecule—possibly some particular grouping of certain amino-acids—on which the catalytic activity depends. A careful study of the same enzyme isolated from several different sources might throw considerable light on the nature of enzymic catalysis. Catalase, which has now been isolated pure from so many different sources, should be a suitable enzyme to choose for such an investigation.

Another point of interest arising from this work is the remarkably high concentration of catalase found in *M. lysodeikticus*. This can be calculated from the $Kat.\text{-}f.$ values of the pure enzyme (95,000) and the lyzed bacteria (800–1800 in different batches), giving a catalase content for this organism of 1–2 % of its dry weight. This is about ten times the catalase content of human red blood corpuscles (Herbert & Pinsent, 1948). It can also be calculated that a single bacterial cell (dry weight taken as $2\cdot5 \times 10^{-13}$ g.) contains 10–20×10^3 enzyme molecules.

Such calculations raise the question of the function of catalase in *M. lysodeikticus*. The above concentrations of catalase would enable each bacterial cell to decompose c. 35–70 times its own weight of hydrogen peroxide/min. (at $0°$ and hydrogen peroxide concentration of $0\cdot01\text{M}$). Such large amounts of peroxide could scarcely be formed as a result of cell metabolism, and it is difficult to devise any teleological explanation for this high enzyme concentration unless, as the discovery of 'coupled oxidation' by Keilin & Hartree (1936, 1945b) suggests, catalase has other functions besides the simple decomposition of hydrogen peroxide.

SUMMARY

1. The use of lysozyme in the study of intracellular bacterial enzymes and some phenomena noticed when lysozyme acts on concentrated bacterial suspensions are discussed.

2. Using lysozyme to liberate the enzyme from the bacterial cell, catalase has been isolated from *Micrococcus lysodeikticus* in crystalline form.

3. Bacterial catalase is in many respects similar to the catalases of animal tissues. The crystalline enzyme contains c. $1·1\%$ of haematin, identical with ordinary blood haematin.

4. It differs from liver catalases, but resembles erythrocyte catalases, in containing no verdohaematin.

5. Haematin content and ultracentrifugal data indicate a molecular weight of c. 230,000, with four haematin groups/molecule.

6. The catalytic activity is considerably higher than that of mammalian tissue catalases; the difference is to be attributed to the protein component of the enzyme.

Our thanks are due to Dr D. W. Henderson, Chief Superintendent of the Microbiological Research Department, Porton, and his staff, for their invaluable assistance in growing the large quantities of bacteria necessary for this work.

REFERENCES

Agner, K. (1938). *Biochem. J.* **32**, 1702.
Agner, K. (1942). *Ark. Kemi Min. Geol.* **16** A, no. 6.
Agner, K. & Theorell, H. (1946). *Arch. Biochem.* **10**, 321.
Alderton, G. & Fevold, H. L. (1946). *J. biol. Chem.* **164**, 1.
Alderton, G., Ward, W. H. & Fevold, H. L. (1945). *J. biol. Chem.* **157**, 43.
Anson, M. L. & Mirsky, A. E. (1929–30). *J. gen. Physiol.* **13**, 469.
Bonnichsen, R. K. (1947). *Arch. Biochem.* **12**, 83.
Booth, V. & Green, D. E. (1938). *Biochem. J.* **32**, 855.
Campbell, D. H. & Fourt, L. (1939). *J. biol. Chem.* **129**, 385.
Cecil, R. & Ogston, A. G. (1948). *Biochem. J.* **43**, 205.
Curran, H. R. & Evans, F. R. (1942). *J. Bact.* **43**, 125.
Epps, H. M. R. & Gale, E. F. (1942). *Biochem. J.* **36**, 619.
Euler, H. von & Josephson, K. (1927). *Liebigs Ann.* **452**, 158.
Fleming, A. (1922). *Proc. Roy. Soc. B,* **93**, 306.
Fleming, A. (1929). *Lancet,* **216**, 217.
Gladstone, G. P. & Fildes, P. (1940). *Brit. J. exp. Path.* **21**, 161.
Gottstein, A. (1893). *Virchows Arch.* **133**, 295.
Herbert, D. & Pinsent, J. (1948). *Biochem. J.* **43**, 203.
Kalnitsky, G., Utter, M. F. & Werkman, C. H. (1945). *J. Bact.* **49**, 595.
Keilin, D. & Hartree, E. F. (1936). *Proc. Roy. Soc. B,* **119**, 141.
Keilin, D. & Hartree, E. F. (1937). *Proc. Roy. Soc. B,* **121**, 173.

Keilin, D. & Hartree, E. F. (1945a). *Biochem. J.* **39**, 148.
Keilin, D. & Hartree, E. F. (1945b). *Biochem. J.* **39**, 293.
King, E. J. & Gilchrist, M. (1947). *Lancet,* **253**, 201.
Krampitz, L. O. & Werkman, C. H. (1941). *Biochem. J.* **35**, 595.
Laskowski, M. & Sumner, J. B. (1941). *Science,* **94**, 615.
Lemberg, R. & Legge, J. W. (1943). *Biochem. J.* **37**, 117.
Penrose, M. & Quastel, J. H. (1930). *Proc. Roy. Soc. B,* **107**, 168.
Pressman, D. (1943). *Industr. Engng Chem.* (Anal. ed.), **15**, 357.
Quastel, J. H. (1937). *Enzymologia,* **2**, 37.
Rimington, C. (1942). *Brit. med. J.* **1**, 177.
Scott Blair, G. W., Folley, S. J., Malpress, F. M. & Coppen, F. M. V. (1941). *Biochem. J.* **35**, 1039.
Stumpf, P. K., Green, D. E. & Smith, F. W. (1946). *J. Bact.* **51**, 487.
Sumner, J. B. (1941). *Advanc. Enzymol.* **1**, 163.
Sumner, J. B. & Dounce, A. L. (1937). *J. biol. Chem.* **121**, 417.
Sumner, J. B. & Dounce, A. L. (1939). *J. biol. Chem.* **127**, 439.
Sumner, J. B., Dounce, A. L. & Frampton, O. D. (1940). *J. biol. Chem.* **136**, 343.
Sumner, J. B. & Gralén, J. (1938). *J. biol. Chem.* **125**, 33.
Tria, E. (1939). *J. biol. Chem.* **129**, 377.
Warburg, O. & Christian, W. (1933). *Biochem. Z.* **266**, 377.

Part III

OXIDATIVE PHOSPHORYLATION

Editor's Comments
on Papers 16, 17, and 18

ERA OF THE "CHEMICAL INTERMEDIATE" HYPOTHESIS

We have so far examined the development of concepts of terminal electron transport during microbial respiration without considering mechanisms through which the energy thereby liberated is biologically conserved. This question is central to our understanding of respiration. The phenomenon of oxidative phosphorylation—the esterification of inorganic phosphate energized by respiration—has been known for nearly forty years, but the intimate chemical mechanism by which it occurs still resists resolution. Several hypotheses to explain such a reaction have been advanced, but only the major theories are offered here, since they dominated the period immediately following their publication. The theories seek to describe the mechanism by which respiratory energy is trapped prior to its conservation in the form of a phosphate anhydride bond in adenosine 5'-triphosphate. The first hypothesis, conceived by analogy with "substrate-level" phosphorylation, was advanced by E. C. Slater in Paper 16. This is the so-called "chemical intermediate" hypothesis. Its strength lay in the fact that it was based upon the precedent of soluble enzymes synthesizing ATP, most notably glyceraldehyde-3-phosphate dehydrogenase-1,3-diphosphoglycerate phosphokinase; its weakness (as we now know) lay in its lack of consideration of the role of the membrane in biological energy conservation.

In the period during which the chemical intermediate hypothesis predominated, the study of microbial oxidative phosphorylation began. The earliest demonstration of oxidative phosphorylation in a subcellular preparation was that reported by Gifford Pinchot and Efraim Racker in Paper 17.

The so-called "partial" reactions of oxidative phosphorylation were also identified in subcellular preparations from bacteria. Furthermore, in Paper 18, Asano, Imai, and Sato provided a description of energy-dependent reversed electron transport in a *Micrococcus* and several investigators independently observed the energy-dependent reduction $NADP^+$ by NADH (see reference 1 and Paper 30). These reactions had been previously demonstrated in mitochondria.

Chemoautotrophy is a phenomenon peculiar to the procaryotes. Having attained a high degree of biochemical sophistication, such organisms survive at the expense of only inorganic sources of energy, reducing equivalents and carbon. Except for the hydrogen oxidizers, autotrophic energy conservation proceeds through the oxidation of electron donors (e.g. NH_4^+, NO_2^-, Fe^{2+}, $S_2O_3^{2-}$) considerably more electropositive than the NAD^+/NADH couple, and it is to be expected that energy would be required for net NADH production for purposes of biosynthesis. Several hypotheses of "obligate" chemoautotrophy have invoked anomalous NADH oxidation as the explanation for the apparent inability of these bacteria to grow at the expense of organic compounds, even though the same organic compounds may be incorporated into cell material.

The first comprehensive studies of respiration in chemoautotrophic bacteria were performed by W. W. Umbreit and his associates at Wisconsin, who established that respiratory mechanisms were operative in the thiobacilli similar to those of heterotrophic microorganisms (see, for example, reference 2). L. Kiesow examined the special properties of the respiratory apparatus of nitrite-oxidizing *Nitrobacter*, and brought forward the notion of partitioning of respiratory energy between ATP synthesis and energy-requiring reversed-electron transport bringing about NAD^+ reduction for biosynthesis (see, for example, reference 3). Recently, a chemiosmotic treatment of these phenomena has been presented.[4]

Using intact thiobacilli, Roth, Hempfling, Conners, and Vishniac[5] showed that energy-dependent reversed-electron transport is the major, if not the sole, pathway of net NADH formation during thiosulfate or sulfide oxidation. This is perhaps the only example of an essential biological function of energy-dependent reversed electron transport.

REFERENCES

1. Murthy, P. S., and A. F. Brodie. *J. Biol. Chem.*, **239**, 4292–4297, 1964.
2. Vogler, K., G. LePage, and W. W. Umbreit. *J. Gen. Physiol.*, **26**, 89–102, 1942.
3. Kiesow, L., *Proc. Nat. Acad. Sci.* (U.S.), **52**, 980–988, 1964.
4. Cobley, J. G. *Biochem. J.*, **156,** 481–491, 493–498, 1976.
5. Roth, C. W., W. P. Hempfling, J. N. Conners, and W. V. Vishniac. *J. Bact.*, **114**, 592–599, 1973.

16

Reprinted from *Nature* (London) **172**:975–978 (1953)

MECHANISM OF PHOSPHORYLATION IN THE RESPIRATORY CHAIN

By Dr. E. C. SLATER

Molteno Institute, University of Cambridge

WHEN Belitzer and Tsibakowa[1] and Ochoa[2] found that more than one atom of phosphorus was esterified for each atom of oxygen consumed by respiring tissue preparations, they suggested that the phosphorylation must occur not only when the substrate was dehydrogenated, but also during the passage of the hydrogen atoms over the intermediate carriers to oxygen. This was demonstrated experimentally by Lehninger[3], who showed that phosphorylation accompanied the oxidation of reduced diphosphopyridine nucleotide by oxygen. In fact, it was shown that when β-hydroxybutyrate was substrate, all the phosphorylation occurred in the reaction between reduced diphosphopyridine nucleotide and oxygen, and none between substrate and diphosphopyridine nucleotide. With α-ketoglutarate[4], glyceraldehydephosphate[5] or pyruvate[6] (in certain micro-organisms only) as substrate, there is also phosphorylation linked with the initial dehydrogenation of the substrate. It is convenient to distinguish between oxidative phosphorylation of this type ('substrate-linked phosphorylation') and that associated with the further transfer of hydrogen atoms over the respiratory chain ('respiratory chain phosphorylation'). While considerable progress has been made in recent years with the elucidation of the mechanism of substrate-linked phosphorylation, little success has yet been met with in the case of respiratory chain phosphorylation. In fact, the particular hydrogen- or electron-transferring reactions in the respiratory chain which are associated with phosphorylation have not yet been identified. A detailed description of the mechanism of respiratory chain phosphorylation must await this identification. However, some recent findings have made it possible to suggest in general terms a mechanism in which the actual hydrogen-carriers are not specified.

Proposed Mechanism

The suggested mechanism is based on the following observations.

(a) In intact mitochondria, the passage of each pair of hydrogen atoms over the respiratory chain is coupled with the esterification of one, two or perhaps three atoms of inorganic phosphorus. The respiration appears to be compulsorily linked with phosphorylation[7], in the sense that inorganic phosphate and adenosine diphosphate are necessary for respiration.

(b) It is possible to obtain tissue preparations (for example, the Keilin and Hartree heart-muscle preparation[8]) which actively catalyse the aerobic oxidation of succinate or reduced diphosphopyridine nucleotide, without carrying out oxidative phosphorylation. Inorganic phosphate is not necessary for these reactions[8,9]. It has been suggested that these preparations consist of disrupted sarcosomal or mitochondrial membrane[10].

(c) A number of substances of widely different chemical structure can 'uncouple' phosphorylation from oxidation. In some cases (liver mitochondria[7], heart sarcosomes[11]), the rate of oxidation in the presence of inorganic phosphate, adenosine diphosphate, hexokinase and glucose is scarcely affected by the addition of a typical uncoupling agent, dinitrophenol; in the case of sarcosomes prepared from the flight muscles of the blowfly, the rate of oxidation is greatly increased[11]. The latter sarcosomes have an unusually low phosphorus to oxygen ratio.

(d) Some of the substances which 'uncouple' phosphorylation from respiration increase the rate of hydrolysis of adenosine triphosphate[12].

A common feature of the mechanisms of the substrate-linked phosphorylations (Racker[5]; Kaufman[4]) is that the dehydrogenated substrate is not immediately liberated, but remains bound to a grouping in the dehydrogenase molecule, from which it is freed by phosphorolysis reactions. In the present state of our knowledge, it seems worth while to see if the same general type of mechanism can explain respiratory chain phosphorylation. A mechanism along these lines is embodied in the following equations:

(1) $AH_2 + B + C \rightleftharpoons A{\sim}C + BH_2$

(2) $A{\sim}C + ADP + H_3PO_4 \rightleftharpoons A + C + ATP$

(3) $A{\sim}C + H_2O \rightarrow A + C.$

AH_2 and B are adjacent members of the respiratory chain and C is an additional component or grouping required for their interaction. A and C must be regenerated from the compound $A{\sim}C$ before hydrogen-transfer can proceed. In the intact mitochondria or sarcosome, this is brought about primarily by the transphosphorylating reaction (2), which leads to the esterification of inorganic phosphate. It is suggested that reaction (3) is relatively slow in the intact mitochondria, but can be greatly increased by dinitrophenol or other uncoupling agents. In this way, $A \sim C$ would be hydrolysed and be unavailable for the synthesis of adenosine triphosphate by reaction (2).

The idea that a compound like C mediates the conversion of the energy of an oxido-reduction into phosphate bond energy was first suggested in 1946 by Lipmann[13], whose mechanism may be described as :

$$AH_2 + C \rightarrow A + CH_2$$
$$CH_2 + H_3PO_4 \rightarrow CH_2.H_2PO_3 \text{ } (CH_2 \text{ is first dehydrated})$$
$$CH_2.H_2PO_3 + B \rightarrow C \sim H_2PO_3 + BH_2$$
$$C \sim H_2PO_3 + ADP \rightarrow C + ATP.$$

An essential difference between the two mechanisms is that in Lipmann's scheme phosphate enters before, and in the scheme described in reactions (1)–(3) it enters after, the formation of an energy-rich bond. The latter scheme is suggested by the work carried out since 1946 in a field largely opened up by Lipmann's discovery of coenzyme A.

Since phosphorylation occurs more than once during the passage of hydrogen atoms through the respiratory chain, more than one set of reactions described by equations (1)–(3) will occur, in which AH_2 and B are different. It is possible, however, that a common mediator C occurs in all sets of reactions. This would not be the case with Lipmann's mechanism, since the $C \rightleftharpoons CH_2$ oxidation-reduction potential must be suitably related to those of the $A \rightleftharpoons AH_2$ and $B \rightleftharpoons BH_2$ systems[13].

Equations (1) and (2) are probably the sums of a number of partial reactions, which are not specified in full, because it is impossible to choose between alternatives. For example, the intermediate in reaction (2) could be A-phosphate, C-phosphate, A-adenosine diphosphate or C-adenosine diphosphate.

Effect of Dinitrophenol

The uncoupling action of dinitrophenol is explained if it promotes the hydrolytic reaction of $A \sim C$, thereby decreasing the amount of the latter available for the phosphorolytic reaction.

The different behaviour of liver mitochondria and heart sarcosomes, on one hand, and of blowfly sarcosomes, on the other (see paragraph (c) above), can be readily explained in the following way. The high phosphorus to oxygen ratio of heart-muscle sarcosomes and the relative insensitivity of the ratio to treatments which affect the rate of hydrogen-transfer[14] suggest that reaction (2) can proceed much faster than reaction (1); that is, the regeneration of A and C from $A \sim C$ is not a rate-limiting step. The addition of dinitrophenol, by promoting reaction (3), will stop the esterification of phosphate; but since it increases the rate of a process which is not rate-limiting, it will not increase the rate of hydrogen-transfer to any extent. The low phosphorus to oxygen ratio of blowfly sarcosomes, on the other hand, suggests that reaction (2) is relatively weak. The rate of hydrogen-transfer will, therefore, be increased by increasing the rate of breakdown of $A \sim C$, for example, by the addition of dinitrophenol. It is also understandable on this basis why lower concentrations of dinitrophenol are required to uncouple phosphorylation with the blowfly sarcosomes than with heart-muscle sarcosomes[11].

The different behaviour of heart and blowfly sarcosomes to the addition of dinitrophenol could also be explained by Lipmann's mechanism, if it is assumed that dinitrophenol increases the rate of hydrolysis of $C \sim H_2PO_3$. However, the mechanism described by reactions (1)–(3) is more successful in explaining the discovery of Loomis and Lipmann[15] that dinitrophenol abolishes the requirement of respiration for inorganic phosphate, since in the presence of dinitrophenol respiration proceeds by reactions (1) and (3), which do not involve phosphate.

The stimulation of reaction (3) by dinitrophenol not only explains the uncoupling of phosphorylation, but also the stimulation of the rate of hydrolysis of adenosine triphosphate, since the back-reaction of equation (2), followed by a rapid reaction (3), would cause the hydrolysis of adenosine triphosphate. This idea is essentially that of Hunter and of Lardy and Wellman[12], except that they suggest a phosphorylated compound (corresponding to $C \sim H_2PO_3$ in the above formulation of Lipmann's mechanism) as the intermediate the hydrolysis of which is stimulated by dinitrophenol (see also Green[16]).

In considering the possible mechanism of the stimulation of reaction (3) by inhibitors of oxidative phosphorylation, it is necessary to take account of the wide range of substances of varying chemical composition which can act as inhibitors. This strongly suggests that most of these substances if not all, act by a relatively non-specific mechanism. It is likely that the enzyme catalysing reaction (3) is present even in the intact mitochondria in the absence of inhibitors, but it may be inaccessible to $A \sim C$, and the inhibitor acts by making the enzyme and its substrate accessible to one another. An explanation of this type is supported by the fact that incubation of mitochondria or sarcosomes, which causes well-defined changes in the morphology of the granules, brings about a loss of respiratory chain phosphorylation; for example, that associated with the oxidation of succinate or β-hydroxybutyrate. This explanation would not exclude the possibility that some inhibitors of oxidative phosphorylation might react by a more specific mechanism, for example, by actual participation in reaction (3) (see Lardy and Wellman[12]).

Respiratory Chain Activity in the Absence of Inorganic Phosphate

The oxidation of succinate or of reduced diphospho-pyridine nucleotide by the Keilin and Hartree heart-muscle preparation in the absence of inorganic phosphate can be explained in two ways : (i) during the preparation of these particles from the sarcosomes, the mutual accessibilities of the components of the respiratory chain are altered in such a way that reactions (1), (2) and (3) are replaced by the simple hydrogen-transferring reaction :

$$(4) \quad AH_2 + B \rightarrow A + BH_2 \ ;$$

or (ii) even in this preparation, C is necessary for the reaction between AH_2 and B, and the preparation also contains the enzyme catalysing reaction (3). This would mean that this hydrolytic enzyme is, like all the components of the respiratory chain, firmly bound to the insoluble portion of the sarcosome, which resists the disintegration treatment. However, the enzyme catalysing reaction (2) may be lost during the preparation.

While the first explanation is adequate for studies with the Keilin and Hartree heart-muscle preparation of hydrogen-transfer without accompanying phosphorylation, the second has the advantage that it eliminates the necessity of postulating that C is essential for the reaction between AH_2 and B in the intact sarcosome, but is not required in the disintegrated sarcosome, which still contains all the components of the respiratory chain firmly bound to the particles. It is simpler to assume that the reactions which are retained in the disintegrated sarcosomes follow the same course as in the intact sarcosomes.

In any event, reaction (4) does not take account of an important difficulty in any formulation of the

185

mechanism of the respiratory chain. Although kinetic studies[17] suggest that the components react together by binary collision, the independence of the rate of reaction on the degree of dilution shows that the components are very firmly bound to the particles. This suggests that the mechanism may, in fact, be much more complicated than indicated by reaction (4).

Utilization of Respiratory Energy

An essential feature of the proposed mechanism is that the free-energy change in the reaction $AH_2 + B \rightarrow A + BH_2$ is not immediately liberated as heat, but remains chemically available in the compound $A \sim C$. Thus an essentially irreversible oxido-reduction reaction could become easily reversible. The energy in $A \sim C$ may either be utilized in reaction (2) to synthesize adenosine triphosphate, another reversible reaction, or be lost as heat in the irreversible hydrolytic reaction (3). But it would be unwise to assume that adenosine triphosphate is the only energy-rich compound which the cell can utilize. It is possible that $A \sim C$ might itself be used in some reactions. Woolley[18] has recently directed attention to the possibility of the utilization in the cell of energy-rich bonds, other than the pyrophosphate bond. If the $A \sim C$ bond can be used in this way, it is important to note that it can be formed in two ways, either by the respiratory chain reaction (1) without the intervention of phosphorus, or from adenosine triphosphate by reversal of reaction (2). This is exactly analogous to the case of acetyl–coenzyme A, the general acetylating agent in the cell. Acetyl–coenzyme A may be formed either by the oxidative decarboxylation of pyruvate in the complete absence of phosphorus[19], or by the reaction of coenzyme A, acetate and adenosine triphosphate[20].

If $A \sim C$ is concerned in certain energy-requiring processes in the cell, the reverse of reaction (2) might be a way in which adenosine triphosphate produced by fermentation or glycolysis could be utilized under anaerobic conditions by cells possessing the necessary enzymes. These processes would be expected to be prevented by any substance, for example, dinitrophenol, causing the breakdown of $A \sim C$. Thus, dinitrophenol would prevent the utilization, not the synthesis, of adenosine triphosphate. This would also be the case if the adenosine triphosphate formed anaerobically were utilized by another mechanism, since dinitrophenol causes its hydrolysis. Either of these possibilities might be the explanation of one puzzling action of dinitrophenol. It has been shown with extracts that the reactions in glycolysis or fermentation which bring about the formation of adenosine triphosphate are not susceptible to dinitrophenol[21]. Nevertheless, energy-requiring processes such as enzyme adaptation in yeast[22], or uptake of glutamate by *Staphylococcus aureus*[23], are inhibited by dinitrophenol, even under anaerobic conditions. On the other hand, the transport of ions by erythrocytes, a process also receiving its energy from glycolysis, is not affected by dinitrophenol[24]. This is understandable on the basis of the above explanation, since erythrocytes do not contain a complete respiratory chain, that is, they may not contain A.

The suggestion that $A \sim C$ might itself be used directly for certain energy-requiring processes raises the possibility that the energy of certain steps of the respiratory chain is normally utilized in this way and not via phosphorylation. The measurement of the yield of phosphorylation in respiration might not be a complete measure of the efficiency of utilization of the energy potentially available from respiration.

Conclusion

In conclusion, it should be emphasized that many of the features of the proposed mechanism are based on analogy with reaction schemes describing the participation of coenzyme A or the sulphydryl group of glyceraldehydephosphate dehydrogenase in substrate-linked phosphorylation which have recently been worked out by Racker[5] and Kaufman[4]. While there is no reason why similar reactions should necessarily operate in respiratory chain phosphorylation, the fact that the suggested mechanism offers possible explanations of some puzzling findings is some justification for believing that this might be the case. However, much more experimental evidence is required. It is obvious without considering any particular mechanism that the identification of AH_2 and B from among the comparatively few and well-studied components of the respiratory chain remains an urgent task. But it could be important to recognize that a third substance might be required for their interaction. A fat-soluble substance is a possibility to be kept in mind, since about 40 per cent of the dry weight of the Keilin and Hartree preparation is phospholipid.

I wish to thank Prof. D. Keilin for his interest and advice. This work was carried out on behalf of the Agricultural Research Council.

[1] Belitzer, V. A., and Tsibakowa, E. T., *Biokhimiya*, **4**, 516 (1939).

[2] Ochoa, S., *Nature*, **146**, 267 (1940) ; *J. Biol. Chem.*, **138**, 751 (1941).

[3] Friedkin, M., and Lehninger, A. L., *J. Biol. Chem.*, **178**, 611 (1949). Lehninger, A. L., *J. Biol. Chem.*, **178**, 625 (1949). Lehninger, A. L., and Smith, S. W., *J. Biol. Chem.*, **181**, 415 (1949). Lehninger, A. L., *J. Biol. Chem.*, **190**, 345 (1951).

[4] Hunter, F. E., and Hixon, W. H., *J. Biol. Chem.*, **181**, 67 (1949). Kaufman, S., in "Phosphorus Metabolism", **1**, 370 (Johns Hopkins Press, Baltimore, Md., 1951).

[5] Warburg, O., and Christian, W., *Biochem. Z.*, **303**, 40 (1939). Racker E., and Krimsky, I., *J. Biol. Chem.*, **198**, 731 (1952).

[6] Lipmann, F., *J. Biol. Chem.*, **155**, 55 (1944).

[7] Lardy, H. A., and Wellman, H., *J. Biol. Chem.*, **195**, 215 (1952).

[8] Keilin, D., and Hartree, E. F., *Biochem. J.*, **41**, 500 (1947).

[9] Bonner, W. D., *Biochem. J.*, **49**, viii (1951).

[10] Cleland, K. W., and Slater, E. C., *Biochem. J.*, **53**, 547 (1953).

[11] Lewis, S. E., and Slater, E. C., *Biochem. J.* (in the press). Slater, E. C., and Lewis, S. E., *Biochem. J.* (in the press).

[12] Ronzoni, E., and Ehrenfest, E., *J. Biol. Chem.*, **115**, 749 (1936). Lardy, H. A., and Elvehjem, C. A., "Ann. Rev. Biochem.", **14**, 1 (1945). Potter, V. R., and Recknagel, R. O., in "Phosphorus Metabolism", **1**, 377 (Johns Hopkins Press, Baltimore, Md., 1951). Hunter, F. E., in "Phosphorus Metabolism", **1**, 297 (1951). Lardy, H., and Wellman, H., *J. Biol. Chem.*, **201**, 357 (1953).

[13] Lipmann, F., in "Currents in Biochemical Research", p. 137 (Intersci. Pub., Inc., New York, 1946).

[14] Slater, E. C., and Cleland, K. W., *Biochem. J.*, **53**, 557 (1953).

[15] Loomis, W. F., and Lipmann, F., *J. Biol. Chem.*, **173**, 807 (1948),

[16] Green, D. E., *Biol. Rev.*, **26**, 410 (1951).

[17] Chance, B., *Nature*, **169**, 215 (1952). Slater, E. C., in "Biologie und Wirkung der Fermente", 4. Colloquium der Gesellschaft für physiologische Chemie, p. 64 (Springer-Verlag, Heidelberg, 1953).

[18] Woolley, D. W., *Nature*, **171**, 323 (1953).

[19] Korkes, S., Campillo, A. del, Gunsalus, I. C., and Ochoa, S., *J. Biol. Chem.*, **193**, 721 (1951). Korkes, S., Campillo, A. del, and Ochoa, S., *J. Biol. Chem.*, **195**, 541 (1952).

[20] Lipmann, F., Jones, M. E., Black, S., and Flynn, R. M., *J. Amer. Chem. Soc.*, **74**, 2384 (1952).

[21] Greville, G. D., and Rowsell, E. V., unpublished experiments (1949), quoted by Judah, J. D., *Biochem. J.*, **49**, 271 (1951).

[22] Spiegelman, S., *J. Cell. Comp. Physiol.*, **30**, 315 (1947).

[23] Gale, E. F., *Biochem. J.*, **48**, 286 (1951).

[24] Maizels, M., *J. Physiol.*, **112**, 59 (1951).

17

Reprinted from pp. 366–369 of *Phosphorous Metabolism*, W. D. McElroy and
B. Glass, eds., The Johns Hopkins Press, 1951, 762pp.

ETHYL ALCOHOL OXIDATION AND PHOSPHORYLATION IN EXTRACTS OF *E. COLI*

G. B. PINCHOT AND E. RACKER

Department of Microbiology
New York University College of Medicine, New York

AN ENZYME system has been found in *E. coli* extracts which is capable of esterification of inorganic phosphate during alcohol oxidation. The crude extract can be stored for several weeks in the deep freeze without marked loss of activity. When centrifuged for 3 hours at 18,000 g, most of the activity remains in the supernatant.

The crude enzyme preparation was made from strain B *E. coli* cells, grown in neopeptone broth for 18 hours. The organisms were washed twice in distilled water and broken with a Raytheon sonic disintegrator, after which the cellular debris was removed by a short period of high-speed centrifugation.

DPNH oxidase activity was determined spectrophotometrically by measuring the disappearance of DPNH absorption at 340 mμ. The specific activity of extracts made from cells grown on neopeptone broth was three to five times that of preparations made from organisms grown on a defined medium with glucose as the carbon source. Oxidation of reduced DPN was not inhibited by 2×10^{-3} M KCN, whereas 2×10^{-4} M caused 80% inhibition in a pigeon heart muscle preparation prepared according to the method of Keilin and Hartree

(2). 2×10^{-2} molar BAL did not inhibit the bacterial enzyme, while according to Slater this concentration causes complete inhibition of heart muscle preparations (4). These findings demonstrate some of the differences between the bacterial and animal oxidizing systems.

Phosphorylation was studied by following oxygen and phosphate uptake in a mixture of glycylglycine and phosphate buffer at pH 7.2. 100 micromoles of alcohol, an excess of crystalline yeast alcohol dehydrogenase, and 0.75 micromoles of DPN were added to the enzyme preparation. The high energy phosphate formed was trapped by adding 100 micromoles of glucose, purified yeast hexokinase, MgCl₂

TABLE 1

THE DEPENDENCE OF PHOSPHORYLATION ON THE ADDITION OF DPN

Enzyme Preparation Substrate	Crude Extract Alcohol	Crude Extract Alcohol
DPN	—	+
Oxygen consumption in microatoms	2.80	11.25
Phosphate taken up in micromoles	3.01	11.84
P/O ratio	1.07	1.05

The complete system contained in each vessel: 0.5 ml. *E. coli* extract, 0.5 ml. of 0.5 M glycylglycine buffer, pH 7.2; 20 micromoles of inorganic phosphate, 100 micromoles of alcohol, 0.75 micromoles of DPN, excess alcohol dehydrogenase, MgCl₂ (7 x 10⁻³ M), and water to make a final volume of 3.0 ml. In the side arm were placed excess hexokinase, 100 micromoles of glucose, 1.5 micromoles of ATP and NaF (10⁻² M f.c.). The center well contained 0.2 ml. of 40% KOH.

$(7 \times 10^{-3} \text{ M})$, and 1.5 micromoles of ATP. 10^{-2} M NaF was added to inhibited ATPase and enolase. At the end of the experiment the reaction was stopped with trichloroacetic acid, and the disappearance of inorganic phosphate was measured. The oxidation and phosphorylation were largely dependent on the addition of DPN to the reaction mixture, as shown in Table 1.

It was then observed that the oxidation of acetaldehyde contributed considerably to the phosphate uptake, resulting in P/O ratios often as high as 1.5. This was found to be due to an aldehyde dehydrogenase which is present in the *E. coli* extracts, similar to the enzyme in *Clostridium kluyveri* described by Stadtman and Barker (5). As shown in Table 2, this enzyme in *E. coli* is dependent on the presence of coenzyme A preparations for its activity in respect to hydrogen transfer as well as acetyl phosphate formation. Treatment with

Dowex 1 according to the method of Chantrenne and Lipmann (1) resulted in nearly complete loss of dehydrogenase activity, which was fully restored by the addition of coenzyme A preparations (kindly supplied by Dr. S. Korkes). The large amounts of acetyl phosphate formed relative to oxygen uptake was probably due to a dismutation, since these crude *E. coli* preparations contain some alcohol dehydrogenase activity.

TABLE 2

EFFECT OF COENZYME A PREPARATION ON ACETALDEHYDE DEHYDROGENASE OF *E. coli*

	Micromoles	
	O_2 uptake	Acetyl-phosphate formed
Dowex-treated enzyme	0	<0.3
Dowex-treated enzyme + acetaldehyde	0.2	<0.3
Dowex-treated enzyme + acetaldehyde and Co A	6.15	9.5
Dowex-treated enzyme + Co A	0.15	<0.3

The system contained in each vessel 0.5 ml. of the *E. coli* enzyme, 0.2 ml. of 1 M K phosphate buffer, pH 7.4 and 0.75 micromoles of DPN; where indicated 8.4 units of coenzyme A and 30 micromoles of acetaldehyde. Final volume was 3 ml. and the center well contained 0.2 ml. of 40% KOH.

When the crude *E. coli* enzyme was treated with Dowex-1, then precipitated at 50% ammonium sulfate saturation, and dialyzed for 2 hours, the preparation was still capable of esterification of inorganic phosphate if an alcohol dehydrogenase preparation and alcohol were added (Table 3). Pretreatment of the *E. coli* extract with iodoacetate (10^{-3} M) effectively depressed endogenous glycolysis of such preparations without impairing significantly the uptake of inorganic phosphate. Although treatment of the extracts with Dowex-1 and iodoacetate would seem to eliminate acetyl phosphate and glycolysis as donors of energy-rich phosphate, a final conclusion cannot yet be drawn from these preliminary observations.

Several findings which still obscure the picture should be mentioned. Dinitrophenol, known to inhibit phosphorylation in animal tissues, has no effect on the bacterial system. Two attempts, in which large amounts of reduced DPN have been used to determine whether phosphate uptake occurs during its oxidation, have been negative.

However, in view of Lehninger's findings (3) of a toxic factor in DPNH preparations, these experiments cannot be considered conclusive. Furthermore, with some preparations of alcohol dehydrogenase and hexokinase no phosphate esterification was obtained. This could have been due to an inhibitor present in the preparation. Such an inhibitor of phosphorylation was actually found to be present in fractions of baker's yeast obtained during hexokinase purification. On the other hand, it is equally possible that the positive results may have been due to contamination of the " crystalline enzyme preparations " with small amounts of glycolytic enzymes. Since treatment

TABLE 3

The Effect of Dowex-1 Treatment on Phosphorylation and Acetaldehyde Oxidation

Enzyme preparation	0.50% Dowex, 1	Ammonium 2	Sulfate Precipitate 3
Substrate added	None	Alcohol	Acetaldehyde
Oxygen uptake in microatoms	1.43	6.63	1.46
Phosphate uptake in micromoles	0	4.91	0
P/O ratio	0	0.74	0

The vessels contained the complete system as outlined in Table 1. Vessel #3 contained 30 micromoles of acetaldehyde, and no alcohol dehydrogenase was added in vessels #1 and #3.

of the alcohol dehydrogenase with iodoacetate was avoided because of the known sensitivity of this enzyme to the poison, glycolysis still remains a possibility to explain the phosphorylating activity after Dowex-1 treatment.

In conclusion, it may be said that two phosphorylating reactions can be demonstrated in *E. coli* extracts both of which are dependent on the addition of DPN. One was shown to be due to the formation of acetyl phosphate. The other may be due to the oxidation of reduced DPN, but a more rigid exclusion of a glycolytic mechanism or another unknown pathway of phosphorylation must be awaited, in view of the negative results with reduced DPN.

REFERENCES

1. Chantrenne, H., and F. Lipmann. 1950. *J. biol. Chem.*, 187: 757.
2. Keilin, D., and E. F. Hartree. 1947. *Biochem. J.*, 41: 500.
3. Lehninger, A. L 1951. *J. biol. Chem.*, 190: 345.
4. Slater, E. C. 1950. *Biochem. J.*, 46: 484.
5. Stadtman, E. R., and H. A. Barker. 1948. *J. biol. Chem.*, 174: 1039.

18

Reprinted from J. Biochem. (Tokyo) 62:210–214 (1967)

Oxidative Phosphorylation in *Micrococcus denitrificans*

III. ATP-supported Reduction of NAD+ by Succinate

By Akira Asano, Katsuyuki Imai and Ryo Sato

(*From the Division of Physiology, Institute for Protein Research,
Osaka University, Osaka*)

(Received for publication, February 20, 1967)

Evidence accumulated in recent years has suggested close similarity between the mechanism of oxidative phosphorylation in mammalian mitochondria and that in certain bacterial preparations, though some differences have also been noted (*1—3*). From the viewpoint of the evolution of energy-yielding process in living orgaisms, it is of interest to study the extent of the similarity between the mitochondrial and bacterial phosphorylation systems. Our previous studies (*4*) have described the properties of the oxidative phosphorylation system in membrane fragments obtained from *Micrococcus denitrificans* grown under aerobic conditions. It has also been reported that the membrane fragments, like mammalian mitochondria, catalyzed an energy-linked NAD(P) transhydrogenase [EC 1.6.1.1] reaction (*5*), which is a reversal of a part of the energy-transfer pathway of oxidative phosphorylation.

Another energy-linked process, *i.e.*, the ATP-linked reduction of NAD+ by succinate, has also been detected in mammalian mitochondria (*1*) and shown to represent a reversal of oxidative phosphorylation at the NADH-cytochrome *b* segment of the respiratory chain.

In this paper we report that this ATP-linked process could also be demonstrated in the membrane fragments of *M. denitrificans*.

MATERIALS AND METHODS

Materials—Phosphorylating membrane fragments of aerobically grown *Micrococcus denitrificans* were prepared as described previously (*4*). Acetylpyridine NAD+ (acetylpyridine-adenine dinucleotide) was kindly supplied from Dr. T. Kawasaki of Kyoto Prefectural University, Medical School. Other chemicals and biochemicals were the same as described previously (*4—5*).

Measurement of ATP-supported Reduction of NAD+ by Succinate—The reaction system consisted of 100 μmoles of Tris-HCl buffer (pH 8.2), 190 μmoles of sucrose, 2.5 mg. of bovine serum albumin, 20 μmoles of $MgCl_2$, 4 μmoles of NAD+, 5 μmoles of potassium cyanide, 15 μmoles of succinate (pH 7.4), 2.5 μmoles of inorganic phosphate (pH 8.2), and water to a final volume of 2.0 ml. ATP (2.5 μmoles, 50 μl.) was added to start the reaction. The reaction was performed at 20°C to 24°C in a cuvette with 1.0 cm. light-path. Increase in optical density at 340 mμ was followed in a Cary Model 14 recording spectrophotometer.

RESULTS

Demonstration of ATP-supported Reduction of NAD+ by Succinate—Addition of ATP to the

[*Editor's Note:* Corrections in ink were made to the original reprint by the authors of this article.]

TABLE I

ATP-supported Reduction of NAD⁺ by Succinate

Experiment number	Reaction medium	NADH formed (mμmoles/min./mg. protein)
1	Complete	4. 40
	−ATP+AMP	0. 18
	−NAD⁺+NADP⁺	0. 05
	−Succinate	0. 00
	−Succ.+Formate	0. 36
	−Succ.+Fumarate	0. 00
	−Succ.+L-Malate	0. 00
2	Complete	5. 00
	−Inorganic phosphate	3. 20
	−Serum albumin	4. 60

Conditions employed were as described in "MATERIALS AND METHODS" except that 3.6 mg. and 2.9 mg. protein of the membrane fragments were used in experiments 1 and 2, respectively, and omissions and additions were made as indicated.

cyanide-inhibited membrane fragments of *M. denitrificans* in the presence of succinate and NAD⁺ caused, after a short lag time, about a 4-fold increase in the rate of reduction of NAD⁺ as measured at 340 mμ. As shown in Table I, this effect of ATP could not be replaced by AMP. Moreover, succinate had to be present in the system to obtain this stimulation. With the washed membrane fragments, formate, fumarate and L-malate did not affect the rate of endogenous reduction of NAD⁺, nor that in the presence of ATP. NADP⁺ was not reduced by succinate plus ATP. These results strongly suggested that the preparation possessed the ability to reverse the electron flow from succinate to NAD⁺, utilizing the energy derived from ATP.

Conditions Affecting NAD⁺ Reduction by Succinate—As will be seen from Fig. 1, a value of 220 μM was obtained for the apparent Michaelis constant (K_m) for ATP. The K_m value for NAD⁺, on the other hand, was rather high and was determined to be 4.0 mM under the conditions employed. Acetylpyridine NAD⁺, which has a higher oxidation-reduction potential than NAD⁺, was a very poor acceptor in this system. The reaction proceeded optimally in the pH range between 8.0 and 8.2. The addition of 1.25 mM inorganic phosphate

to the reaction medium shortened the lag phase of reaction (Fig. 2) and further stimulated the rate of reaction by about 55% (Table I). However, the stimulation of NAD⁺ reduction by inorganic phosphate was not as clear as that observed in the ATP-supported NAD(P) transhydrogenase reaction (5). This difference was probably due to the high concentration of the membrane fragments employed for the measurement of the former reaction. In other words, inorganic phosphate produced

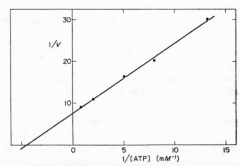

FIG. 1.   Effects of ATP concentration on ATP-supported reduction of NAD⁺ by succinate.

Conditions employed were as described in "MATERIALS AND METHODS" except that 3.9 mg. protein of the membrane fragments were used and ATP concentration was varied as indicated.

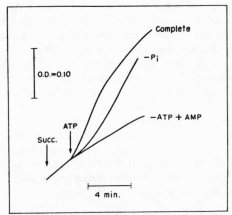

FIG. 2. Effect of inorganic phosphate on ATP-supported reduction of NAD+ by succinate.

Reaction conditions employed were as described in "MATERIALS AND METHODS" except that 2.9 mg. protein of the membrane fragments were used and omissions and additions were made as indicated.

TABLE II

Effects of Sucrose, Mannitol and Salts on the Rate of ATP-supported Reduction of NAD+ by Succinate

Medium	Concentration (M)	O.D. at 340 mμ/4 min.
Sucrose	0.30	0.074
Sucrose	0.05	0.062
Mannitol	0.28	0.072
KCl	0.15	0.003
NaCl	0.15	0.008
Sucrose+KCl	0.30+0.15	0.007

Conditions employed were as described in "MATERIALS AND METHODS" except that 3.8 mg. protein of the membrane fragments were used and sucrose was replaced by mannitol or salts when indicated.

during the lag phase by the ATPase [EC 3.6.1.3] activity of the membrane fragments might have obscured the stimulation effect of the added inorganic phosphate. The medium employed also affected the rate of NAD+ reduction; sucrose and mannitol were equally good as the reaction medium, whereas KCl and NaCl were strongly inhibitory (Table II).

Effect of Uncouplers—As shown in Fig. 3, the ATP-supported reversal of electron transfer from succinate to NAD+ was inhibited by

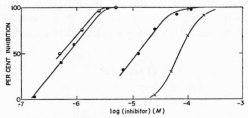

FIG. 3. Effects of uncouplers and energy-transfer inhibitors on ATP-supported reduction of NAD+ by succinate.

Reaction conditions employed were as described in "MATERIALS AND METHODS" except that 3.9 mg. protein of the membrane fragments were used and inhibitors were added as indicated.
—○—: m-Cl CCP   —■—: Tributyltin chloride
—●—: Oligomycin   —×—: Pentachlorophenol

uncouplers and energy-transfer inhibitors of oxidative phosphorylation in mitochondria. Tributyltin chloride and m-Cl CCP* were effective at micromolar concentrations, but higher concentrations of oligomycin and pentachlorophenol were required for complete inhibition. The concentrations of these inhibitors required for the NAD+ reduction by succinate were somewhat higher than those required for the ATP-supported NAD(P) transhydrogenase reaction (5). This could also be due to the higher concentration of the membrane fragments employed for the measurement of the former reaction. At any rate, these inhibitions of the NAD+ reduction by uncouplers and energy-transfer inhibitors suggested that the reaction actually involved a reversal of the energy transfer associated with oxidative phosphorylation.

Effects of Electron-transfer Inhibitors—The electron-transfer pathway in the ATP-supported reduction of NAD+ by succinate was studied by means of electron-transfer inhibitors of the bacterial NADH and succinate oxidations. As shown in Table III, an inhibitor of the succinate-cytochrome *b* segment (malonate) and those of the NADH-cytochrome *b* segment (rotenone, *o*-phenanthroline) of the respiratory chain also inhibited the ATP-supported reduction of NAD+ at concentrations similar to

---

* *m*-Cl CCP; Carbonyl cyanide *m*-chlorophenyl-hydrazone.

those required for the succinate and NADH oxidase activities. Antimycin A at a concentration 100 times higher than that required

TABLE III

Effect of Inhibitors on ATP-supported Reduction of NAD⁺ by Succinate

Addition	Concentration	% Inhibition
Malonate	$2.0\,mM$	96
Malonate	$5.0\,mM$	100
Rotenone	$25.4\,\mu M$	1
Rotenone	$50.8\,\mu M$	69
Rotenone	$127\,\mu M$	96
Antimycin A	$7.4\,\mu M$	25
Antimycin A	$18.2\,\mu M$	36
o-Phenanthroline	$1.5\,mM$	68
o-Phenanthroline	$4.5\,mM$	99
Irradiation at $360\,m\mu$	60 min.	96

Conditions employed were as described in "MATERIALS AND METHODS" except that 3.1 mg. protein of the membrane fragments were used and inhibitors were added as indicated. Irradiation of the membrane fragments by $360\,m\mu$ light was performed as described previously (4).

for the inhibition of succinate and NADH oxidations also inhibited the ATP-supported reaction. Partial inhibition of the ATP-supported succinate-NAD⁺ reaction by higher concentrations of antimycin A has been also reported for the mitochondrial system (6), though the reason for this inhibition is not yet clear. Irradiation by $360\,m\mu$ light which destroys coenzyme Q also inhibited the ATP-supported reduction of NAD⁺ by succinate. These results strongly supported that the ATP-linked reaction involved the reversal of electron transfer of the NADH-cytochrome b segment of the respiratory chain.

DISCUSSION

Our previous findings on oxidative phosphorylation, ATP- and succinate-supported NAD(P) transhydrogenase reactions, and ATPase activity (4—5) of the membrane fragments of *M. denitrificans* have been shown to be explicable by the operation of electron- and energy-transfer pathways depicted in Fig. 4. The data presented in this paper, indicating the occurrence of an ATP-linked reduction of NAD⁺ by succinate in the membrane fragments may also be accounted for by the

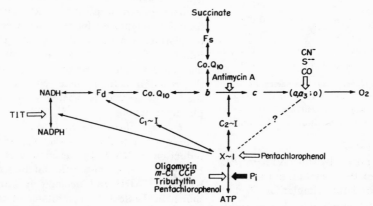

FIG. 4. Electron- and energy-transfer systems of phosphorylating membrane fragments of *Micrococcus denitrificans*.

Postulated scheme of the electron- and energy-transfer system in membrane fragments of *Micrococcus denitrificans*. → indicates the flow of electron or transfer of energy. ⇨ shows the site of inhibition and ⇥ shows the site of activation.

Abbreviations:

TIT: 3, 5, 3′-Triiodothyronine F_d: NADH dehydrogenase [EC 1.6.99.3]

F_s : Succinate dehydrogenase [EC 1.3.99.1]

C∼I and X∼I, high energy intermediates.

same scheme. Thus, the reduction observed seems to involve an energy-dependent reversal of electron flow from cytochrome b to NAD^+. A support to this view comes from the finding that the reaction is inhibited by the addition of rotenone and irradiation by 360 mμ light, which have been shown to be effective inhibitors of the electron transfer from NADH to cytochrome b in the membrane fragments (7). o-Phenanthroline, which inhibits the NADH oxidase at alkaline pH's (7), is also a potent inhibitor of the ATP-supported reduction of NAD^+ under similar conditions. The sensitivity of the reaction to various energy-transfer inhibitors further suggests the involvement of a reversal of energy transfer from ATP. This reversal of electron flow from cytochrome b to NAD^+, driven by the energy derived from ATP, may be taken as the first conclusive evidence for the occurrence of phosphorylation at site I (the NADH-flavoprotein segment) in bacterial systems. More direct studies on phosphorylation at this site are now in progress in our laboratory.

The rate of reduction of NAD^+ by succinate in the ATP-supported reaction determined in the present study is rather slow (5.0 mμmoles/min./mg. protein) as compared with those of NADH and succinate oxidations by the same preparation (98 and 167 mμmoles/min./mg. protein, respectively). This slow rate of NAD^+ reduction is, however, comparative with that of reaction in opposite direction, i.e., the reduction of fumarate by NADH (6.2 mμmoles/min./mg. protein). It seems that the link between the NADH chain and the succinate chain has been damaged to certain extents during the preparation of the membrane fragments.

As already pointed out (4—5), the electron- and energy-transfer mechanisms shown in Fig. 4 closely resemble those reported for mammalian mitochondria. It is indeed remarkable that such similar mechanisms of the energy-yielding process are operative in a bacterium on one hand and in mammals on the other.

Indications of ATP-supported reversal of electron flow have also been reported in certain other bacterial preparations. Thus, an ATP-dependent stimulation of the reduction of NAD^+ by succinate has been observed with small particles prepared from Escherichia coli W (8). However, this system has not yet been fully identified as the reversal of oxidative phosphorylation. Recently, Aleem (9—10) has reported the energy-linked reduction of nicotinamide nucleotides by reduced cytochrome c in Thiobacillus novellus and Nitrobactor europaea. Since these autotrophic organisms utilize inorganic compounds having redox potentials higher than that of nicotinamide nucleotides as energy sources, this reaction may be of vital importance for the generation of reducing power. However, oxidative phosphorylation coupled to the oxidation of reduced nicotinamide nucleotides has not yet been studied. If Aleem's claim that the above energy-linked process in T. novellus is catalyzed by the soluble fraction of the cells is correct, this preparation would be an interesting and important system for the study of oxidative phosphorylation.

After completion of this manuscript, we have became aware of Aleem's recent paper (11) reporting the occurrence of ATP-linked reduction of NAD^+ by succinate in the soluble fraction of T. novellus.

REFERENCES

(1) Chance, B., and Hollunger, G., Nature, 185, 666 (1960)

(2) Klingenberg, M., and Slenczka, J., Biochem. Z., 331, 786 (1959)

(3) Asano, A., and Brodie, A.F., J. Biol. Chem., 240, 4002 (1965)

(4) Imai, K., Asano, A., and Sato, R., Biochim. et Biophys. Acta, submitted for publication

(5) Asano, A., Imai, K., and Sato, R., Biochim. et Biophys. Acta, submitted for publication

(6) Sanadi, D.R., Fluharty, A.L., and Andreoli, T.E., Biochem. Biophys. Research Communs., 8, 200 (1962)

(7) Imai, K., Asano, A., and Sato, R., Symposium on Enzyme Chemistry (in Japanese), 18, 187 (1966)

(8) Kashket, E.R., and Brodie, A.F., J. Biol. Chem., 238, 2564 (1963)

(9) Aleem, M.I.H., J. Bacteriol., 91, 729 (1966)

(10) Aleem, M.I.H., Biochim. et Biophys. Acta, 113, 216 (1966)

(11) Aleem, M.I.H., Biochim. et Biophys. Acta, 128, 1 (1966)

Editor's Comments
on Paper 19

19   PECK
*Phosphorylation Coupled with Electron Transfer in Extracts
of the Sulfate Reducing Bacterium,* Desulphovibrio gigas

Those properties of a phosphate esterification system dependent upon sulfate reduction sufficient to classify it as oxidative phosphorylation are described by H. D. Peck, Jr., in Paper 19. Even though the extracts bringing about respiration-dependent phosphate esterification are obtained from an obligately anaerobic bacteria using sulfate as terminal electron acceptor, the characteristics of the reaction described by Peck are those shared by nearly all other cell-free microbial systems carrying out oxidative phosphorylation. Subcellular preparations from bacteria, moreover, esterify phosphate with poor efficiency (low P/2e⁻ value) as compared with the phosphorylation efficiency of mitochondrial suspensions oxidizing the same electron donors, although painstaking optimization of preparative and assay conditions may sometimes enhance the ratio of phosphate esterified to oxidant consumed.[1]

Unlike extracts from less oxygen-sensitive microorganisms, those from *Methanobacterium* do not esterify phosphate during net electron transport to CO_2 as terminal oxidant, Roberton and Wolfe[2] were able, however, to show that ATP synthesis did in fact occur during CO_2 reduction to CH_4 by suspensions of *intact* cells. Although these workers did not estimate the P/2e⁻ value of oxidative phosphorylation, it was demonstrated that true uncoupler-sensitive phosphate esterification occurred.

Inability to achieve reasonable efficiencies of oxidative phosphorylation in cell-free bacterial extracts prompted several investigators to devise procedures whereby P/2e⁻ values might be estimated in intact bacteria. [3,4,5,6,7,8] Although the phosphorylation efficiencies observed frequently approach 3 moles of phosphate esterified per g atom of oxygen reduced, the reproducibility with which that P/O value is found is as yet inadequate to conclude that all bacteria oxidizing NAD^+-linked substrates are capable of such high efficiencies.

REFERENCES

1. Estabrook, R. W., and M. E. Pullman, eds. *Meth. Enzymol.,* vol X, Academic Press, New York, 1967, pp. 147–175.
2. Roberton, A. M., and R. S. Wolfe. *J. Bact.,* **102**, 43–51, 1970.
3. Ramirez, J., and L. Smith. *Biochim. Biophys. Acta,* **153**, 466–475, 1968.
4. Hempfling, W. P. *Biochim. Biophys. Acta,* **205**, 169–182, 1970.
5. Van Der Beek, E. G., and A. H. Stouthamer, *Arch. Microbiol.,* **89**, 327–339, 1973.
6. Van Verseveld, H. W., and A. H. Stouthamer. *Arch. Microbiol.,* **107**, 241–247, 1976.
7. Gadkari, D., and H. Stolp. *Arch. Microbiol.,* **108**, 125–132, 1976.
8. Hempfling, W. P., and E. L. Hertzberg. In S. Fleischer and L. Packer, eds. *Meth. Enzymol.,* **55**(Part F):164–175 (1979).

19

Reprinted from *Biochem. Biophys. Res. Commun.* **22**:112–118 (1966)

PHOSPHORYLATION COUPLED WITH ELECTRON TRANSFER IN EXTRACTS OF

THE SULFATE REDUCING BACTERIUM, DESULFOVIBRIO GIGAS

Harry D. Peck, Jr.[1,2]

Laboratoire de Chimie Bacterienne
Centre National de la Recherche
Scientifique, Marseille

The occurrence of an oxidative phosphorylation in the anaerobic respiration of the "sulfate-reducing bacteria" has been postulated from a consideration of the energetics of sulfate respiration (Peck, 1960; Senez, 1962). The reduction of sulfate with molecular hydrogen requires a source of ATP (2 P/$SO_4^=$) for the activation of sulfate (Ishimoto and Fujimoto, 1961; Peck, 1961) that neither of the substrates, $SO_4^=$ or H_2, can obviously provide by means of a substrate phosphorylation. An alternative source of the required ATP could be from oxidative phosphorylation coupled with the oxidation of hydrogen. This idea is further supported by the observation that DNP inhibits the reduction of sulfate (Peck, 1960) but not the reduction of sulfite or thiosulfate that does not directly involve ATP.

With lactate as electron donor, the necessity for oxidative phosphorylation during growth is indicated because, theoretically, there does not appear to be a net production of ATP from substrate phosphorylation

---

[1]Senior Post Doctoral Fellow of the National Science Foundation, 1964–65.

[2]Present address: Department of Biochemistry, University of Georgia, Athens.

(Peck, 1960). Furthermore, Senez (1962) has pointed out that the growth
yields obtained with lactate and pyruvate can not be explained by summation of the reactions involved in the metabolism of lactate or pyruvate
and sulfate.

It has now been possilbe to demonstrate in extracts of one of these
anaerobic bacteria, Desulfovibrio gigas, an esterification of orthophosphate
dependent upon the oxidation of hydrogen with either sulfite or thiosulfate
as electron acceptor. The requirements for this esterification and its
inhibition by uncoupling agents indicate that the esterification is due to
an oxidative phosphorylation system comparable to that found in aerobic
bacteria.

METHODS

D. gigas (Le Gall, 1963) was grown on the medium described by Le Gall
et al. (1965) at 30°C. Log phase cells were harvested from 40 liters of
medium (30 gm. wet weight) and suspended in 75 ml. of a solution containing
0.25 M sucrose, 0.02 M Tris-HCl (pH 7.8) and 0.01 M $MgCl_2$. The extract
is prepared by passing the suspension once through the French pressure
cell at 3,000 p.s.i. A few crystals of DNase are added to reduce the
viscosity of the extract and, after 5-10 minutes, the preparation centrifuged for 15 minutes in a Spinco Model L at 70,000 x G. The pellet is
discarded and the preparation recentrifuged at 140,000 x G for 2 hr.
This pellet is suspended in 15 ml. of the previously mentioned sucrose
solution and serves as the source of particles. Soluble protein is
prepared in the same manner but from a 50% suspension of cells (based on
wet weight) from which the soluble cytochrome has been extracted (Le Gall
et al, 1965). Hydrogen utilization was determined by means of the conventional Warburg apparatus and P_i esterification by the procedure of
Nielson and Lenninger (1955).

201

RESULTS

Sulfite can function as the terminal electron acceptor in the normal respiration of the "sulfate-reducing bacteria" and the overall reaction for the reduction of sulfite with molecular hydrogen is shown in equation I.

1) $3H_2 + SO_3^= \longrightarrow S^= + 3H_2O$

As this type of respiration does not involve molecular oxygen, the usual P/O ratio has been expressed as a P/H_2 ratio. The actual number of phosphorylations is unknown; however, $\Delta \overset{\bullet}{F}$ calculations (Postgate, 1956) indicate that the maximum number of phosphorylations involved in the reduction of $SO_3^=$ (Eq. 1) is 3, or possibly 4, and would result in a theoretical maximum P/H_2 ratio of 1.0 and a minimum P/H_2 ratio of 0.33.

Although centrifuged extracts of D. desulfuricans usually reduce $SO_3^=$ with H_2 and activity is stimulated by exogenous cytochrome c_3 (however, see Postgate, 1961), similar extracts from D. gigas do not reduce $SO_3^=$ even when supplemented with cytochrome from either organism. In order to obtain the reduction of $SO_3^=$ with H_2 by extracts of D. gigas, it is necessary to supplement the soluble protein with the dye, methyl viologen, or with particulate protein as shown in Table I. Similarly, with a glucose-hexokinase trap, the esterification of orthophosphate was observed and shown to be completely dependent upon the presence of both protein fractions. The P/H_2 ratio was routinely found to be between 0.1 and 0.2, but values as high as 0.4 have been observed. The phosphorylation required both H_2 and $SO_3^=$ and was destroyed by boiling either the particles or the soluble protein. Thiosulfate would partially substitute for $SO_3^=$ in both the oxidation and phosphorylation.

The omission of ADP had little effect upon the phosphorylation but the omission of ADP plus the glucose-hexokinase trap completely eliminated detectable phosphorylation. In the presence of the trap, it was possible to demonstrate a complete dependence of the phosphorylation on ADP by treating the soluble protein with small amounts of norite to remove exo-

TABLE I

REQUIREMENTS FOR PHOSPHORYLATION COUPLED WITH

SULFITE REDUCTION

Reaction Mixture	P_i Esterified (μmoles)	H_2 Utilized (μmoles)	P/H_2
Complete	1.77	9.9	0.12[1]
minus soluble protein	0.22	0.0	-
minus particles	0.39	0.0	-
minus H_2	0.58	0.0	-
minus Na_2SO_3	0.60	0.0	-
minus ADP	1.63	12.7	0.08[1]
minus ADP, hexokinase and glucose	0.00	10.0	-
minus hexokinase and glucose	0.89[2]	10.6	0.08
minus glucose, plus mannose	1.05[2]	8.7	0.12
Boiled Particles	0.66	0.0	-
Boiled Soluble Protein	0.37	0.0	-

The complete reaction mixture contained in umoles: Tris-HCl, pH 7.3, 40; $MgCl_2$, 40; glucose (or mannose where indicated) 100; p32 (9.8 x 10^5 cpm.) pH 7.3, 5; ADP, 5; Na_2SO_3, 20; NaF, 50 and hexokinase, 0.1 mg; soluble protein, 30 mg. ; and particle protein, 39.5 mg. , in a total volume of 3.0 ml. Center wells contained 0.1 ml. of 10% $CdSO_4$ and the gas phase was H_2 or N_2 where indicated. Temperature, 37°. time, 15 min.

    1. Calculated from the difference between H_2 and N_2 control indicated above as "minus H_2".
    2. Calculated from the difference between H_2 and N_2 control not included in the above data.

genous nucleotides. In the absence of a trapping system, phosphorylation

was observed, but the amount of phosphorylation was smaller and more

variable than that observed with the hexokinase-glucose trap. In addition,

the control or blank values were considerably greater with ADP alone than

with ADP plus glucose and hexokinase. The phosphorylation does not appear
to result from the metabolism of glucose because glucose is not fermented
by $\underline{D}$. $\underline{gigas}$, mannose replaces glucose in the trapping system and phosphorylation is observed with ADP alone. These results indicate that both
electron transfer and a system for accepting phosphate are required for
the phosphorylation.

In Table 2, the effect of uncoupling agents on the phosphorylation
is shown. Both gramicidin and pentachlorophenol completely inhibited the
esterification of phosphate and generally had little effect upon the
amount of H_2 utilized. Although, in this experiment, there appeared to
be some inhibition of H_2 utilization by these uncoupling agents, in other
experiments, employing these agents at different concentrations, a small,
stimulation of H_2 utilization was normally observed. DNP also inhibited
the phosphorylation but an exact calculation of the effectiveness of this
inhibitor is not possible as it is reduced in the presence of H_2 to amino-
phenols by extracts of this organism. Oligomycin had no inhibitory effect
on the system but usually caused by slight stimulation of oxidative activity
similar to that described in some bacterial systems (Ishikana and Lehninger,
1962). Both with respect to the dependence of the phosphorylation on
electron transfer and the uncoupling of phosphorylation from electron
transfer by known uncoupling agents, this system meets the requirements
suggested by Chance and Williams (1956), for the demonstration of oxidative
phosphorylation.

The soluble protein is stable when stored at -20° and can be fractionated by $(NH_4)_2 SO_4$ into two protein fractions, both of which are
required for phosphorylation as well as electron transfer. Passage of
the soluble protein through a short DEAE column (5 x 2.5 cm) renders
the protein inactive, but recombination of the dialyzed protein (eluted
from the DEAE by 3 M NaCl) with the inactive protein, restores activity
for both electron transfer and phosphorylation. The fraction contains

TABLE 2

THE EFFECT OF UNCOUPLING AGENTS ON PHOSPHORYLATION

Additions	Concentration	H_2 Utilized (μmoles)	P_i Esterified (μmoles)	P/H_2
None		13.9	1.82	0.13
Gramicidin	5.2×10^{-5} M	8.05	0.16	0.02
Pentachloro-phenol	3×10^{-5} M	9.12	0.08	0.01
DNP	2×10^{-4} M	8.60	0.58	0.07
Oligomycin	42 γ/ml	13.3	2.34	0.18

Each reaction mixture contained in umoles; Tris-HCl, 40; $MgCl_2$, 20; Na_2SO_3, 20; p^{32} (600,000 cpm) 5; ADP, 5; glucose, 100, NaF, 50; and hexokinase, 1 mg; particle protein, 19.8 mg; soluble protein, 39 mg in a total volume of 3.0 ml. Reaction mixtures were incubated at 37° under H_2 or N_2 and stopped by the addition of 1.0 ml of 10% TCA. The center well contained 0.1 ml of 10% $CdSO_4$. P_i esterified represents the difference between identical flasks incubated under atmospheres of H_2 and N_2. Gramicidin, pentachlorophenol and oligomycin were added in ethanol and the other flasks received an equivalent amount of ethanol (0.025 ml).

large amounts of ferredoxin and the possible role of this electron transfer protein in the system is being investigated.

The particle fraction rapidly looses activity when stored at 0° but does retain activity for several weeks when stored at -20°. Only one cytochrome has been detected on the particles and it is probably identical with the cytochrome isolated from these organisms by Le Gall et al (1965).

Although this system was obtained from a strictly anaerobic bacterium, it appears to be similar to oxidative phosphorylation systems extracted from other bacteria with regard to the effectiveness of uncoupling agents and the requirements of both soluble and particulate components for the oxidation and phosphorylation. Reversal of this oxidative phosphorylation should effect an ATP-dependent evolution of H_2 perhaps similar to that described by Bulen et al (1965) in Azotobacter and Clostridium pasteurianum (Hardy et al, 1965) and implicated in the fixation of nitrogen.

The observation that this organism possesses a single cytochrome suggests

the unique possibility that it also carries out a single oxidative phos-

phorylation.

ACKNOWLEDGMENTS

I wish to thank Dr. Jacques C. Senez for extending the hospitality of his
laboratory and for many stimulating discussions.   The advice and interest
of Dr. Jean Le Gall was essential in the development of the problem and is
gratefully acknowledged.

REFERENCES

Bulen, W. A., Burns, R. C. and LeComte, J. R.   Proc. Natl. Acad. Sci.
     53, 532 (1965).
Chance, B. and Williams, G. R.   Adv. in Enzymol. 17, 65 (1956).
Hardy, R. W. F., Knight, E., Jr., and D'Eustachio, A. J.   Biochem.
     Biophys. Res. Commun 20, 539 (1965).
Ishikawa, S. and Lehninger, A. I   J. Biol. Chem. 237, 2401 (1962).
Ishimoto, M. and Fujimoto, J J.   J. Biochem. (Tokyo) 50, 229 (1961).
Le Gall, J.   J. Bacteriol 86, 1120 (1963).
Le Gall, J., Mazza, G. and Dragoni, N.   Biochem. Biophys. Acta 99,
     385 (1965).
Nielson, S. O. and Lenninger A. L.   J. Biol. Chem. 215, 555 (1955).
Peck, H. D., Jr.   J. Biol. Chem. 235, 2734 (1960).
Peck, H. D., Jr.   J. Biol. Chem. 273, 198 (1961).
Postgate, J. R.   J. Gen. Microbiol. 14, 545 (1956).
Postgate, J. R.   in "Symposium on Hematin Enzymes C.J.E. Falk, R. Lemberg
     and R. K. Morton, eds.   Pergamon Press, New York (1961).
Senez, J. D.   Bacteriol Rev. 26, 95 (1962).

Editor's Comments
on Papers 20, 21, and 22

ERA OF THE "CHEMIOSMOTIC" HYPOTHESIS

Peter Mitchell offered in Paper 20 a fresh view of respiration-dependent energy conservation which at once accommodated the membrane association of respiratory components, energy-dependent transport processes, and oxidative phosphorylation. Although the initial experiments testing his "chemiosmotic" hypothesis were done with mitochondria and were strongly supported by Andre Jagendorf's chloroplast work, it was reasonable to expect that similar phenomena would be observed in procaryotes.

Scholes and Mitchell went on in Paper 21 to demonstrate the feasibility of Mitchell's model in a *Micrococcus,* at least with regard to the ability of respiration to drive proton extrusion under certain conditions. Several investigators have since repeated the substance of the observations reported in Paper 21 using other organisms (see, for example, references 1 and 2).

Proton extrusion values are far more easily measured than is the phosphorylation efficiency of oxidative phosphorylation, and the assumption that H^+/O values bear a constant relation to P/O values seems to have become an unfortunate consequence of Mitchell's theory. Until a rigorous demonstration of the stoichiometric relationship between those parameters is established, proton extrusion data should be interpreted with caution. Nevertheless, Maloney, Kashket, and Wilson have demonstrated that an externally imposed proton gradient can elicit ATP synthesis in intact bacteria.[3]

Membrane vesicles derived from bacteria have been shown to extrude or take up protons in a respiration-dependent manner. Vesicles that are "inside-out" as compared with the original orientation of the membrane ("everted" vesicles) have been prepared by Elliot Hertzberg and Peter Hinkle as outlined in Paper 22. Such vesicles are capable of oxidative phosphorylation unlike the vesicles prepared according to the procedure of H. R. Kaback.[4] Tsuchiya[5] has succeeded in preparing "right-side out" vesicles that preserve some phosphorylating activity, and a proton gradient also drives ATP synthesis in such preparations.[6]

REFERENCES

1. Lawford, H., G., and B. A. Haddock. *Biochem. J.,* **136**, 217–220, 1973.
2. Farmer, I. S., and C. W. Jones. *Eur. J. Biochem.,* **67**, 115–122, 1976.
3. Maloney, P. C., E. R. Kashket, and T. H. Wilson. *Proc. Nat. Acad. Sci.* (U.S.), **71**, 3898–3900, 1974.
4. Kaback, H. R. *Science,* **186**, 882–892, 1974.
5. Tsuchiya, T. *J. Biol. Chem.,* **251**, 5315–5320, 1976.
6. Tsuchiya, T., and B. P. Rosen. *Biochem. Biophys. Res. Commun.,* **68**, 497–502, 1976.

20

Reprinted from *Nature* (London) **191**:144–148 (1961)

COUPLING OF PHOSPHORYLATION TO ELECTRON AND HYDROGEN TRANSFER BY A CHEMI-OSMOTIC TYPE OF MECHANISM

By Dr. PETER MITCHELL

Chemical Biology Unit, Zoology Department, University of Edinburgh

AT present, the orthodox view of the coupling of phosphorylation to electron and hydrogen transfer in oxidative and photosynthetic phosphorylation stems from knowledge of substrate-level phosphorylation[1,2]. It is based, consequently, on the idea that water is expelled spontaneously between two chemical groups, A and B, by the formation of a strong bond (of low hydrolysis energy), and that subsequent or simultaneous oxidation or reduction of $A–B$ to $A–B^*$ can result in a weakening of the bond, popularly written $A \sim B^*$, so that adenosine triphosphate (ATP) can be synthesized by coupling the opening of $A \sim B^*$ to the closing of the 'high-energy bond' between adenosine diphosphate (ADP) and phosphorus through group transfer systems of appropriate substrate and oxido-reduction-carrier specificities[3–5]. There are a number of facts about the systems catalysing oxidative and photosynthetic phosphorylation that are generally acknowledged to be difficult to reconcile with this orthodox (chemical) view of the mechanism of coupling. For example: (a) The hypothetical 'high-energy' intermediates (for example, reduced diphosphopyridine nucleotide (DPNH) $\sim$?, reduced flavin adenine dinucleotide (FADH) $\sim$?, cytochrome $\sim$?) are elusive to identification[4,6]. (b) It is not clear why phosphorylation should be so closely associated with membranous structures[7–9]. It has sometimes been assumed that digitonin-treated mitochondrial 'particles' can couple oxidation to phosphorylation without membranes[10]; but it is doubtful whether this assumption can be justified, for such 'particles' give only poor respiratory control and contain much lipid[11], which may well exist as a leaky membrane[12]. (c) Coupling may vary with the stress, causing variation of respiratory control without corresponding variation in phosphorus/oxygen quotient[4,13]—a phenomenon difficult to explain in terms of molecular stoichio-

209

metry. (*d*) Hydrolysis of external ATP by mitochondria causes reduction of internal DPN, accentuated by the oxidation of succinate[14]. There is disagreement as to what complex assumptions offer the better explanation[15]. (*e*) Uncoupling can be caused at all three hypothetical oxido-reduction sites in mitochondria by agents that do not share an identifiable specific chemical characteristic[4] (for example, dinitrophenol, dicoumarol, salicylate, azide). (*f*) Unexplained swelling and shrinkage phenomena accompany the activity of the phosphorylation systems[7,9a,11,16].

Structural features have been invoked as the causes of the departure of the phosphorylation systems from 'ideal' behaviour[4,14,17]; but, as Green has pointed out in a far-sighted paper[18], although the structural features have been recognized as playing an important part in the catalytic activity of multi-enzyme systems, they have so far been treated rather conservatively. The structural (or supramolecular) features have, in fact, generally been regarded only as modifiers of the basic chemical type of coupling process outlined above. The general conception of enzyme-catalysed group translocation that we have been developing in my laboratory for some years[19] offers a more radical approach to the problem; but this has not, so far, been made use of by those working in the field of oxidative and photosynthetic phosphorylation.

The purpose of this article is to suggest that in view of the difficulties confronting the orthodox chemical conception of coupling in oxidative and photosynthetic phosphorylation, one might now profitably consider the basic requirements and potentialities of a type of mechanism that is based directly on the group translocation conception. This type of mechanism differs fundamentally from the orthodox one in that it depends absolutely on a supramolecular organization of the enzyme systems concerned. Such supramolecularly organized systems can exhibit what I have called chemi-osmotic coupling[19c,20], because the driving force on a given chemical reaction can be due to the spatially directed channelling of the diffusion of a chemical component or group along a pathway specified in space by the physical organization of the system[20]. We shall consider chemi-osmotic coupling between the so-called ATPases on one hand and the electron and hydrogen transfer chain on the other: mediated by the translocation of electrons and the elements of water across the membrane of mitochondria, chloroplast grana, and chromatophores.

The first basic feature of the chemiosmotic coupling conception is a membrane-located reversible 'ATPase'

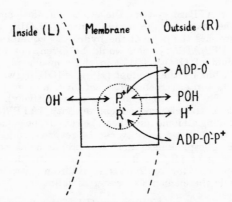

Fig. 1.   Anisotropic reversible 'ATPase' system located in an ion-impermeable membrane between aqueous phases L and R

system[20b] shown very diagrammatically in Fig. 1. This system, which may include lipids and other components as well as proteins, is assumed to be anisotropic so that the active centre region (indicated by the dotted circle) is accessible to OH′ ions but not H+ ions from the left (inside organelle), and to H+ ions but not OH′ ions from the right (cytoplasm side of organelle). The active centre, like that of phosphokinases in general, is assumed to be relatively inaccessible to water as water. To illustrate the hydrolytic activity of the system, the OH′ ion is depicted as diffusing from left to right and finally combining at the active centre region with the terminal phosphorylium (P+) derived from the ATP (ADP—O′—P+) giving inorganic phosphate (POH) and ADP having a terminal ionized oxygen (ADP—O′), assuming the right-hand phase to be at about pH 7 and at electrical neutrality. The elegant conception of the transfer of phosphoryl as phosphorylium ion is due to Lipmann[21]. The system, of course, catalyses hydrolysis equilibrium, and the reverse or phosphokinetic activity of the 'ATPase' is indicated by the single barbs on the arrows of Fig. 1. In the case of the phosphokinetic activity, the OH′ ion is depicted as passing down a free-energy gradient towards the left from an inorganic phosphate group (POH) that passes to the active centre region from the right. The phosphorylium ion (P+), created by the withdrawal of the OH′, is attacked by the negative atom (− R′) in the active centre region, and the phosphorylium ion is then donated to the terminal oxygen of ADP—O′ to give ATP. The chemi-osmotic coupling hypothesis depends thermodynamically on the fact that in such an anisotropic ATPase system, the electrochemical activity of the water at the active centre ($[H_2O]_c$), which determines the poise of the hydrolysis equilibrium in the ATP/ADP system, would be given, not by the product of $[H^+] \times [OH']$ in the aqueous phases L or R, but by the product $[H^+]_R \times [OH']_L$ (where [] stands for electrochemical activity, and R and L for right- and left-hand phases respectively). The ratio of the electrochemical activity $[ATP]/[ADP]$ (including all ionic forms) can be raised, consequently, and the ATPase activity can be reversed to give an ADP phosphokinase activity proportional to the lowering of $[H_2O]_c$, in accordance with the mass-action law for hydrolysis equilibrium, written to include the elements of water as follows:

$$\frac{[ATP]}{[ADP]} = \frac{[P]}{K_1[H_2O]_c} \qquad (1)$$

The electrochemical activity of a component in a certain place defines absolutely the escaping tendency of the particles of the component due both to the chemical and to the electrical pressure to which the particles are subject in that place at equilibrium. Since

$$K_2 = \frac{[OH']_L \times [H^+]_L}{[H_2O]_L} \qquad (2)$$

and K_2 is independent of the medium because we are using electrochemical activities, we can describe the electrochemical activity of the water at the active centre of the 'ATPase' system as follows:

$$[H_2O]_c = [H_2O]_{aq.} \times \frac{[H^+]_R}{[H^+]_L} \qquad (3)$$

where $[H_2O]_{aq.}$ stands for the electrochemical activity of water in the aqueous physiological media of phases L or R, and is equivalent to about $55 \cdot 5$ M water.

By the definition of the electrochemical activity:

$$\frac{[H^+]_L}{[H^+]_R} = 10^{\,pH_{R-L}} \times 10^{\,(mV._{L-R})\frac{F}{2303\,RT}} \qquad (4)$$

where pH_{R-L} is the pH of phase R minus that of phase L; $mV._{L-R}$ is the membrane potential in millivolts, positive in phase L; R is the gas constant; F is the faraday; and the factor $\frac{F}{2303\,RT}$ is approximately $1/60$. It can be seen from equation (4) that the ratio $[H^+]_L/[H^+]_R$ is multiplied by a factor of 10 for each pH unit more negative on the left, relative to the right, and for each 60 mV. membrane potential, positive on the left.   Equations 1 and 3 show that the ratio [ATP]/[ADP] at equilibrium is determined by $[H^+]_L/[H^+]_R$ as follows:

$$\frac{[ATP]}{[ADP]} = \frac{[P]}{K_1[H_2O]_{aq.}} \times \frac{[H^+]_L}{[H^+]_R} \qquad (5a)$$

When the right-hand phase (representing the cytoplasm) is the region of the zero or reference potential, the electrochemical activity ratio of total ATP to ADP will be nearly the same as the corresponding concentration ratio, and [P] will correspond approximately to the inorganic phosphate concentration. Thermodynamic data[22] show that at *p*H 7 and at physiological temperatures the 'hydrolysis constant' as usually defined or the product $K_1[H_2O]_{aq.}$ is approximately 10^5; and when [P] is at the physiological level of 10^{-2} *M*, equation (5a) can be written:

$$\frac{[ATP]}{[ADP]} \simeq 10^{-7} \frac{[H^+]_L}{[H^+]_R} \qquad (5b)$$

Thus, the [ATP]/[ADP] equilibrium can be poised centrally through the anisotropic 'ATPase' by making the ratio $[H^+]_L/[H^+]_R$ about 10^7.   Equation 3 shows that this could be done, for example, by poising the left side 2 *p*H units below and 300 mV. above the right side.   Such is the basic thermodynamic conception of the mechanism of reversal of the 'ATPase' activity.   In kinetic terms, the reversal of the 'ATPase' activity can be understood by regarding the electrochemical activity gradient of hydrogen and hydroxyl ions across the active centre region of the 'ATPase' as the cause of the donation of the phosphorylium ion to the negative acceptor atom $(-R')$ by the simultaneous withdrawal of an OH' ion from the inorganic phosphate down a steep gradient to the left and of an H^+ ion from $-R$H to the right to ionize $-R$H or to prevent H^+ from competing with phosphorylium ion for the acceptor $-R'$.   Dehydration is accomplished by using the high $[H^+]$ region as a sink for OH' and the high [OH'] region as a sink for H^+. It should be understood that the phosphorylation of ADP can be strictly described as dehydration only when the standard state is less than *p*H 6 (see Lipmann[21]).   Since, however, the hydrogen atom of the terminal hydroxyl group of ADP, involved in phosphorylation, is dissociated reversibly as an H^+ ion, when the standard state is taken as *p*H 7, the phosphorylation process is mainly that of dehydroxylation. From the kinetic point of view, the fundamental processes involved are dehydroxylation + deprotonation, or dehydroxylation.   It is relevant to note that phosphorylation is not directly caused by raising

Peter Mitchell

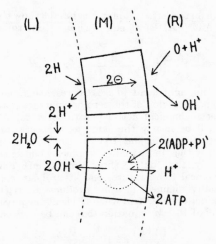

Fig. 2. Electron transport system (above) and reversible 'ATPase' system (below) chemiosmotically coupled in a charge-impermeable membrane (*M*) enclosing aqueous phase *L* in aqueous phase *R*

[H⁺], but is due to depression of [OH′]. For this reason, the hydrogen ion depicted in phase R of Fig. 1 (and correspondingly in Figs. 2 and 3) is shown as equilibrating with the active centre region of the 'ATPase' system, but not as being withdrawn stoichiometrically in relation to the withdrawal of OH′.

The second basic feature of the chemi-osmotic coupling conception is the electron and hydrogen translocation system, which is assumed to create the gradient of electrochemical activity of H⁺ and OH′. Unlike the conception of the anisotropic 'ATPase', the idea of the anisotropic o/r system is not new, but stems from the work of Lund[23], and Stiehler and Flexner[24], and was first stated explicitly by Lundegårdh[25] more than 20 years ago. Lundegårdh's idea was more exactly defined in relation to ion transport by Davies and Ogston[26], and was elaborated by Conway[27]. It has been excellently reviewed by Robertson[28].

Fig. 2 illustrates how the electron transfer can affect the ratio $[H^+]_L/[H^+]_R$. The electron translocation and 'ATPase' systems are depicted as being placed in opposition in a charge-impermeable membrane. The hydrogen ions generated on the left and the hydroxyl ions generated on the right by the electron translocation system dehydrate ADP and inorganic phosphate (now simply denoted by P) to form ATP by withdrawing hydroxyl ions to the left and hydrogen ions to the right through specific

214

translocation paths in the 'ATPase' system as described here. Conversely, of course, the effect of the back pressure of ATP hydrolysis is to force the o/r system towards reduction on the left (inside the organelle). Note that the stoichiometry is 2 ATP per O, as in succinate oxidation by mitochondria. As shown in this simple diagram, the dehydrating force driving the phosphokinetic activity of the 'ATPase' system would be due largely to the chemical potential differential of the H^+ and OH' ions across the membrane, which would have to show as a pH difference of some 7 units across the membrane, acid on the left when the [ATP]/[ADP] equilibrium was poised centrally (see equations (5b) and (4)). We assume, however, that exchange diffusion carriers, as defined by Ussing[29], are present in the membrane and that they will allow strictly coupled one-to-one exchange of H^+ against K^+ or of OH' against Cl', for example. The pH differential would thus tend to be reduced to a relatively small figure and would be equivalently replaced by a membrane potential as described by equation (4).

When the oxido-reduction and phosphorylation systems are in chemi-osmotic equilibrium, one ATP molecule will be produced per electron translocated across the membrane. The relationship between the o/r potential span (ΔE) of the electron and hydrogen translocation system and the poise of the [ATP]/[ADP] equilibrium will be given as follows:

$$\frac{[ATP]}{[ADP]} = \frac{[P]}{K_1[H_2O]_{aq.}} \times 10^{\frac{\Delta E.F}{2303\,RT}} \qquad (6a)$$

or approximately:

$$\frac{[ATP]}{[ADP]} = \frac{[P]}{10^5} \times 10^{\Delta E/60} \qquad (6b)$$

ΔE being in millivolts. It should be understood that ΔE, as defined here, is equivalent to the free-energy change in the electron-translocating system per electron translocated. Assuming that ATP synthesis were occurring when the [ATP]/[ADP] ratio was poised centrally at pH 7 and in the presence of 10^{-2} M inorganic phosphate, the o/r span, ΔE, would have to be about 420 mV. This, of course, being the equilibrium potential, represents the minimum o/r span of the electron and hydrogen translocation system required to drive ATP synthesis under the conditions specified above. The span between the succinate–fumarate couple and oxygen at 76 mm. mercury pressure is about 750 mV.—well above the minimum ΔE of 420 mV.

In practice, the mitochondrial or chloroplast

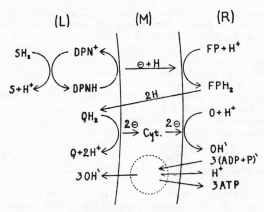

Fig. 3. Diagram of chemi-osmotic system for coupling phosphorylation to the oxidation of substrate (SH₂) through DPN, *FP* (tentatively identified with flavoprotein), *Q* (tentatively identified with a quinone) and the cytochromes (*Cyt.*). The other conventions are as in Figs. 1 and 2

membrane across which the chemi-osmotic coupling may be organized would allow a certain amount of ion leakage, and the translocation paths for H⁺ and OH′, connecting the internal and external phases (*L* and *R*) with the active centre region of the 'ATP-ase', would not be expected to have absolute specificity for H⁺ and OH′ respectively. Consequently, equations (6*a*) and (6*b*) would represent the practical state of affairs in the most tightly coupled systems. On 'loosening' the membrane system, or if 'uncoupling' were effected by catalysing the equilibration of H⁺ and charge across the lipid of the membrane with reagents like dinitrophenol or salicylate, the relationship between the poise of the [ATP]/[ADP] ratio and ΔE in the steady state would be described by the inequality:

$$\frac{[P]}{K_1[H_2O]_{aq.}} \leqslant \frac{[ATP]}{[ADP]} \leqslant \frac{[P]}{K_1[H_2O]_{aq.}} \times 10^{\frac{\Delta E.F}{2303\,RT}} \quad (6c)$$

The outer terms of equation (6*c*) represent the extreme values of the [ATP]/[ADP] ratio from complete uncoupling on the left to complete coupling on the right.

Fig. 3 shows, in principle, a rather fuller description of oxidative phosphorylation, in which I have included the o/r components *FP* and *Q*, tentatively identified with flavoprotein and quinol–quinone systems respectively. The main aim is to illustrate how a stoichiometry of 3 ATP per O can readily be obtained for substrate (SH₂) oxidation through DPN, by the obligatory transport of one (net) hydrogen atom inwards per O, owing to the spatial arrangement of the electron and hydrogen transfer chain and the zero, one, or two hydrogen-transfer characteristics of the carriers involved. In this system, the span of both parts of the o/r chain across the membrane would have to be poised against the same ratio $[H^+]_L/[H^+]_R$ at equilibrium, according to equation (5a). Using the conventions of Dixon[2], the $-\Delta F$ value for the DPN/DPNH couple at about pH 5 would be some 3,000 cal. and the $-\Delta F$ for FP (corresponding to an E'_0 (pH 7) of -60 mV.) (ref. 30) would be about 17,000 cal., giving a span of 14,000 cal.; equivalent to a ΔE of 600 mV. Assuming the $-\Delta F$ of the Q system to be about 24,000 cal., corresponding to an E'_0 (pH 7) of $+100$ mV., as in the ubiquinone system[31], the span from the Q system to oxygen at 76 mm. mercury pressure would be equivalent to a ΔE of about $750-100 = 650$ mV. The tendency of the two o/r values to drift together and the exact magnitude of the composite o/r potential would, of course, depend on many factors that it would be premature to consider here. It will suffice to point out at present that the value of 600–650 mV. for ΔE is appropriately above the required minimum of 420 mV. and that the proposed system is thus in accord with the thermodynamic facts.

The above basic chemi-osmotic conception can be applied to photosynthetic phosphorylation with the difference that the electron and hydrogen translocation are seen as being driven, not by the affinity of oxygen for the hydrogen atoms and electrons, but by the energy of the absorbed photons, according to the type of mechanism described by Calvin[9b]. It can readily be shown that in a chemi-osmotically coupled system for non-cyclic photophosphorylation, the photon-activated movement of 2 electrons and 2 hydrogen atoms outwards through the membrane of the grana would produce one O_2 and 2 ATP molecules. Similarly, in non-cyclic photophosphorylation, the skew of $[H^+]_L/[H^+]_R$, and thus the synthesis of ATP, could be caused by the photon-activated passage of equal numbers of hydrogen atoms and electrons in opposite directions across the membrane of the grana or chromatophores.

The facts that were listed at the beginning of this article as being difficult to reconcile with the orthodox chemical conception of the mechanism of coupling phosphorylation to electron and hydrogen transfer can now be reconsidered in relation to the chemi-osmotic coupling hypothesis: (a) The elusive character of the 'energy-rich' intermediates of the orthodox chemical coupling hypothesis would be explained by the fact that these intermediates do not exist. (*b*) According to the chemi-osmotic coupling hypothesis, the differential of the electrochemical activity of the hydrogen and hydroxyl ions across the membrane, generated by electron transport, causes the specific translocation of hydroxyl and hydrogen ions from the active centre of the so-called ATPase system, thus effectively dehydrating ADP + P. The charge-impermeable membrane would therefore be an absolute requirement for tight coupling. (*c*) Coupling would be expected to vary with the extent of leakiness or strain in the membrane, determined, of course, by the osmotic and electrical stress. (*d*) The internal components of mitochondria such as DPN would tend to be reduced by the high electrochemical activity of H^+ caused by hydrolysis of external ATP, which would withdraw OH' ions from the inside in competition with the electron-transport system. This effect would be accentuated by oxidation of succinate (which would raise the internal value of $[H^+]$) but not, of course, by substrates such as acetoacetate that directly oxidize DPNH. (*e*) Uncoupling would be caused by lipid-soluble reagents, such as DNP, salicylate, azide, and ammonia, catalysing equilibration of H^+ or OH' and charge across the membrane. (*f*) According to the chemi-osmotic type of hypothesis, the coupling of phosphorylation to electron and hydrogen translocation would cause considerable electrical and mechanical stress in the membrane across which coupling was effected. Complex swelling and shrinkage effects would therefore be expected to accompany the activity of the system.

It is evident that the basic features of the chemi-osmotic coupling conception described here and elsewhere[20] are in accord with much of the circumstantial evidence at present available from studies of oxidative and photosynthetic phosphorylation. This simple hypothesis also has the merit that it represents the result of carrying to its logical conclusion the present trend towards recognizing the equivalent status of supramolecular and molecular features in the channelling of chemical processes in living organisms[18]. Further experimental support for the chemi-osmotic coupling conception may best be sought by attempting to characterize separately each of the three hypothetical basic elements of which the system is thought to be built: (1) the anisotropic 'ATPase' system which I have defined above; (2) the anisotropic *o/r* system of the type originally defined by Lundegårdh; (3) the specific charge-impermeable membrane in which the systems 1 and 2 are supposed to be orientated in opposition. Work along these three lines is proceeding in my laboratory.

In the exact sciences, cause and effect are no more than events linked in sequence. Biochemists now generally accept the idea that metabolism is the cause of membrane transport. The underlying thesis of the hypothesis put forward here is that if the processes that we call metabolism and transport represent events in a sequence, not only can metabolism be the cause of transport, but also transport can be the cause of metabolism. Thus, we might be inclined to recognize that transport and metabolism, as usually understood by biochemists, may be conceived advantageously as different aspects of one and the same process of vectorial metabolism[20a,32].

I am indebted to the Nuffield Foundation for grants in aid of this work. It is also a pleasure to thank Dr. G. D. Greville, Prof. D. Keilin, Dr. R. Hill, Dr. Jennifer Moyle, Sir Rudolph Peters, and other colleagues for very helpful discussion and criticism.

[1] Lipmann, F., *Adv. Enzymol.*, **1**, 99 (1941); *Currents in Biochemical Research*, edit. by Green, D. E., 137 (Intersci. Pub., Inc., New York, 1946).

[2] Dixon, M., *Multienzyme Systems* (Cambridge Univ. Press, 1949).

[3] Slater, E. C., *Nature*, **172**, 975 (1953). Chance, B., and Williams, G. R., *Adv. Enzymol.*, **17**, 65 (1956). Myers, D. K., and Slater, E. C., *Nature*, **179**, 363 (1957). Dawkins, M. J. R., Judah, J. D., and Rees, K. R., *ibid.*, **182**, 875 (1958).

[4] Slater, E. C., and Hülsmann, W. C.; Chance, B.; Lehninger, A. L., Wadkins, C. L., and Remmert, LeM. F., in *Ciba Found. Symp. Regulation Metabolism*, edit. by Wolstenholme, G. E. W., and O'Connor, C. M., 58, 91 and 130, and associated discussion (Churchill, Ltd., London, 1959).

[5] Arnon, D. I., *Nature*, **184**, 10 (1959). Hill, R., and Bendall, F., *ibid.*, **186**, 136 (1960).

[6] Slater, E. C., in *Biological Structure and Function*, First IUB/IUBS Joint Symp., Stockholm, September 1960, edit. by Goodwin, T. W. (Academic Press, Inc., New York, in the press).

[7] Slater, E. C., *Symp. Soc. Exp. Biol.*, **10**, 110 (1957).

[8] Zeigler, D. M., Linnane, A. W., and Green, D. E., *Biochim. Biophys. Acta*, **28**, 524 (1958).

[9] (a) Lehninger, A. L., in *Biophysical Science: A Study Program*, edit. by Oncley, J. L., *et al.*, 136 (John Wiley and Sons, Inc., New York, 1959). (b) Calvin, M., *ibid.*, 147. (c) Vatter, A. E., and Wolfe, R. S., *J. Bacteriol.*, **75**, 480 (1958).

[10] Cooper, C., and Lehninger, A. L., *J. Biol. Chem.*, **219**, 489 (1956).

[11] Lehninger, A. L., *et al.*, *Science*, **128**, 450 (1958).

[12] Lehninger, A. L. (personal communication, 1960).

[13] Hoch, F. L., and Lipmann, F., *Proc. U.S. Nat. Acad. Sci.*, **40**, 909 (1954). Lipmann, F., in *Enzymes: Units of Biological Structure and Function*, edit. by Gaebler, O. H., 444 (Academic Press, Inc., New York, 1956).

[14] Chance, B., *Nature*, **189**, 719 (1961).

[15] Krebs, H. A., Hopkins Memorial Lecture, March 1961, *Biochem. J.* (in the press).

[16] Ernster, L., and Lindberg, O., *Ann. Rev. Physiol.*, **20**, 13 (1958). Beechey, R. B., and Holton, F. A., *Biochem. J.*, **73**, 29 P (1959). Lehninger, A. L., *Ann. N.Y. Acad. Sci.*, **86**, 484 (1960). Emmelot, P., *et al.*, *Nature*, **186**, 556 (1960). Emmelot, P., *ibid.*, **188**, 1197 (1960).

[17] Green, D. E., *Adv. Enzymol.*, **21**, 73 (1959). Lehninger, A. L., in *Biological Structure and Function*, First IUB/IUBS Joint Symp., Stockholm, September 1960, edit. by Goodwin, T. W. (Academic Press, Inc., New York, in the press).

[18] Green, D. E., *Symp. Soc. Exp. Biol.*, **10**, 30 (1957).

[19] (a) Mitchell, P., *Symp. Soc. Exp. Biol.*, **8**, 254 (1954), (b) *Nature* **180**, 134 (1957); (c) in *Structure and Function of Subcellular Components*, Sixteenth Symp. Biochem. Soc., February 1957, edit. by Crook, E. M., 73 (Cambridge Univ. Press, 1959). (d) Mitchell, P., and Moyle, J., *Nature*, **182**, 372 (1958); (e) *Proc. Roy. Phys. Soc., Edinburgh*, **27**, 61 (1958).

[20] (a) Mitchell, P., in *Biological Structure and Function*, First IUB/IUBS Joint Symp., Stockholm, September 1960, edit. by Goodwin, T. W. (Academic Press, Inc., New York, in the press); (b) *Biochem. J.*, **79**, 23 P (1961).

[21] Lipmann, F., in *Molecular Biology*, edit. by Nachmansohn, D., **37** (Academic Press, Inc., New York, 1960).

[22] Atkinson, M. R., Johnson, E., and Morton, R. K., *Nature*, **184**, 1925 (1959).

[23] Lund, E. J., *J. Exp. Zool.*, **51**, 327 (1928).

[24] Stiehler, R. D., and Flexner, L. B., *J. Biol. Chem.*, **126**, 603 (1938).

[25] Lundegårdh, H., *Lantbr. Hogsk. Ann.*, **8**, 233 (1940).

[26] Davies, R. E., and Ogston, A. G., *Biochem. J.*, **46**, 324 (1950).

[27] Conway, E. J., *Internat. Rev. Cytol.*, **2**, 419 (1953).

[28] Robertson, R. N., *Biol. Rev.*, **35**, 231 (1960).

[29] Ussing, H. H., *Nature*, **160**, 262 (1947); *Physiol. Rev.*, **29**, 127 (1949).

[30] Kuhn, R., and Boulanger, P., *Ber.*, **69**, 1557 (1936).

[31] Morton, R. A., *Nature*, **182**, 1764 (1958).

[32] Mitchell, P., in *Membrane Transport and Metabolism*, Symposium, Prague, August 1960, edit. by Kleinzeller, A., and Kotyk, A (Academic Press, Inc., New York, in the press).

21

Reprinted from *J. Bioenerg.* 1:309–323 (1970)

Respiration-Driven Proton Translocation in Micrococcus Denitrificans

Peter Scholes and Peter Mitchell

Glynn Research Laboratories, Bodmin, Cornwall, England

Abstract

The polarity and stoichiometry of respiration-driven proton translocation was studied by electrometric and spectrophotometric techniques in *Micrococcus denitrificans* in the context of the energy transduction mechanism in bacterial oxidative phosphorylation.

1. Protons are ejected through the plasma membrane during respiratory pulses and thereafter diffuse slowly back.

2. In presence of ionic species mobile across the membrane (K^+-valinomycin, K^+-gramicidin, or SCN^-), limiting $\rightarrow H^+/O$ quotients of 8 were obtained with endogenous respiratory substrates, and the rate of translocation (14·3 μg ions of H^+/sec g cell dry weight) was commensurate with that of respiration optimally stimulated by FCCP* at an $\rightarrow H^+/O$ quotient of 8.

3. The rate of decay of the proton pulses was greatly increased by FCCP, but there was little or no effect on the $\rightarrow H^+/O$ quotient characteristic of the respiratory system.

4. Various interpretations of the observations are discussed, and it is concluded that respiration is probably coupled directly or indirectly to electrogenic proton translocation. The observations are compatible with the chemiosmotic hypothesis of coupling between respiration and phosphorylation.

Introduction

Mitchell[1] observed that during the oxidation of endogenous substrates or of ethanol by *Micrococcus lysodeikticus*, there was an outward translocation of protons. More recently, proton translocation has been observed in whole photosynthetic bacteria and blue-green algae.[2-7] It was found that these organisms, like rat liver mitochondria,[8] translocated protons outwards.

The object of the work described in this paper was to investigate the conditions required for obtaining stoichiometric proton translocation during the rapid reduction of small pulses of oxygen by endogenous substrates in *Micrococcus denitrificans*; and to obtain information that would help to shed light on the possible mechanisms by which activity of the respiratory chain is coupled to proton translocation.

As the $\rightarrow H^+/O$ quotient has been found to be equal to the product of the P/O quotient and the $\rightarrow H^+/P$ quotient in rat liver mitochondria,[8-10] and the P/O stoichiometry of bacterial oxidative phosphorylation cannot readily be measured, except in comparatively uncoupled subcellular membrane preparations,[11] the $\rightarrow H^+/O$ quotients estimated in

---

* Abbreviations: FCCP, carbonylcyanide *p*-trifluoromethoxy phenylhydrazone; BCP, bromocresol purple; BTB, bromothymol blue; BSA, bovine serum albumin; $t_{1/2}$, time for half equilibration or half reaction; pH_0, the pH of the outer or suspension medium.

whole bacteria may provide valuable information concerning the possible energy-transducing characteristics of the bacterial respiratory chain system.

There is an obvious disadvantage in using endogenous substrates as reductants in studies of characteristics of the respiratory chain system such as the $\rightarrow H^+/O$ quotient (or the P/O quotient), because such characteristics depend on the point or points from which reducing equivalents travel down the respiratory chain during oxygen reduction. There is, however, the advantage that the participation of substrate porter systems that may themselves be linked to proton translocation[12] is avoided. Moreover, it has been shown that the respiratory chain system of *M. denitrificans* is very similar to that of mitochondria[11, 13, 14] and includes NAD- and NADP-linked dehydrogenase systems; and observations on the absorbance difference $A_{374-340}$ have indicated oxidoreduction of nicotinamide adenine nucleotides during respiratory pulse experiments similar to those described in the present paper (P. Scholes and P. Hinkle, unpublished data). Thus, with the knowledge that the respiratory chain and the nicotinamide adenine nucleotides were reduced by the endogenous substrates under appropriate conditions, we expected to be able to obtain $\rightarrow H^+/O$ quotients characteristic of all or of most of the respiratory chain.

Materials and Methods

Reagents

FCCP and valinomycin were gifts from Dr. P. G. Heytler of E. I. du Pont de Nemours and Co., Inc. (Wilmington, Delaware, U.S.A.) and Dr. J. C. MacDonald of Prairie Research Laboratory (Saskatoon, Saskatchewan, Canada) respectively. Gramicidin (mixture of A, B, and C, predominantly A) was obtained from Koch-Light Laboratories Ltd. (Colnbrook, Bucks.). Bromocresol purple (BCP) and glycylglycine were obtained from Hopkin and Williams Ltd. (Chadwell Heath, Essex). Crystalline bovine serum albumin and carbonic anhydrase were obtained from Sigma London Chemical Co. Ltd. (London, S.W.6).

Simple organic and inorganic reagents were of Analar grade where available, or otherwise of the highest purity obtainable commercially.

Carbonic anhydrase was freshly prepared (10 mg/ml) in 150 mM KCl. Standard acid and alkali, and ethanolic solutions of FCCP, valinomycin, and gramicidin were prepared and made oxygen-free as described previously.[15]

Growth and Harvesting of Bacteria

M. denitrificans ATCC 13543 was grown and maintained as previously described.[15] The bacteria were harvested at $15,000 \times g$ in a M.S.E. High Speed 18 centrifuge (Measuring and Scientific Equipment Ltd., 25–28 Buckingham Gate, London, S.W.1). After two washes in 150 mM KCl-3 mM glycylglycine buffer at pH 7·0, the cells to be used in experiments at outer pH (pH_0) 7·0–7·1 were suspended in the same medium at approximately 50 mg cell dry weight/ml, but cells to be used in experiments at pH_0 6·0–6·1 were suspended in 150 mM KCl–10 mM glycylglycine buffer at pH 7·0. All washing and suspending media were de-oxygenated by bubbling with a stream of oxygen-free nitrogen gas, and the temperature was maintained at about 4° during the preparation of the washed cell suspensions.

Measurement of Respiration-Driven Proton Translocation

The reaction cell and electrode system was as described by Mitchell and Moyle.[16] The degassed media of 150 mM KCl–3 mM glycylglycine for experiments at pH_0 7·0–7·1 or 150 mM KCl–10 mM glycylglycine for experiments at pH_0 6·0–6·1 was introduced into the reaction chamber (volume 4 ml) under a stream of nitrogen gas. About 25 mg dry weight of bacterial cells in 0·5 ml of the appropriate anaerobic medium were then added with the stirrer running, and the volume enclosed by the vessel was returned to 4 ml by lowering the piston of the reaction cell. Residual oxygen was rapidy used up, and thereafter the organisms were maintained under strictly anaerobic conditions. The cells were allowed to equilibrate for 1–2 h before experiments were started. After this time any baseline drift of the pH_0 was very slow. Carbonic anhydrase was added to suspension media as described previously.[15]

Known quantities of oxygen in air-saturated 150 mM KCl were introduced into the anaerobic suspension, and the resulting respiration-driven acidification of the medium was compared with calibrations of pH_0 displacement due to addition of standard acid or alkali to permit estimation of the quantity of protons translocated per oxygen atom reduced, referred to as the $\rightarrow H^+/O$ quotient, as described before.[8]

Corrections for Response-Time of the pH-Measuring System

The rationale for correcting respiration-driven proton pulses has been discussed previously.[8] When the $t_{1/2}$ of decay is 100 times greater than the response-time of the electrode, the error introduced by extrapolating the value of the observed outer pH change (ΔpH_0) is about 1%. In most experiments described in this paper the decay rate of ΔpH_0 was slow, and corrections have been made by the previous method[8] only in the experiments of Fig. 10 where rapid decay rates were observed.

Extrapolation of ΔpH_0 to Give Initial Quantity of Protons Translocated

In mitochondria, it has been shown that the rate of proton translocation at the beginning of a pulse of respiration is faster than the State 3 rate of respiration under conditions where the membrane potential is neutralized.[17] The $\rightarrow H^+/O$ quotients were measured by extrapolation of the ΔpH_0 decay curve, which may be scaled to read as an $\rightarrow H^+/O$ curve, back to a time corresponding to 50% reduction of the oxygen in the pulse.[8,18] In *M. denitrificans*, the rate of respiration, stimulated by FCCP (corresponding to the State 3 rate), is 1·39 μg atoms of O/sec g cell dry weight,[15] while the rate of respiration estimated from the rate of proton translocation during a respiratory pulse in presence of valinomycin, measured using BCP (Fig. 11) and assuming an $\rightarrow H^+/O$ quotient of 8, was 1·79 μg atoms of O/sec g cell dry weight. We have accordingly estimated the time for half reduction ($t_{1/2}$) of 1 μg atom of O/g cell dry weight in the pulsed respiration experiments as 0·3 sec, and have extrapolated the decay of the proton pulses back to this time. In practice extrapolation to zero time did not differ significantly from extrapolation to 0·3 sec except when the $t_{1/2}$ of decay of the proton pulses was less than 30 sec.

Measurement of the Rate of Proton Translocation

Changes of pH_0 occurring within 2 sec cannot be closely followed using the glass electrode system described here, because the observed changes are dominated by the response-time of the electrode, which corresponded to a $t_{1/2}$ of 0·33 sec. We have therefore followed the pH_0 change spectrophotometrically, using BCP (ref. 19).

The problems associated with the use of BTB (refs. 20–23) for measuring the pH of a particular phase of three-phase systems, such as mitochondrial or bacterial suspensions, apply also to the structurally similar, but rather less lipid-soluble, BCP. We found that some 15% of BCP (20 mM) added to a bacterial suspension (5 mg cell dry weight/ml) records the pH of the inner phase. However, when BCP was adsorbed on bovine serum albumin (BSA), present as a 1% solution in the suspension medium, the equilibrium pH_0 changes measured with a glass electrode were identical to those measured by the change of absorbance of BCP, but the apparent rate of pH_0 change recorded by the latter technique during respiratory pulses was the more rapid, as expected.

The absorbance changes of BCP were measured using a dual wavelength spectrophotometer of conventional design, fitted with a toothed light-chopping wheel giving alternation between the reference and measuring beams at 5000 cycles/sec. A measuring wavelength of 580 nm and reference wavelength of 620 nm were used. The cuvette and the arrangement of the pH electrode and stirrer were as described previously.[20] Recordings of signals from the pH electrode and spectrophotometer were fed into a multichannel strip-chart recorder (Oscillograph type 5-127 of Bell and Howell Ltd., Basingstoke, Hants.). The measurements were done in the pH_0 range 6·0–6·1 in bacterial suspensions (5 mg cell dry weight/ml) in 150 mM KCl–10 mM glycylglycine (total volume 5·5 ml) with addition of 1% BSA, 450 μg of carbonic anhydrase and a final concentration of 20 μM BCP.

The concentration of BCP was maintained constant by incorporating 20 μM BCP in the calibrating acid, alkali and air-saturated KCl solutions which were otherwise as described previously.[8]

Rationale of the Measurement of →H^+/O Quotients in Bacteria

The conclusions drawn from the measurements of →H^+/O quotients in mitochondria,[8] that it is important to use the smallest oxygen pulses consistent with the accurate measurement of the corresponding pH_0 displacement, and that conditions should be arranged so as to minimize the build up of an opposing pH difference or electric potential difference across the coupling membrane, have been used in the measurements on the bacterial suspensions described in this paper.

Results

The Displacement of pH_0 During Pulses of Respiratory Activity

Figure 1 shows the time-course of the observed outer pH change (ΔpH_0) when anaerobic suspensions of *M. denitrificans* in a medium containing 150 mM KCl buffered with 3 mM glycylglycine at pH_0 7·0–7·1 or 10 mM glycylglycine at pH_0 6·0–6·1 were pulsed with small amounts of oxygen (about 1 μg atom/g cell dry weight, as indicated in legend). The medium was slowly acidified, and the subsequent decay of ΔpH_0 was extremely slow in both pH_0 ranges. When the effective proton conductance of the plasma membrane was increased by the presence of 2·5 μM FCCP (ref. 15), the respiration-driven changes in pH_0 were much decreased. These observations indicate that the changes in pH_0 are the result of proton translocation.

The change of pH_0 is sluggish compared with respiratory activity, for, under similar experimental conditions, the cycle of oxidation and reduction of cytochrome $(a + a_3)$, estimated by the absorbance difference $A_{607-630}$, occurs within 1 sec (P. Hinkle and P. Scholes, unpublished data).

When the size of the injected oxygen pulse was decreased from about 1 μg atom/g cell dry weight, as in Fig. 1, to 0·1 μg atom/g cell dry weight, there was an increase in the $\rightarrow$H$^+$/O quotient, and in some cases values greater than 4 were recorded.

Figure 2 shows that when the oxygen was added at different constant rates to anaerobic cell suspensions at pH_0 7·0–7·1, the $\rightarrow$H$^+$/O quotient was higher at the slower rates, but the decay rate of ΔpH_0 was apparently unaffected. At pH_0 6·0–6·1, there was a relatively greater increase in the $\rightarrow$H$^+$/O quotient at slower rates of oxygen utilization, and the decay of ΔpH_0 was more rapid. The $\rightarrow$H$^+$/O quotients obtained by extrapolation of the time-course of ΔpH_0 (see Materials and Methods) are given under the curves of Fig. 2.

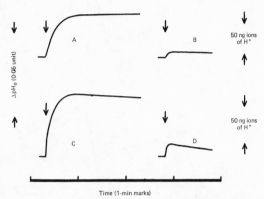

Figure 1. Time-course of respiration-driven ΔpH_0 in presence and absence of FCCP. Bacteria (5·25 mg cell dry weight/ml) were equilibrated under anaerobic conditions at 25° in 150 mM KCl-3 mM glycylglycine for measurements (A and B) in the pH_0 range 7·0–7·1, and in 150 mM KCl-10 mM glycylglycine for measurements (C and D) in the pH_0 range 6·0–6·1. Oxygen (23·5 ng atoms) was added as air-saturated 150 mM KCl at the arrows. FCCP (2·5 μM) was present in B and D. The quantity of H$^+$ ions equivalent to the recorded pH_0 changes is given for the 4 ml of suspension. Increase in acidity of the outer phase is shown upwards.

The Effect of Valinomycin on ΔpH_0 During Pulses of Respiration

Figure 3 shows the quantity of protons translocated outwards per oxygen atom reduced when a cell suspension in the range pH_0 6·0–6·1 was pulsed with air-saturated saline at several time intervals after the addition of valinomycin (0·75 mg/g cell dry weight). Under these conditions, proton translocation occurred very rapidly and, as shown in the semilogarithmic plots of Fig. 4A to C, the subsequent decay of the pulses was exponential. Over a period of 1–3 h incubation with valinomycin, an increase was observed both in the extrapolated $\rightarrow$H$^+$/O quotient and in the subsequent rate of ΔpH_0 decay (Fig. 4). The extrapolated $\rightarrow$H$^+$/O quotients obtained after 2 h preincubation with valinomycin in the range pH_0 6·0–6·1 gave an average of 7·5 $\pm$ 0·3 in 12 experiments. The $t_{1/2}$ of decay was between 120 and 150 sec, after preincubation with about 0·75 mg valinomycin/g cell dry weight. However, after preincubation of 2 h with larger amounts of valinomycin (about 2·0 mg/g cell dry weight), the $t_{1/2}$ of decay fell to 75 sec.

Experiments in the pH_0 range 7·0–7·1 gave qualitatively similar results to those of Fig. 3, although longer preincubation in the presence of valinomycin was required in the higher pH_0 range to obtain the transition from the type of proton pulse shown in Fig. 1 to that shown in Fig. 3. The limiting $\rightarrow$H$^+$/O quotient was usually lower after preincubation at neutral than at acid pH_0. The average value for six experiments was 6·0 $\pm$ 1·2, but values between 7 and 8 were recorded in some experiments. An important difference between experiments carried out in the two pH_0 ranges is seen in the decay of ΔpH_0, which was not exponential (Fig. 4D) at pH_0 7·0–7·1. A non-exponential decay of ΔpH_0 was obtained in the range pH_0 7·0–7·1, when preincubation of the anaerobic suspension with valinomycin was carried out at either acid or neutral pH_0 ranges.

Under the conditions where high stoichiometries were obtained in the presence of valinomycin, the extrapolated $\rightarrow H^+/O$ quotient remained constant over a wide range of oxygen quantities added. In one series of experiments at pH_0 6·0–6·1, the value of

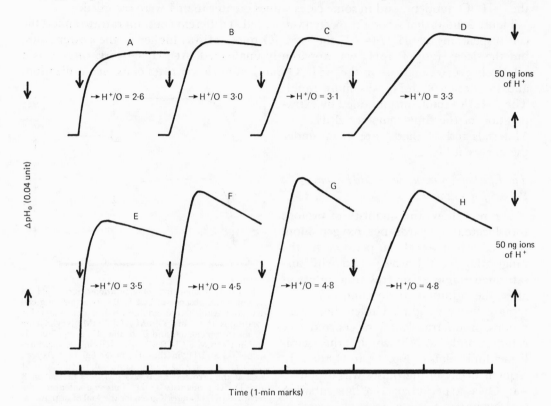

Figure 2. The effect of respiration rate on the time-course of respiration-driven ΔpH_0. Experiments were done at pH_0 7·0–7·1 (A, B, C, D) with a cell suspension containing 5·1 mg cell dry weight/ml; and at pH_0 6·0–6·1 (E, F, G, H) with a cell suspension containing 5·9 mg cell dry weight/ml under the same conditions as for Fig. 1. The oxygen (23·5 ng atoms O) as air-saturated 150 mM KCl was injected (commencing at the arrows) during the following times: A, about 0·2 sec; B, 18 sec; C, 29 sec; D, 68 sec; E, about 0·2 sec; F, 16 sec; G, 32 sec; H, 50 sec. The quantity of H^+ ions equivalent to the recorded pH_0 changes is given for the 4 ml of suspension. The values of $\rightarrow H^+/O$ given for each trace are calculated by extrapolating the decay of ΔpH_0 to the $t_{1/2}$ of oxygen reduction. Outward proton translocation is represented upwards.

the extrapolated $\rightarrow H^+/O$ quotient was 7·5 when the amount of oxygen reduced was between 0·4 and 2·0 μg atoms/g cell dry weight.

The Effect of Gramicidin on ΔpH_0 During Pulses of Respiration

The change in the characteristics of the time-course of ΔpH_0, and in the observed maximum values of $\rightarrow H^+/O$, after preincubation with gramicidin in the pH_0 ranges 6·0–6·1 and 7·0–7·1, are illustrated in Fig. 5. In both cases there was a considerable increase in the observed maximum $\rightarrow H^+/O$ values compared with corresponding respiratory pulses in the absence of gramicidin (Fig. 1). In the pH_0 range 6·0–6·1 the average maximum extrapolated →H^+/O quotient was 7·3 ± 0·6 (two experiments) but

the value obtained at pH_0 7·0–7·1 was only 5·0 ± 1·1 (four experiments). In both pH_0 ranges the decay of ΔpH_0 was not exponential (Fig. 6), but the initial decay rate was dependent on the quantity of gramicidin present. Maximum extrapolated →H^+/O quotients were observed with a lower concentration of gramicidin in experiments at pH_0 7·0–7·1 than at pH_0 6·0–6·1, and the initial $t_{1/2}$ of decay was near 30 sec in either pH_0 range. However, for a given amount of gramicidin, the initial decay rate was faster in the pH_0 range 7·0–7·1 than in the range 6·0–6·1.

The Effect of Potassium Thiocyanate on ΔpH_0 During Pulses of Respiration

After cells of *M. denitrificans* were equilibrated for 15 min with potassium thiocyanate, respiratory pulses were accompanied by rapid outward proton translocation, followed by a relatively slow decay towards equilibrium (Fig. 7). Maximum values of the extrapolated →H^+/O quotients were 7·4 ± 0·3 (three experiments) and 8·0 ± 0·1 (three experiments) at pH_0 6·0–6·1 and pH_0 7·0–7·1 respectively. The maximum extrapolated →H^+/O quotient at pH_0 6·0–6·1 required 17·5 mM thiocyanate, while the maximum value at pH_0 7·0–7·1 required 100 mM thiocyanate. As shown in Fig. 8, the decay of the ΔpH_0 was initially exponential at pH_0 6·0–6·1 when the SCN^- concentration was at least 17·5 mM; but at pH_0 7·0–7·1 the decay was not exponential even at 100 mM SCN^-. When the concentration of thiocyanate was increased above the level giving maximum extrapolated →H^+/O quotients, the $t_{1/2}$ of decay was more rapid. This effect was more pronounced in the range pH_0 6·0–6·1; and

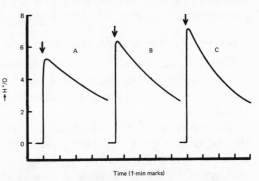

Figure 3. The effect of valinomycin on the time-course of respiration-driven proton translocation. Oxygen (23·5 ng atoms) in air-saturated 150 mM KCl was injected (at the arrows) into the anaerobic bacterial suspension under the conditions used in Fig. 1 for the pH_0 range 6·0–6·1. The bacterial suspension (4 ml) containing 5·03 mg cell dry weight/ml was preincubated, at pH_0 6·0–6·1 with valinomycin (0·75 mg/g cell dry weight) for: A, 45 min; B, 90 min; C, 120 min. The traces represent ΔpH_0 scaled to read as →H^+/O, outward proton translocation being represented upwards.

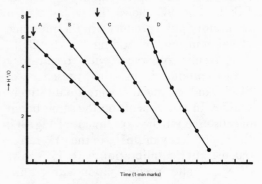

Figure 4. Semi-logarithmic plot of the decay of respiration-driven proton translocation. Data of Fig. 3 are plotted as curves A, B and C. For comparison, D is plotted from an identical experiment carried out in the pH_0 range 7·0–7·1. In D, the bacterial suspension (4 ml) containing 4·3 mg cell dry weight/ml was preincubated at pH_0 6·0–6·1 for 3 h with valinomycin (0·9 mg/g cell dry weight) and was reequilibrated at pH_0 7·0–7·1 prior to injection of 23·5 ng atoms of oxygen as air-saturated 150 mM KCl. The arrows indicate the time to which the observed →H^+/O value (obtained by scaling ΔpH_0) should be extrapolated to obtain the →H^+/O quotient corrected for decay.

at thiocyanate levels of 100 mM (corresponding to that required for maximum extrapolated →H^+/O quotients at pH_0 7·0–7·1) the $t_{1/2}$ of decay was about 20 sec, but the extrapolated →H^+/O quotient was only slightly depressed.

In rat liver mitochondria, Ca^{2+} ions release respiration-driven proton translocation when pulses of oxygen are added in excess of the normal backlash.[8] In contrast, the addition of $CaCl_2$ (60 μmoles/g cell dry weight) had no effect on respiration-driven proton translocation in *M. denitrificans*.

The Effect of FCCP on ΔpH_0 During Pulses of Respiration

Figure 9 shows the effect of the proton-conducting uncoupler FCCP on the decay of respiratory pulses in the normal suspension medium or with the addition of valinomycin, potassium thiocyanate or gramicidin.

The addition of 2·5 μM FCCP to untreated cells after a respiratory pulse increased the decay rate of ΔpH_0. In an experiment (A) where oxygen was added rapidly (0·2 sec) or (B) at a slow constant rate, the $t_{1/2}$ of decay was about 100 sec. Subsequent respiratory pulses were very small, as described in Fig. 1.

In the presence of valinomycin, SCN^- or gramicidin at pH_0 6·0–6·1, the large values of ΔpH_0 induced by pulses of respiration were collapsed rapidly on adding FCCP. Fig. 9C shows the collapse of a respiratory pulse produced in the presence of valinomycin, by adding 1 μM FCCP. The results observed with respiratory pulses produced in the presence of SCN^- and gramicidin were qualitatively similar. In experiments on the same batch of cells used for the experiment of Fig. 9C, the $t_{1/2}$ of decay of ΔpH_0 in the pH_0 range 6·0–6·1 after equilibration with 17·5 mM SCN^-, or after preincubation with gramicidin (0·8 mg/g cell dry weight) or valinomycin (2·0 mg/g cell dry weight) was 55

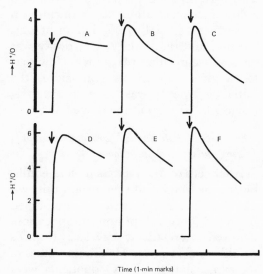

Time (1-min marks)

Figure 5. The effect of gramicidin on the time-course of respiration-driven proton translocation. Oxygen (23·5 ng atoms) was injected as air-saturated 150 mM KCl at the arrows. The conditions in the pH_0 range 6·0–6·1 or 7·0–7·1 were as described in Fig. 1. At pH_0 7·0–7·1 (A, B, C) the cell suspension (4 ml) contained 5·3 mg cell dry weight/ml with addition of gramicidin: A, 2·5 μg; B, 5·0 μg; C, 10 μg. At pH_0 6·0–6·1 (D, E, F) the cell suspension (4 ml) contained 5·2 mg cell dry weight/ml with the addition of gramicidin: D, 4 μg; E, 8 μg; F, 15 μg. The traces are shown as $\rightarrow H^+/O$ as in Fig. 3.

sec, 25 sec, and 75 sec respectively; and the addition of 1 μM FCCP decreased the $t_{1/2}$ to 20 sec, 12 sec and 3·5 sec respectively. When subsequent pulses were done in the presence of these reagents and FCCP, a considerable pH_0 displacement was still observed with a similar short $t_{1/2}$ of decay.

When respiratory pulses were done in the presence of 100 mM SCN^- at pH_0 7·0–7·1, ΔpH_0 was completely collapsed by 1 μM FCCP, and the $t_{1/2}$ decreased from 70 sec to 12 sec (Fig. 9D). On the other hand, in the presence of gramicidin at pH_0 7·0–7·1, ΔpH_0 did not decay to the baseline after the addition of 1 μM FCCP (Fig. 9E), and in some instances this effect was also observed with valinomycin at pH_0 7·0–7·1. However, subsequent respiratory pulses in the presence of FCCP and gramicidin, SCN^- or valinomycin gave large values of ΔpH_0 that decayed rapidly to the baseline.

Figure 10 shows the effect of increasing concentrations of FCCP on the decay rate and stoichiometry of respiratory pulses in the presence of KSCN at pH_0 7·0–7·1. In these experiments the points have been corrected for the response-time of the electrode. The values extrapolated back to the time of half reduction of the oxygen pulse show that the stoichiometry remains high until the $t_{1/2}$ of decay becomes less than 5 sec.

The Rate of Proton Translocation in the Presence of Valinomycin

Figure 11 illustrates a typical experiment in which the pH_0 was followed by measuring the change in absorbance of BCP and compared with measurements using the glass electrode system. Control injections of HCl and KOH under the conditions used in these experiments showed that the injection and mixing times did not exceed 0·1 sec. The rate of pH_0 change and the corresponding rate of proton translocation given by the spectrophotometric method in the type of experiment described by Fig. 11 was constant for the first 4/5 of the pH_0 excursion or for about 0·4 sec. The rate of proton translocation calculated for this part of the pulse was 14·3 μg ions of H^+/sec g cell dry weight.

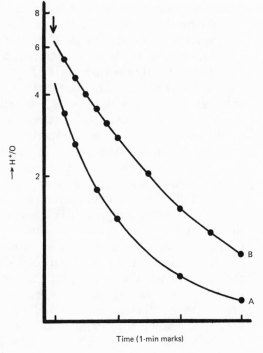

Time (1-min marks)

Figure 6. Semi-logarithmic plot of the decay of respiration-driven proton translocation. Data of Fig. 5C and F, are plotted as A and B respectively. Arrow convention as in Fig. 4.

Discussion and Conclusions

The results show that when transitory respiratory activity is induced in anaerobic suspensions of *M. denitrificans* with pulses of oxygen, protons are translocated outwards. The polarity of proton translocation during activity of the respiratory chain is thus the same as in mitochondria,[8] prokaryotic photosynthetic microorganisms,[2, 3] and other aerobic bacteria.[1]

In contrast to rat liver mitochondria, in absence of ion-conducting agents such as valinomycin or permeant ions such as SCN^-, the observed change of pH_0 during pulses of respiration-driven proton translocation in *M. denitrificans* was sluggish and did not give a stoichiometric value of $\rightarrow H^+/O$. When the size of the oxygen pulse was decreased from 1·0 μg atom of oxygen to 0·1 μg atom of oxygen/g cell dry weight, the stoichiometry of proton translocation increased and values greater than 4 were recorded in some cases. Under similar conditions in mitochondria the $\rightarrow H^+/O$ quotient during the oxidation of β-hydroxybutyrate and succinate is very close to 6 and 4 respectively.[8]

As discussed previously for the case of mitochondria,[18] if no charge leakage occurred across the M phase, the translocation of a small quantity of H^+ would produce a large membrane potential. Mitochondria and bacteria appear to be alike in that the conductance of the coupling membrane to the major ions usually present is low[15, 16, 24, 25] so that a membrane potential is rapidly produced by the chemically coupled translocation of ions, and ATP synthesis (resulting in net alkalinization) may occur. The fact that in *M. denitrificans* low $\rightarrow H^+/O$ quotients are observed in the normal KCl media, and the stoichiometry increases at lower respiratory rates, when the extent of reversal of the ATPase reaction should be less, is thus to be expected. The contrast between the bacteria and rat liver mitochondria in this respect is explained (see ref. 26) by the fact that in the mitochondria endogenous Ca^{2+} ions are mobile across the membrane and can electrically neutralize the translocation of up to some 10 μg ions of H^+/g of protein. The specific translocation of Ca^{2+} ions across the membrane of mammalian mitochondria evidently does not apply to the plasma membrane of *M. denitrificans*; for although proton translocation is released by the ion-conducting reagents valinomycin and gramicidin or the permeant anion SCN^- in the bacteria as in mitochondria, it is not released by Ca^{2+} ions.

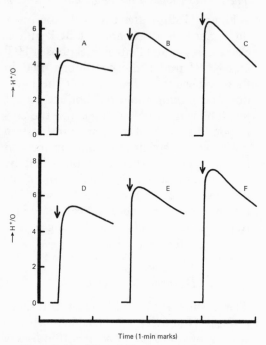

Some comment is required on the relative ineffectiveness of valinomycin as an ion-conducting reagent near pH_0 7, and on the long preincubation times required to release proton translocation near either pH_0 6 or 7. When the preincubation with the antibiotic was done near pH_0 6 it was more effective in releasing respiration-driven proton translocation tested near pH_0 7 than when the preincubation was done near pH_0 7. Our earlier observations on the effect of valinomycin on acid-base titration across the M phase of *M. denitrificans*[15] indicated that the K^+ ion conductance of the membrane was increased by valinomycin on incubation at acid pH_0,

Figure 7. The effect of thiocyanate on the time-course of respiration-driven proton translocation. Oxygen (23·5 ng atoms) was injected as air-saturated 150 mM KCl at the arrows. The conditions of the experiments in the pH_0 range 6·0–6·1 and 7·0–7·1 were as described in Fig. 1. At pH_0 6·0–6·1 (A, B, C), the cell suspension (4 ml) contained 5·1 mg cell dry weight/ml with addition of: A, 2·5 mM KSCN; B, 7·5 mM KSCN; C, 17·5 mM KSCN. At pH_0 7·0–7·1 (D, E, F) the cell suspension (4 ml), contained 4·7 mg cell dry weight/ml with addition of: D, 25 mM KSCN; E, 55 mM KSCN; F, 100 mM KSCN. The traces are shown as $\rightarrow H^+/O$, as in Fig. 3.

but that incubation with valinomycin at neutral or alkaline pH_0 had relatively much less effect. The slowness of development of K^+ ion permeability in *M. denitrificans* on incubation with valinomycin, and the pH-dependence of this process probably reflect the resistance of the cell wall and plasma membrane structure to the penetration and mobility of the valinomycin molecules, as in the case of other reagents studied in bacterial suspensions.[27–29] It is noteworthy, incidentally, that the release of respiration-driven proton translocation by SCN^- did not require preincubation beyond the time (15 min) permitting equilibration of the permeant SCN^- ion across the plasma membrane of the anaerobic cell suspensions. This was consistent with osmotic swelling experiments, using spheroplasts of *M. denitrificans* (P. Scholes, unpublished data) under conditions corresponding to those employed with mitochondrial suspensions,[30] which showed that the plasma membrane of *M. denitrificans* like that of staphylococci,[24] has a relatively high permeability to SCN^- ions. The increase in the rate of decay of the respiration-driven proton pulses at SCN^- concentrations approaching 100 mM, particularly at acid pH_0, are probably attributable to changes in the charge distribution in the lipid phase of the plasma membrane of the cells by the lipid-soluble SCN^- ion.

The effects of gramicidin in releasing proton translocation were qualitatively similar to those of valinomycin, but the maximum $\rightarrow H^+/O$ quotients obtained were lower than in the case of valinomycin. This, and other differences in the effects of gramicidin are probably attributable to the fact that gramicidin conducts not only alkali metal ions but also protons across lipid membranes.[15,31]

The extrapolated $\rightarrow H^+/O$ quotients obtained under different conditions in the pH_0 ranges 6·0–6·1 and 7·0–7·1 are summarized in Table I. The highest stoichiometries were obtained with valinomycin at pH_0 6·0–6·1 and with thiocyanate at pH_0 7·0–7·1. The lower stoichiometries observed can be ascribed to a decreased efficiency of the electrical potential-collapsing agent or to an increased conductance of the membrane to protons, induced by the reagent used, or to both causes.

The results of these and previous experiments on *M. denitrificans*[15] show clearly that FCCP enhances the proton conductance of the membrane. When the FCCP is added after termination of the respiration-driven proton translocation, the rapid collapse of the pulse requires the presence

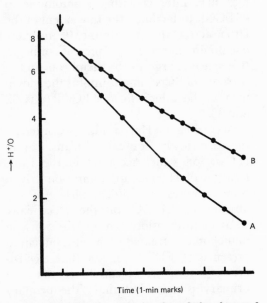

Figure 8. Semi-logarithmic plot of the decay of respiration-driven proton translocation. Data of Fig. 7C and F are plotted as A and B respectively. Arrow convention as in Fig. 4.

of the ion-conducting reagents valinomycin or gramicidin, or the permeant ion SCN^-, presumably because the respiration-driven proton translocation must be accompanied by the passage of an equivalent quantity of ionic charge across the membrane under the influence of the membrane potential. When conditions are such that the neutralizing ions do not permeate readily, the displacement of ions (such as Cl^-) across the membrane, under the influence of the high membrane potential developed during the respiratory pulse, would be expected to subside relatively slowly, even when the proton conductance of the membrane was moderately high. Thus, pH equilibration should be retarded in absence of ion-conducting reagents or permeant ions as in acid-base titrations with HCl or KOH (ref. 15).

As demonstrated in Fig. 10, increasing amounts of FCCP have little effect on the $\rightarrow H^+/O$ quotient until the $t_{1/2}$ of decay is as low as 5 sec. Similar observations in mitochondria have been discussed previously.[8] One may conclude that the membrane conductance to SCN$^-$ is much greater than that to H$^+$, induced by FCCP, under these conditions.

When experiments similar to those of Fig. 10 were carried out in presence of valino-mycin or gramicidin, qualitatively similar results were obtained, although for a given amount of FCCP the decay of the proton pulses was more rapid and was not ex-ponential. These findings are difficult to interpret in detail, but we suggest that the positively charged valinomycin-K$^+$ com-plex may interact with the anionic form of FCCP to facilitate the movement of the latter across the membrane. Conversely one might expect that an increase of nega-tive space-charge in the membrane in the presence of SCN$^-$ might inhibit the move-ment of the anionic form of FCCP (refs. 32 and 33).

According to Harris and co-workers,[34] the electrically equivalent translocation of Ca^{2+} ions which accompanies the trans-location of H$^+$ ions in respiration-driven proton pulses in mitochondria (in the absence of EDTA) or the electrically equivalent translocation of K$^+$ ions in mitochondria treated with valinomycin in presence of EDTA suggest that electro-genic proton translocation is not the primary process, but that "the primary event in proton pulse production is an energy-driven cation exchange." Evidence that is incompatible with this interpreta-tion in rat liver mitochondria has been discussed.[35] It might be suggested that the proton pulses observed in suspensions of *M. denitrificans* should be similarly interpreted. This interpretation is not, however, ac-ceptable because proton pulses with an →H$^+$/O quotient approaching 8 have been observed under conditions in which the anion SCN$^-$ is the charge-neutralizing

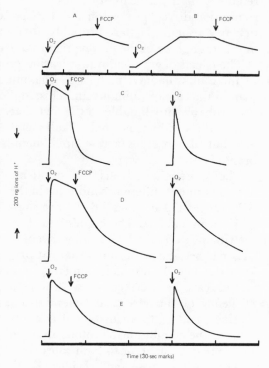

Figure 9. The effect of FCCP on the time-course of respiration-driven ΔpH$_0$ under various conditions. Oxygen (23·5 ng atoms) was injected as air-saturated 150 mM KCl, commencing at arrows, and taking 0·2 sec except in (B), when it was injected at a slow constant rate. The media were as described for Fig. 1. A, pre-incubation was at pH$_0$ 7·0–7·1 with no addition, and 2·5 μM FCCP was added at arrow. B, was as A, but the duration of the oxygen pulse was 60 sec. In C, D, and E, the cells were preincubated respectively: with valino-mycin (2·0 mg/g cell dry weight) at pH$_0$ 6·0–6·1; with KSCN (100 mM) at pH$_0$ 7·0–7·1; and with gramicidin (0·29 mg/g cell dry weight) at pH$_0$ 7·0–7·1. After pre-incubation, an initial oxygen pulse, FCCP (1 μM), and a final oxygen pulse were added at arrows. In all experiments the cell suspension contained about 5 mg dry weight/ml. Upward deflection of traces indicates acidification of the medium. The quantity of H$^+$ equivalent to the recorded pH$_0$ changes is given for the 4 ml of suspension.

ion species and there is no evidence to support the suggestion that proton/cation exchange occurs under these conditions. Moreover, if non-electrogenic proton/cation exchange were the primary process, since the data of Fig. 10 show that 3 μM FCCP in presence of SCN$^-$ does not prevent proton translocation (e.g. by hydrolysing an energy-rich intermediate) but only facilitates conduction of H$^+$ ions back across the membrane (as discussed below), FCCP alone at this or at a lower concentration should not largely prevent the appearance of the respiration-driven proton pulses, as observed (Fig. 1).

The $\rightarrow H^+/O$ quotients approaching 8, observed in both acid and neutral pH_0 ranges (Table I), are especially interesting, since the highest $\rightarrow H^+/O$ quotient obtained from respiratory pulses in rat liver mitochondria (oxidizing β-hydroxybutyrate) was 6. Two main alternative mechanisms of primary proton translocation coupled to oxidoreduction have been suggested. According to the chemiosmotic view of the coupling mechanism, protons are produced at the outer surface and taken up at the inner surface of the M phase by the oxidation of H atoms and reduction of H^+ ions respectively at junctions between hydrogen-carrying and electron-carrying members of the respiratory chain, supposed to be arranged in a "looped" configuration in the membrane.[9] According to a version of the chemical hypothesis of the coupling mechanism,[36] the protons are translocated outwards across the membrane by a squiggle-actuated pump which drives $2H^+$ outwards per squiggle derived from the hypothetical coupling sites in the respiratory chain. The chemical or the chemiosmotic mechanism respectively could also utilize ATP, derived from substrate-level phosphorylation, either by driving the squiggle-actuated proton pump (via the ATPase system) or by driving the proton-translocating ATPase. Thus, an $\rightarrow H^+/O$ quotient of 8 demands either four oxidoreduction loops, or the generation of four squiggle bonds (including ATP generated by a substrate-level mechanism), or some combination. It appears to be unlikely that substrate-level phosphorylation could

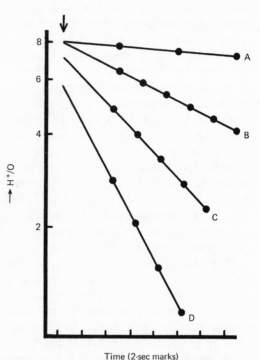

Figure 10. The effect of increasing concentrations of FCCP on the $\rightarrow H^+/O$ quotient and the rate of decay of respiration-driven proton translocation. Oxygen (23·5 ng atoms) was injected as air-saturated 150 mM KCl. The conditions were as described in Fig. 1 for experiments at pH_0 7·0–7·1. Additional reagents present were: A, 100 mM KSCN; B, 100 mM KSCN + 1 μM FCCP; C, 100 mM KSCN + 3 μM FCCP; D, 100 mM KSCN + 7 μM FCCP. The cell suspension (4 ml) contained 6·8 mg cell dry weight/ml. The $\rightarrow H^+/O$ values plotted on the vertical axis represent appropriately scaled ΔpH_0 values obtained by correcting the observed ΔpH_0 values for the response-time of the electrode (see Materials and Methods). Arrow convention as in Fig. 4.

be involved because the translocation of only $2H^+$ of the observed $8H^+$ in the pulses would require some 1 μmole of ATP/g cell dry weight, and it is known that, at this ATP level in *M. denitrificans*, hydrolysis is slow (P. Scholes and F. Welsch, unpublished data) compared with the rate of appearance of the H^+ ions observed in the respiration-driven pulses. The observations described here do not permit a decision between the chemiosmotic and chemical types of proton-translocation mechanisms; but the fact that FCCP causes an increase in the rate of decay of the respiration-driven proton pulses, but does not cause a decrease in the quantity of protons initially translocated during the pulse of respiration shows that, if a squiggle-intermediate is involved, it is relatively insensitive to destruction by the uncoupling agent. _M. denitrificans_ behaves like rat liver mitochondria in this respect.[8]

The circumstances under which the $\rightarrow$H$^+$/O quotients approaching 8 have been observed in _M. denitrificans_ were arranged so as to minimize thermodynamic back-pressure on the proton-translocation reaction. This high stoichiometry may not therefore be characteristic of the system in the near-equilibrium state during ATP synthesis. Assuming, however, that the $\rightarrow$H$^+$/O quotient of 8 may be physiologically normal, the probable implication would be that the P/O quotient is 4, whether by chemiosmotic or by chemical coupling. This is thermodynamically feasible, since total P/O quotients of 4 (including the substrate-level phosphorylation) are characteristic of α-oxoglutarate oxidation in mitochondria.[37]

The characteristics of the transhydrogenase reaction, described by Asano _et al._[13], suggest that the respiratory chain of _M. denitrificans_ may possibly consist of four oxidoreduction loops similar to those previously postulated for mitochondria;[9] but that, unlike mitochondria, Loop 0, corresponding to the transhydrogenase reaction system, may catalyse the oxidation of NADPH, at least under the special conditions of the experiments described here.

Figure 11 shows that the rate of proton translocation in presence of valinomycin

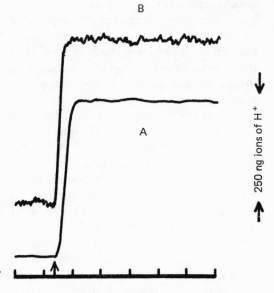

Time (2-sec marks)

Figure 11. Time-course of respiration-driven proton translocation in the presence of valinomycin. Traces A and B respectively show the observed proton translocation measured simultaneously with the pH electrode system, and by observing the absorbance changes of BCP in the pH$_0$ range 6·0–6·1. For experimental details see Materials and Methods. Oxygen (47 ng atoms) was injected as air-saturated 150 mM KCl at the arrow. Upward deflection of traces represents acidification of medium. The quantity of H$^+$ ions equivalent to the recorded pH$_0$ changes is given for the 5·5 ml of suspension.

TABLE I. Summary of the extrapolated $\rightarrow$H$^+$/O quotients obtained in presence of valinomycin, gramicidin, and SCN$^-$.

Membrane potential-collapsing agent	Extrapolated $\rightarrow$H$^+$/O quotient	
	pH$_0$ 6·0–6·1	pH$_0$ 7·0–7·1
Valinomycin	7·5 ± 0·3 (12)	6·0 ± 1·2 (6)
Gramicidin	7·3 ± 0·6 (2)	5·0 ± 1·1 (4)
Potassium thiocyanate	7·4 ± 0·3 (3)	8·0 ± 0·1 (3)

The conditions were as described for Figs. 3, 5, and 7.

was 14·3 μg ions of H$^+$/sec g cell dry weight. At an →H$^+$/O quotient of 8 this would correspond to a respiration rate of 1·79 μg atoms of O/sec g cell dry weight. The steady-state rate of respiration optimally stimulated by FCCP is 1·39 μg atoms of O/sec g cell dry weight,[15] and it follows that the proton flux rate is high enough to account for coupling between respiration and phosphorylation by an intermediary current of protons.[9]

Acknowledgments

We are grateful to Dr. Jennifer Moyle for helpful discussion and criticism. We thank Glynn Research Ltd. for general financial support, and record our indebtedness to Mr. Roy Mitchell, Mr. Robert Harper, Mr. Michael Pearse, and Miss Stephanie Phillips for expert assistance. One of us (Peter Scholes) holds the Royal Society Horace le Marquand and Dudley Bigg Fellowship.

References

1. P. Mitchell, in: *Cell Interface Reactions*, H. D. Brown, (ed.), Scholar's Library, New York, 1963, p. 33.
2. P. Scholes, P. Mitchell, and J. Moyle, *European J. Biochem.*, **8** (1969) 450.
3. G. E. Edwards and C. R. Bovell, *Biochim. Biophys. Acta*, **172** (1969) 126.
4. H. Baltscheffsky and L. -V. Von Stedingk, in: *Currents in Photosynthesis*, J. B. Thomas and J. C. Goedheer (eds.), Ad. Donker, Rotterdam, 1966, p. 253.
5. L. -V. Von Stedingk and H. Baltscheffsky, *Arch. Biochem. Biophys.*, **117** (1966) 400.
6. B. Chance, M. Nishimura, M. Avron, and M. Baltscheffsky, *Arch. Biochem. Biophys.*, **117** (1966) 158.
7. J. B. Jackson, A. R. Crofts, and L. -V. Von Stedingk, *European J. Biochem.*, **6**, (1968) 41.
8. P. Mitchell and J. Moyle, *Biochem. J.*, **105** (1967) 1147.
9. P. Mitchell, *Chemiosmotic Coupling in Oxidative and Photosynthetic Phosphorylation*, Glynn Research, Bodmin, Cornwall, 1966.
10. P. Mitchell and J. Moyle, *European J. Biochem.*, **4** (1968) 530.
11. K. Imai, A. Asano, and R. Sato, *Biochim. Biophys. Acta*, **143** (1967) 462.
12. P. Mitchell, *Symp. Soc. Gen. Microbiol.*, **20** (1970) 121.
13. A. Asano, K. Imai, and R. Sato, *Biochim. Biophys. Acta*, **143** (1967) 477.
14. P. Scholes and L. Smith, *Biochim. Biophys. Acta*, **153** (1968) 363.
15. P. Scholes and P. Mitchell, *J. Bioenergetics*, **1** (1970) 61.
16. P. Mitchell and J. Moyle, *Biochem. J.*, **104** (1967) 588.
17. P. Mitchell and J. Moyle, *European J. Biochem.*, **7** (1969) 471.
18. P. Mitchell, *Chemiosmotic Coupling and Energy Transduction*, Glynn Research, Bodmin, Cornwall, 1968.
19. B. Chance and L. Mela, *J. Biol. Chem.*, **241** (1966) 4588.
20. P. Mitchell, J. Moyle, and L. Smith, *European J. Biochem.*, **4** (1968) 9.
21. G. F. Azzone, G. Piemonte, and S. Massari, *European J. Biochem.*, **6** (1968) 207.
22. J. B. Jackson and A. R. Crofts, *European J. Biochem.*, **10** (1969) 226.
23. Z. Gromet-Elhanan and S. Briller, *Biochem. Biophys. Res. Commun.*, **37** (1969) 261.
24. P. Mitchell and J. Moyle, *Symp. Soc. Gen. Microbiol.*, **6** (1956) 150.
25. J. B. Chappell and K. N. Haarhoff, in: *Biochemistry of Mitochondria*, E. C. Slater, Z. Kaniuga, and L. Wojtczak (eds.), Academic Press, London, 1967, p. 75.
26. E. Carafoli, *Biochem. J.* **116** (1970), 2 P.
27. B. A. Newton, *Symp. Soc. Gen. Microbiol.*, **8** (1958) 62.
28. W. A. Hamilton, *J. Gen. Microbiol.*, **50** (1968) 441.
29. L. H. Muschel and L. J. Larsen, *J. Bacteriol.*, **98** (1969) 840.
30. P. Mitchell and J. Moyle, *European J. Biochem.*, **9** (1969) 149.
31. P. J. F. Henderson, J. D. McGivan, and J. B. Chappell, *Biochem. J.*, **111** (1969) 521.
32. G. Eisenman, S. M. Ciani, and G. Szabo, *Federation Proc.*, **27** (1968) 1289.
33. E. A. Liberman and V. P. Topaly, *Biochim. Biophys. Acta*, **163** (1968) 125.
34. R. C. Thomas, J. R. Manger, and E. J. Harris, *European J. Biochem.*, **11** (1969) 413.
35. P. Mitchell, in: *The Molecular Basis of Membrane Function*, D. C. Tosteson (ed.), Prentice-Hall, New Jersey, 1969, p. 483.
36. E. C. Slater, *European J. Biochem.*, **1** (1967) 317.
37. E. C. Slater, in: *Comprehensive Biochemistry*, M. Florkin and E. H. Stotz (eds.), Vol. 14, Elsevier, Amsterdam, 1966, p. 327.

22

Reprinted from *Biochem. Biophys. Res. Commun.* **58**:178–184 (1974)

OXIDATIVE PHOSPHORYLATION AND PROTON TRANSLOCATION IN
MEMBRANE VESICLES PREPARED FROM *ESCHERICHIA COLI*

Elliot L. Hertzberg and Peter C. Hinkle

Section of Biochemistry, Molecular and Cell Biology
Cornell University, Ithaca, New York 14850

Received March 8, 1974

SUMMARY

Membrane vesicles have been prepared from *E. coli* which are capable of catalyzing oxidative phosphorylation with several physiological substrates. Phosphorylation efficiencies of 0.62 ± .06 moles ATP formed per gram-atom oxygen consumed have been observed with NADH as substrate. The phosphorylation is sensitive to uncouplers, fulfilling an essential requirement for the study of oxidative phosphorylation in cell-free systems. Since the vesicles also catalyze, either during respiration or ATP hydrolysis, uncoupler sensitive uptake of protons, they are inverted with respect to whole bacteria and allow the study of additional parameters relating to energy coupling.

The discovery of mutants of *Escherichia coli* deficient in oxidative phosphorylation (1) has resulted in a resurgence of interest in the study of energy-linked functions in this bacterium. However, these studies have been confined to secondary energy-linked processes, such as the transhydrogenase (2), reduction of NAD^+ by succinate (3), or substrate transport by the uncoupled mutants (4-8). For the most part, the direct measurement of oxidative phosphorylation has been omitted because of the low efficiencies generally obtained in cell-free systems (9), uncoupled pyridine nucleotide oxidation (10), or lack of sensitivity to uncouplers (11). There is one report of relatively high efficiencies of phosphorylation in the literature, but the authors failed to explore uncoupler sensitivity (12). The possibility of studying proton translocation in an inverted membrane preparation from *E. coli* has also not been pursued.

In this paper we describe the preparation of a particulate fraction from *E. coli* which catalyzes the uncoupler sensitive phosphorylation of ADP with a variety of substrates. In contrast to proton extrusion observed with whole cells (13), the vesicles catalyze the uptake of protons in response to energization by either respiration or ATP, as predicted for an inverted preparation.

METHODS

E. coli W1655 was obtained from the Coli Stock Center, Yale University.

Cells were grown batch-wise, either in an incubator-shaker, or in a New Brunswick Fermentor, in a defined minimal medium, consisting of 30 mM KPi, 9 mM NH$_4$Cl, 3 mM MgCl$_2$, 1 µM FeSO$_4$, 1 µM ZnSO$_4$, pH 7.0, supplemented with methionine to 20 µg/ml. The carbon source was glycerol, at a concentration of 15 mM. Cells were grown to mid-exponential phase and harvested by centrifugation in the cold. The cell pellet was resuspended and washed twice with 50 mM KPi, 5 mM MgCl$_2$, pH 7.0, and resuspended to a 20% (wet weight/volume) suspension in 50 mM KPi, 5 mM MgCl$_2$, 10% (v/v) methanol, 1 mM DTT*, pH 7.0. Cells were broken by a single passage through an Aminco French Pressure Cell (Model 43398-A) at 4500±500 pounds total pressure. Debris and unbroken cells were removed by centrifugation at 39,000 x g for ten minutes in a SS-34 rotor of a Sorvall RC-2B centrifuge. Vesicles were sedimented by centrifugation at 210,000 x g for two hours in a 50 Ti rotor of a Beckman L-2 ultracentrifuge. The pellet was resuspended by gentle homogenization to approximately 5 mg protein per ml in 250 mM sucrose, 10 mM morpholinopropane sulfonate, 5 mM MgCl$_2$, 10% (v/v) methanol, 1 mM DTT, pH 7.5, and the centrifugation repeated. The pellet was finally resuspended to approximately 50 mg/ml in the same buffer. Vesicles prepared by this procedure are stable to freezing and thawing, and remain stable for at least two weeks at -70°. Storage in liquid nitrogen stabilizes virtually all activity for at least two months.

Oxidative phosphorylation was measured by adding approximately 1 mg of vesicle protein to a reaction mixture containing 250 mM sucrose, 5 mM Tris-Cl, 2 mM MgSO$_4$, 0.3 mM EDTA, 32 mM glucose, 10.0 units/ml hexokinase, 1 mM ATP, 1 mg/ml fatty acid free BSA, 20 mM [^{32}P]-KPi, pH 7.4, at a specific activity

---

* Abbreviations used: BSA, bovine serum albumin; CCCP, carbonyl cyanide m-chlorophenylhydrazone; DTT, dithiothreitol.

of 50-100 cpm per nanomole, in a 1.2 ml oxygraph cell maintained at 25°. With

NADH as substrate, the reaction mixture was previously supplemented with 10

units alcohol dehydrogenase (Sigma, Type A-7011) and 10 μl 95% ethanol. After

thirty seconds, substrate in amounts indicated in the legends of the tables

was added and the reaction was generally allowed to proceed until anaerobiosis

occurred, usually in about three minutes. A 0.5 ml aliquot was then withdrawn

and rapidly added to 0.5 ml cold 10% trichloroacetic acid. Protein was sedi-

mented by centrifugation, and esterified phosphate analyzed (14).

   Respiration and ATP driven proton translocation was measured by the pulse

method of Mitchell and Moyle (15,16) using a recording pH meter described by

Thayer and Hinkle (17). In respiration experiments 2-5 mg of protein was added

to nitrogen-bubbled 150 mM KCl, 5 mM $MgCl_2$ and respiration was initiated after

equilibration by injecting microliter quantities of air-saturated 150 mM KCl,

5 mM $MgCl_2$ or oxygen-saturated ethanol. Amounts of proton translocation were

estimated by calibration with pulses of standardized, anaerobic HCl. ATP-driven

proton translocation was measured in a medium of 150 mM KCl, 5 mM $MgCl_2$ at

pH 6.15 in order to prevent net acid or base formation from the hydrolysis of

ATP (17).

   Protein was measured by the biuret procedure (18). CCCP and valinomycin

were obtained from Sigma.

RESULTS AND DISCUSSION

   As shown in Table 1, approximately 25% cell breakage was achieved under

the conditions described. The bulk of the respiratory activity recovered

following removal of unbroken cells and large debris is associated with the

particulate fraction. The remainder is decanted with the supernatant fractions,

and consists of poorly packed material. This procedure probably yields a

fraction contaminated by cell wall debris and ribosomes. However, these are

unlikely to interfere with our measurements.

   Table 2 shows the respiratory rates and phosphorylation efficiencies with

TABLE 1. Cell Breakage and Fractionation of Respiratory Activity

Fraction	Volume ml	Protein mg/ml	Yield total mg	Specific Activity units/mg protein	Total Activity units
Cell Suspension	34.6	36.4	1259	-	-
29,000 x g Supernatant	19	16.2	308	46.6	14,300
210,000 x g Supernatant	18.8	11.4	214	9.4	2,030
210,000 x g Wash	9.5	3.2	30	23.2	74
Particles	1.2	39	47	248	11,700

Respiration was measured utilizing the NADH regenerating system described in the text in the presence of 167 μM NAD^+. The medium was 250 mM sucrose, 5 mM $MgCl_2$, 20 mM KPi, pH 7.4. Units are expressed in ng atoms oxygen consumed per minute.

TABLE 2. Oxidative Phosphorylation in Respiratory Vesicles

Substrate	Specific Activity units/mg protein	Oxygen Uptake ng atoms O	Pi Esterified nmoles Pi	P/O
NAD^+ (Alcohol dehydrogenase limiting)	66	634	463	.73
+ CCCP	68	658	0	0
NAD^+ (Excess alcohol dehydrogenase)	172	624	353	.57
+ CCCP	202	658	11	.02
α-glycerolphosphate	212	627	239	.38
+ CCCP	230	672	3	0
D-lactate	86	620	278	.45
+ CCCP	66	658	1	0
Succinate	30	277	152	.55
+ CCCP	30	249	14	.06

Oxidative phosphorylation was measured as described in the text. NAD^+ was added to 167 μM. The level of alcohol dehydrogenase required for limitation of the respiratory rate due to the regenerating system was determined empirically. All other substrates were used at 12.5 mM. CCCP was used at 83 μM. Units are expressed in ng atoms oxygen consumed per minute.

various substrates. The esterification of inorganic phosphate has been corrected for low levels of respiration-independent incorporation (2-3 nanomoles per minute per mg protein). Interestingly, in the case of NADH, higher coupling efficiencies were obtained if alcohol dehydrogenase was rate limiting in the NADH regenerating system. Such a system showed a mean P/O of 0.66 ± .06, based on four different preparations. With excess alcohol dehydrogenase, fourteen preparations exhibited a mean P/O of 0.62 ± .06. It is significant that the coupling efficiency of NADH was higher than that of the flavoprotein linked substrates, α-glycerolphosphate, D-lactate and succinate. In all cases, phosphorylation was sensitive to the uncoupler CCCP. If BSA was omitted from the oxidative phosphorylation assay mixture, 4.2 μM CCCP resulted in 94% uncoupling. Omission of BSA resulted in a 15% decrease of the P/O.

Experiments carried out by the method of Hempfling (19) (data not shown) indicate a P/O of 2.5 in whole cells. This technique generally utilizes only the initial levels of reduced pyridine nucleotide for determining total electron flow. Since the levels of reduced quinones, flavoproteins and cytochromes are not considered, somewhat high values are obtained, suggesting that there are actually two sites of coupling in this strain. The data in Table 2 also suggest that there is one coupling site between NADH and the point of entry of reducing equivalents from succinate, D-lactate and α-glycerolphosphate, and another between this point and oxygen.

Figures 1 and 2 demonstrate respiration driven proton translocation in this preparation, with limiting and saturating oxygen pulses, respectively. The uptake of protons indicates that the vesicles are inverted with respect to the whole cell. After correcting for the response time of the electrode by a semi-logarithmic plot of the observed pH change versus time (20) (not shown), a ratio of 1.70 protons translocated per gram-atom of oxygen consumed was observed. The uncorrected value was 1.38. Since a stoichiometry of four protons translocated per oxygen is expected for two coupling sites linked to the oxidation of NADH (15), apparently about half of the respiration is not coupled

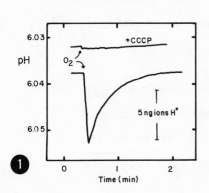

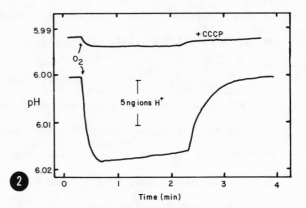

Figure 1. Respiration-driven proton translocation in respiratory vesicles.
A 0.6 ml anaerobic pH cell containing 2.2 mg vesicle protein was used. Valinomycin (0.1 µg) was present during the assay. The substrate was 167 µM NAD^+ in
the presence of the regenerating system described earlier. At the time indicated by the arrow, 10 µl of air-saturated 150 mM KCl, 5 mM $MgCl_2$, corresponding to 4.7 ng atoms of oxygen, was added. Where indicated, CCCP was present at
16.7 µM.

Figure 2. Respiration-driven proton translocation in respiratory vesicles.
The experiment was performed as described in the legend for Figure 1 except
that 2.65 mg vesicle protein was used, and the oxygen pulse consisted of 5 µl
of oxygen-saturated ethanol.

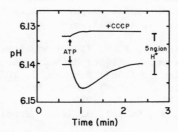

Figure 3. ATP-driven proton translocation in respiratory vesicles. 2.65 mg
vesicle protein suspended in 0.6 ml 150 mM KCl, 2 mM $MgCl_2$ was placed in the
pH cell. Valinomycin (0.1 µg) was also present during the assay. At the time
indicated by the arrow 15 nmoles ATP, pH 6.15 were added. Where indicated,
CCCP was present at 16.7 µM.

---

in this preparation. Preliminary measurements of the proton-to-oxygen ratio

with flavin-linked substrates indicates a proton-to-oxygen ratio approaching

one, consistent with the above interpretation.

Figure 3 demonstrates ATP-driven, uncoupler sensitive uptake of protons in these vesicles. Since coupling efficiencies were low, the data do not yet warrant a detailed analysis of the proton to ATP stoichiometry (17).

ACKNOWLEDGEMENTS

The authors would like to thank Professors A. Jane Gibson and Efraim Racker for many helpful suggestions. This work was supported by research grant HL 11483 from the National Institutes of Health. P.C.H. is the recipient of Career Development Award GM-22427 and E.L.H. of a National Institutes of Health Predoctoral Traineeship.

REFERENCES

1. Butlin, J. D., Cox, G. B. and Gibson, F. (1971) Biochem. J. $\underline{124}$, 75–81.
2. Bragg, P. D. and Hou, C. (1973) Biochem. Biophys. Res. Comm. $\underline{50}$, 729–736.
3. Sweetman, A. J. and Griffiths, D. E. (1971) Biochem. J. $\underline{121}$, 117–124.
4. Simoni, R. D. and Shallenberger, M. K. (1972) Proc. Nat. Acad. Sci. U.S. $\underline{69}$, 2663–2667.
5. Rosen, B. P. (1973) Biochem. Biophys. Res. Comm. $\underline{53}$, 1289–1296.
6. Or, A., Kanner, B. I. and Gutnick, D. L. (1973) FEBS Letters $\underline{35}$, 217–219.
7. Schairer, H. U. and Haddock, B. A. (1972) Biochem. Biophys. Res. Comm. $\underline{48}$, 544–551.
8. Berger, E. A. (1973) Proc. Nat. Acad. Sci. U.S. $\underline{70}$, 1514–1518.
9. Bragg, P. D. and Hou, C. (1968) Can. J. Biochem. $\underline{46}$, 631–641.
10. Kashket, E. R. and Brodie, A. F. (1963) Biochem. Biophys. Acta $\underline{78}$, 52–65.
11. I-shen, Z. (1965) Acta Biochim. Biophys. Sinica $\underline{5}$, 545–547.
12. Turnock, G., Erickson, S., Ackrell, B. C. and Buck, B. (1972) J. Gen. Microbiol. $\underline{70}$, 507–515.
13. Lawford, H. G. and Haddock, B. H. (1973) Biochem. J. $\underline{136}$, 217–220.
14. Lindberg, O. and Ernster, L. (1956) Methods Biochem. Anal. $\underline{3}$, 1–22.
15. Mitchell, P. and Moyle, J. (1967) Biochem. J. $\underline{105}$, 1147–1162.
16. Mitchell, P. and Moyle, J. (1968) Eur. J. Biochem. $\underline{4}$, 530–539.
17. Thayer, W. S. and Hinkle, P. C. (1973) J. Biol. Chem. $\underline{248}$, 5395–5402.
18. Jacobs, E. E., Jacob, M., Sanadi, D. R. and Bradley, L. B. (1956) J. Biol. Chem. $\underline{223}$, 147–156.
19. Hempfling, W. P. (1970) Biochem. Biophys. Res. Comm. $\underline{41}$, 9–15.
20. Hinkle, P. C. and Horstman, L. L. (1971) J. Biol. Chem. $\underline{246}$, 6024–6028.

Editor's Comments
on Papers 23 and 24

23 BOYER
A Model for Conformational Coupling of Membrane Potential and Proton Translocation to ATP Synthesis and to Active Transport

24 ROSING, KAYALAR, and BOYER
Evidence for Energy-dependent Change in Phosphate Binding for Mitochondrial Oxidative Phosphorylation Based on Measurements of Medium and Intermediate Phosphate-Water Exchanges

THE "CONFORMATIONAL" HYPOTHESIS

P. Boyer and his associates have suggested that three kinds of chemical events combine to link ATP formation to electron transport during oxidative phosphorylation[1]: *oxidative transduction,* which comprises electron transfer from one carrier to another more electropositive carrier and the primary trapping of energy released thereby; *energy transmission,* or the conversion of the primary trapped configuration into a state suitable to drive ATP synthesis; and *phosphorylative transduction,* the actual dehydration reaction yielding ATP from ADP and inorganic phosphate catalyzed by membrane ATPase. As described in the series of exchanges between Boyer and Mitchell (references 2, 3, and 4 and Paper 23), the "conformational" hypothesis provides mechanisms for each of these steps, which differ from those employed by the chemiosmotic hypothesis. Where the proton has primacy in the latter model, forming a transmembrane gradient consequent upon respiratory energy and then directly protonating O_2^{2-} derived from phosphate by returning through the ATPase active side, the former mechanism envisages reversible proton ejection and modification of affinities of the ATPase for Pi, ADP, and ATP through respiratory-energy-induced conformational change, thereby leading to ATP synthesis. This model can account for the "exchange" reactions of oxidative phosphorylation, most notably the uncoupler-insensitive ^{18}O-water-Pi exchange, which occurs at a considerably more rapid rate than does ATP synthesis during oxidative phosphorylation. The important findings about that exchange reaction are reported in Paper 24.

The investigations of Boyer's group appear to have led to a model that is capable of accounting for a greater number of the phenomena attending oxidative phosphorylation than that accommodated by the chemiosmotic mechanism. The last word in this controversy has, however, not yet been uttered.

REFERENCES

1. Boyer, P. D., F. J. Smith, J. Rosing, and C. Kayalar. In E. Quagliariello, F. Palmieri, E. C. Slater, and N. Siliprandi, eds. *Electron Transfer Chains and Oxidative Phosphorylation.* North-Holland Publishing Co., Amsterdam, 1975, pp. 361–372.
2. Mitchell, P. *FEBS Lett.,* **43**, 189–194, 1975.
3. Boyer, P. D. *FEBS Lett.,* **50**, 91–94, 1975.
4. Mitchell, P. *FEBS Lett.,* **50**, 95–97, 1975.

A MODEL FOR CONFORMATIONAL COUPLING OF MEMBRANE POTENTIAL AND PROTON TRANSLOCATION TO ATP SYNTHESIS AND TO ACTIVE TRANSPORT

Paul D. BOYER

Molecular Biology Institute and Department of Chemistry, University of California,
Los Angeles, California 90024, USA

Received 21 June 1975

1. Introduction

Important theoretical considerations and experimental findings have led to suggestions that formation of a potential and/or pH gradients across a membrane may serve for transmission of energy from oxidations to the phosphorylating system in oxidative and photophosphorylation, see [1–6]. Resistance to acceptance of this concept has arisen in part from the lack of satisfactory suggestions or evidence as to how energy stored in a membrane potential or proton gradient could be used to drive ATP synthesis. Mitchell has suggested a "chemiosmotic" mechanism involving translocation across the membrane of an 'O_2^{2-}' group derived from P_i at the ATPase catalytic site, driven by specific protonation of phosphate oxygens [7]. I have recently called attention to deficiencies in such proposed chemiosmotic coupling ([8] and footnote*).

Other developments, however, point to an attractive means by which a membrane potential or proton gradient might be coupled to ATP synthesis. Experimental findings have led to the suggestion that ATP synthesis results from energy-linked conformational changes that change the binding of reactants at the catalytic site [10,11]. One prominent use of energy in oxidative phosphorylation has been identified as decreasing the binding of ATP to the catalytic site. More recent findings in my laboratory indicate that

---

* Publication of my criticisms [8] was accompanied by a rebuttal by Mitchell [9] that fails to meet the basic objections. Brief clarifications of his four 'answers' to my criticisms are as follows:

1) The assertion that because F_1 has an alkaline pH optimum, the activity of 'OH⁻ on F_0 side of the active center of F_1 would be very high' is quite illogical. The pH optimum for an enzyme does not govern H⁺ or OH⁻ activity at the catalytic site.

2) and 3) Mitchell states that his 'scheme does not assume the formation of the trinegative species $O=PO_3^{3-}$, as Boyer imagines.' But the appearance of such a species in fig. 1, stage III, of his paper is obviously not a product of my imagination. The contention that I overlooked his suggestion that Mg^{2+} may be close to the bound P_i in turn overlooked my statement, 'Modifications of the nature of the charged species participating in the steps of Mitchell's scheme, as suggested in his concluding remarks, do not obviate the chemical difficulties.' Thus binding to Mg^{2+} could aid formation of a trinegative species, but the highly positive Mg^{2+} would obviously hinder his suggested subsequent proton additions.

4) Mitchell in his paper stressed the formation of -OH⁺₂ group on the phosphorus as a good leaving group. His apparent willingness to abandon this idea in his 4th comment is sound, but his alternate suggestion does not provide a satisfactory manner for driving phosphorylation by protonation.

It must be emphasized that my criticisms of Mitchell's suggestions for how a membrane potential and/or a proton gradient might be used for ATP synthesis are not directed towards his outstanding contributions demonstrating formation of potential and of H⁺ gradients across the mitochondrial inner membrane and his splendid support of the concept that such potential and H⁺ gradients can be used reversibly for ATP formation and for active transport.

(Subsequent to submission of this paper, a recent contribution of R. J. P. Williams, FEBS Lett., 53, 123–125, came to the author's attention. In his paper Professor Williams calls attention to deficiencies in the 'chemiosmotic molecular mechanism' for ATP synthesis suggested by Mitchell.)

energy input also serves to increase affinity for P_i and/or ADP, with the interconversion of bound ADP and P_i to ATP as the step least sensitive to uncouplers [12].

The principal purpose of this paper is to point out how energy-linked conformational changes provide an attractive means for transducing energy of a membrane potential or a proton gradient to the high-energy phosphate of ATP. The suggestions are also applicable to some ATP-linked active transport processes.

The model, although deceptively simple, does not appear to have been presented previously, and readily explains a fixed stoichiometry of proton translocation coupled to ATP formation as well as a summation of membrane potential and proton gradient to drive ATP formation.

2. Charged group migration as a key event in conformational coupling

There is impressive evidence that a negative potential and higher pH in the mitochondrial matrix space [2,3] in the chloroplast intermembrane space [4] or inside bacterial cells [5] can promote ATP formation or be induced by ATP cleavage. A membrane potential can favor movement of a charged group from contact with solvent water on one side of the membrane to the other side**. For example, with mitochondria a positively charged group might be induced to move into the matrix space or a negatively charged group might be induced to depart from the matrix space. A net proton movement may result from return of the uncharged forms. The protonation of the participating groups gives a means by which proton gradients across the membrane can assist in the migration. If the group migration were reversibly linked through protein conformational changes to the events leading to formation or utilization of ATP at the catalytic site, energy-linked coupling of the potential to ATP synthesis or of ATP cleavage to proton translocation and potential generation would result.

The diagram in fig.1 extends and helps illustrate

** In this paper movement of a charged group is indicated, but it should be recognized that a change in position of membrane groups shielding the charged group from solvent would be equally plausible.

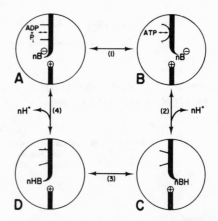

Fig.1. Diagrammatic sketch of conformational coupling of phosphorylation to membrane potential or proton gradient. $-B^{\ominus}$ represents a proton accepting group, a number, n, of which change exposure from the one side to the other of a membrane coupled to conformation and catalytic changes at the phosphorylation site that drive ATP synthesis from ADP and P_i. A positive charge $\oplus$ is depicted at a membrane pore that prevents $H_3O^{\oplus}$ diffusion but allows changes in exposure of $B^{\ominus}$ and free diffusion of H_2O.

Changes in binding and catalytic properties of the phosphorylation site are depicted by transitions from ꓒ,), ⟩ and ⟨ in stages A, B, C and D respectively. The conversion A → B → C → D through steps 1 to 4 respectively serves to drive ATP synthesis coupled to translocation of n protons across the membrane. Operation of the cycle in the opposite direction (D → C → B → A) would couple translocation of n protons across the membrane coupled to ATP cleavage.

the above possibilities. Two functional sites are indicated in the figure, the phosphorylation site for ATP cleavage and synthesis and a site undergoing reversible protonation involved in proton translocation. Four intermediate states, A, B, C, and D, are illustrated, but additional intermediary states must also intervene. For example, events of ATP, ADP and P_i binding and release as well as interconversion are not shown. For ATP synthesis coupled to proton translocation the transitions would occur through steps 1,2,3 and 4. This would be favored by a negative potential and/or higher pH in the left space (the matrix space in the mitochondria). Operation in the reverse direction would couple ATP cleavage to proton transport. This would be favored by a smaller negative or a positive potential and/or a lower pH in the left space.

For reasons indicated below, a negatively charged group, B⁻, is considered to be a likely migratory group. A protein carboxyl group could quite conceivably be involved. For ATP synthesis, the key transition is from state A to state B. For example, in mitochondria, the negative potential in the matrix space is visualized as favoring the movement of the B⁻ group to the opposite side of the membrane. This movement may be conformationally linked to ADP and P_i binding and ATP formation and release. With mitochondria, a low H⁺ activity inside the matrix as compared to the exterior would promote ATP synthesis by making more of the B⁻ form available on the interior.

For proton translocation coupled to ATP cleavage, the binding of ATP in state B is regarded as inducing conformational change favoring movement of the B⁻ group from the right to the left side of the membrane (fig. 1) thus increasing the negative potential on the left side. The change from state B to state A includes cleavage of ATP to ADP and P_i and release of products. The B⁻ group on the left side will be protonated, to the extent determined by the pH, to give state D. The protonated, uncharged group can readily migrate back from left to right through the membrane with formation of state C. The dissociation of the BH group to convert state C to state B results in net proton translocation across the membrane.

The interconversions between each of the 4 states is regarded as resulting in small but vital conformational changes at the phosphorylation catalytic site. These are crudely depicted in the figure by small changes in the shape of the site. The events linked to the conformational changes include changes in affinities of reactants at the catalytic site and modifications in catalytic capacity of the phosphorylation site. The phosphorylation site, for example, must allow ATP cleavage coupled to movement of the H-binding group only when the group is negatively charged and not when it is protonated. Recognition by the ATP site of whether or not the transducing group is protonated provides a simple means of providing the vectorial component necessary for any energy-linked transport.

3. Possible energy-linked movement of a positively charged group

A similar series of events may be considered for movement of a positively charged group, but with some distinct differences. Other means would need to be provided to prevent H_3O^+ migration through the incipient channel. In state A the conformations for mitochondria would be such that the positively charged group is exposed to the opposite side of the phosphorylation site. The membrane potential, negative in the matrix space of mitochondria, would thus favor the movement of the -BH⁺ group to the interior, coupled to the conformational transitions leading to ATP synthesis. Conversely, with ATP cleavage a transition from state B to state A would, by withdrawing a positive charge, add to the negative potential inside the matrix. Dissociation of the proton in the intermembrane space would give the uncharged group that could migrate back to the interior. Protonation of this group, and its expulsion coupled to ATP cleavage would complete a cycle of proton translocation coupled to ATP cleavage.

4. The stoichiometry of the conformational coupling

In fig. 1 an indeterminate number, n, of charged groups is depicted as being coupled to the cleavage of one ATP molecule. Data of Mitchell and Moyle suggest that at least two protons can be translocated for every ATP cleaved [13] and other results have suggested higher equivalents of H⁺ or K⁺ to ATP [14–16]. Higher H⁺/ATP ratios can readily be accommodated by the model, indeed this is one of the attractive features. A protein subunit in a membrane might have several charged groups aligned in the plane of the membrane such that a small movement of the entire subunit would change the exposure from the inner to outer aqueous phase.

An important stoichiometric feature is that the model requires the movement of a fixed number, n, of protons to be transported for each ATP molecule synthesized or used. If the B⁻ group can move only when coupled to ATP synthesis or cleavage, a weak membrane potential and/or proton gradient would diminish the extent or rate of the coupled processes but the stoichiometry would remain the same.

5. A distinction from models based on conformationally-induced changes in p*K*

Electron transport coupled to proton uptake and

release by mitochondrial and chloroplast membranes may involve a change in the pK of membrane groups, or a 'membrane Bohr effect' [17]. Such changes in pK have been discussed as a means of linking proton transport to oxidations and phosphorylations.

The simple suggestion of conformational coupling to proton transport through changes in pK does not readily explain such features as a fixed stoichiometry of proton transfer to ATP formation, a net proton movement in repeated cycles, or the use of membrane potential as a driving force for ATP synthesis. Suitable explanation might be provided by amplification of the suggestion to include features of the model depicted in fig.1. But then the coupled charged group migration and not the change in pK would be vital. It is of course plausible that the B$^-$ group depicted in fig.1 might have a different pK when exposed to opposite sides of the membrane, but such a change in pK is not an essential part of the coupling mechanism.

6. Membrane potential or proton gradient as the primary driving force

The suggested coupling mechanism could under some circumstances involve only membrane potential as the primary driving force. Such potential might be generated by K$^+$ ion migration in presence of valinomycin under suitable conditions as well as by proton translocation. Oxidatively induced proton translocation with buffered media of equal pH on both sides of the membrane would still establish a membrane potential. However, as noted in the above discussion, a pH gradient could promote a distribution of the migrating group so as to favor ATP synthesis. An H$^+$ gradient may play a more important role in chloroplasts than in mitochondria [18]. The protein and charge arrangement may be such that the group B$^-$ once formed by deprotonation tends to move to the opposite side. Proton removal from the BH form would thus provide an important means to drive the cycle. The scheme is thus adaptable to the possibility of ATP synthesis driven by proton gradients even in the absence of a membrane potential.

Because either a membrane potential or a proton gradient or both could drive ATP synthesis, the scheme is quite compatible with Mitchell's valuable suggestion of the addition of potential and proton gradients (the 'protomotive' force) to give the total energy available

for ATP synthesis. But my proposal is not compatible with Mitchell's chemiosmotic coupling mechanism for use of membrane potential and proton gradients for ATP synthesis [7,19], where a migrating proton is regarded as having increased activity usable in some manner for covalent bond synthesis. In a scheme such as presented here protons behave in a normal manner in an equilibrium protonation of basic groups depending on the pH of the surrounding medium.

7. Some molecular characteristics of the transduction

The requisite small magnitude of the conformational changes deserves emphasis. Small movements, even if against a considerable energy barrier, allow efficient energy transduction. If large movements occur, the accompanying molecular reorganization could dissipate energy. Merely for clarity, fig.1 depicts changes that might be taken to imply movements of a group for a considerable distance and major conformational changes. Changes in affinities of reactants at a catalytic site can readily occur with only subtle changes in the Ångström range. The electrogenic migrations of the charged group could transmit the requisite change principally through positional shift of a membrane protein subunit without any major conformational transition. No 'flip-flops' or protein rotations need be involved. The only transition required for the charged group is a relocation so as to have access to solvent water and protons on either side of the membrane. As noted below, water molecules might freely cross the membrane at the transducing site, although this is not vital to the model.

An important requirement might be that the migrating charged group does not move through a space of low dielectric constant such as a hydrophobic portion of the membrane. There is a considerable energy barrier for the desolvation and isolation of the charged group that would be required. It appears more attractive for water to have free access across the transducing site, but with some means of blocking the migration of cations, including protons, through the site. This could readily be achieved by appropriate location of a positive charge or charges. Such a charge is included in the scheme of fig.1. This illustrates one way of meeting the important requirement of maintenance of the negative membrane potential but with water environment for the migrating group.

The likelihood of a positive charge at the transducing pore favors a negatively charged group as the migrating group for the energy transductions. Indeed, the migrating group might have a transitory ionic attraction to the positively charged group during the transition from one state to another but there would be little energy barrier for the key group migration. Other solvent anions could likewise have sufficient access to the positive membrane group to avoid charge isolation. The aqueous pore at the transducing site might well serve as a port of entry and exit for some permeant anions.

8. The coupling to active transport

A series of experiments stimulated by the concepts of Mitchell have given convincing demonstration that potential gradients can be coupled to transport of solutes. The experiments of West and Mitchell [20] demonstrating coupling of lactose transport in *E. coli* to a membrane potential are an excellent example. Obvious extensions of the model depicted in fig.1 could apply to active transport of various metabolites. For example, the charged group translocation could be linked to conformational changes that decrease the apparent affinity of the transported ligand for its binding site at the inner membrane surface.

Only small changes in membrane structure and associated conformational changes need accompany change in access of a bound ligand from the outer to inner aqueous phase. Change in binding of the ligand at the inner membrane phase could result from a higher K_d for binding, see [21], but the possibility of coupling by energy-linked blocking of access to the site once the ligand has dissociated [22] also merits consideration.

Coupling of energy to transport of Ca^{2+}, K^+ and other ions can similarly be readily accommodated by the present model. For bacterial transport systems, where the transport system and the oxidative or ATP energy sources are located in the same membrane, an electrogenic mechanism may operate. Either oxidation or ATP cleavage could create the requisite membrane potential. This could be used to change affinities of ions at different sites of the membrane, similar to changes in affinity for substrates as depicted for ATP synthesis in fig.1. Again, stoichiometry of more than

one ion transported per unit charge dissipated can readily be accommodated. Such a mechanism has additional appeal. It would mean that Nature is using a molecular machine of similar design for both ATP synthesis and active transport.

The specialized transport ATPases such as the microsomal Na^+, K^+-ATPase and the Ca^{2+}, Mg^{2+}-ATPase of the sarcoplasmic reticulum probably function through direct conformational coupling within the membrane ATPase rather than indirectly through membrane potential. For this, the conformational changes accompanying ATP binding and cleavage could be transmitted directly to the affinity sites for ions. A very small change in position of liganding groups could change binding preference from Na^+ to K^+, or from Ca^{2+} to Mg^{2+}. Such changes, accompanied by the minimal transitions necessary for exposure to the aqueous phase on either side of the membrane, would complete the transport process.

The above suggestions for coupling by transport ATPases are in contrast to the suggestions of Mitchell [23] that complexes of ATP and its hydrolysis products bind to the transported ions, and that the water oxygen for ATP cleavage comes from the opposite side of the membrane from the ATP. My suggestions are consistent with and in part derived from other current concepts of membrane structure and transport mechanisms (see Singer, [24]).

9. Coupling of oxidation to ATP synthesis

Brief comment may be appropriate on relationships of conformational coupling as presented here to synthesis of ATP coupled to electron transport by mitochondria and chloroplasts. As mentioned previously, involvement of electrical potential or proton gradients in transmission of energy from oxidations to the phosphorylation complex is regarded as an attractive possibility. But in one sense both proton translocation and protein conformational change could operate in the energy transmissions of oxidative phosphorylation and photophosphorylation. Energy-requiring conformational changes initiated at the sites of electron transfer could be transmitted through protein structures to sites for proton translocation, then transmission to the phosphorylation complexes completed by the potential or proton gradients produced.

Also attractive at this stage is the possibility of direct conformational transfer of energy from electron transport to ATP synthesis in oxidative phosphorylation and photophosphorylation [25]. Indeed, direct conformational interactions appear probable in the ATP-requiring electron transfer reactions occurring in nitrogenase [26].

10. Concluding statement

Acceptance of a membrane potential and/or a proton gradient as a possible means of transmitting energy from oxidations to ATP synthesis rests in part on a satisfactory hypothesis for how the potential or proton gradient could drive ATP synthesis. Recognition that energy input may drive ATP synthesis by change in binding of reactants at the catalytic site has led to the suggestions presented in this paper. These are that in oxidative phosphorylation and photophosphorylation, the requisite conformational changes may be coupled to exposure of charged groups to different sides of the membrane. The cycle of charged group exposure or movement may be driven by the membrane potential or, through protonation and deprotonation, may be coupled to proton translocation across the membrane. Effects of proton gradient and membrane potential may be additive. Similar conformational coupling suggestions may explain proton translocation coupled to ATP cleavage and active transport of metabolites coupled to membrane potential, proton gradients of ATP cleavage.

Acknowledgments

I am indebted to present members of my research group and to other colleagues for helpful discussion of points raised in this letter. Researches in my laboratory pertinent to the views presented have been supported by the Institute of General Medical Sciences, U.S. Public Health Service (GM 11904), the U.S. Atomic Energy Commission (Contract AT-(04-3)), and the National Science Foundation (Grant BMS 75-03019).

References

[1] Robertson, R. N. (1967) Endeavour 26, 134–139.
[2] Skulachev, V. P. (1971) in: Current Topics in Bioenergetics 4, p. 127–190. Academic Press Inc., New York.
[3] Mitchell, P. (1972) Bioenergetics 3, 5–24.
[4] Schuldiner, S., Rottenberg, H. and Avron, M. (1972) FEBS Lett. 28, 173–176.
[5] Racker, E. and Stoeckenius, W. (1974) J. Biol. Chem 249 (2). 662–663.
[6] Witt, H. T. and Zickler, A. (1974) FEBS Lett. 39, 205–208.
[7] Mitchell, P. (1974) FEBS Lett. 43, 189–194.
[8] Boyer, P. D. (1975) FEBS Lett. 50, 91–94.
[9] Mitchell, P. (1975) FEBS Lett. 50, 95–97.
[10] Boyer, P. D., Cross, R. L. and Momsen, W. (1973) Proc. Nat. Acad. Sci. U.S. 70, 2837–2839.
[11] Cross, R. L. and Boyer, P. D. (1975) Biochemistry 14, 392–398.
[12] Rosing, J., Kayalar, C. and Boyer, P. D. 'Structural Basis of Membrane Function' in: Proceedings IUB-IUPAB Symposium (Hatefi, Y., ed.) Tehran, Iran, in press.
[13] Mitchell, P. and Moyle, J. (1968) Eur. J. Biochem. 4, 530–539.
[14] Azzone, C. F. and Massari, S. (1971) Eur. J. Biochem. 19, 97–107.
[15] Junge, H., Rumberg, B. and Schröder, H. (1970) Eur. J. Biochem. 14, 575–581.
[16] Cockrell, R. S., Harris, E. J. and Pressman, B. (1966) Biochemistry 5, 2326–2335.
[17] Chance, B. (1972) FEBS Lett. 23, 3–20.
[18] Pick, U., Rottenberg, H. and Avron, M. (1974) FEBS Lett. 48, 32–36.
[19] Mitchell, P. and Moyle, J. (1974) Biochem. Soc. Spec. Publ. 4, 91–111.
[20] West, I. C. and Mitchell, P. (1974) FEBS Lett. 40, 1–4.
[21] Boos, W. (1974) Ann. Rev. Biochem. 43, 123–147.
[22] Boyer, P. D. and Klein, W. L. (1972) in: Membrane Molecular Biology (Fox, C. F. and Keith, A. D., eds.) Sinauer Assoc., Stamford, Conn., p. 323–345.
[23] Mitchell, P. (1973) FEBS Lett. 33, 267–274.
[24] Singer, S. J. (1974) Ann. Rev. Biochem. 43, 805–833.
[25] Boyer, P. D. (1974) Biochim. Biophys. Acta Library 13, 289–301.
[26] Smith, B. E., Lowe, D. J. and Bray, R. C. (1973) Biochem. J. 135, 331–334.

Copyright © 1977 by The American Society of Biological Chemists, Inc.

Reprinted from *J. Biol. Chem.* **252**:2478–2485 (1977)

Evidence for Energy-dependent Change in Phosphate Binding for Mitochondrial Oxidative Phosphorylation Based on Measurements of Medium and Intermediate Phosphate-Water Exchanges*

(Received for publication, May 3, 1976, and in revised form, December 14, 1976)

Jan Rosing,‡ Celik Kayalar,§ and Paul D. Boyer

From the Department of Chemistry and Molecular Biology Institute, University of California, Los Angeles, California 90024

Characteristics of the exchange reactions catalyzed by beef heart submitochondrial particles give new insight into energy transducing steps of oxidative phosphorylation. The uncoupler-insensitive portion of the total $P_i \rightleftharpoons HOH$ exchange in presence of ATP, ADP, and P_i is the intermediate $P_i \rightleftharpoons HOH$ exchange, that is the exchange occurring with P_i formed by hydrolysis of ATP prior to release of P_i from the catalytic site. The exchange of medium P_i with HOH is as sensitive to uncouplers as the $P_i \rightleftharpoons ATP$ exchange and net oxidative phosphorylation, demonstrating a requirement of an uncoupler-sensitive energized state, probably a transmembrane potential or proton gradient, for bringing medium P_i to the reactive state. The covalent bond forming and breaking step at the catalytic site ($ADP + P_i \rightleftharpoons ATP + HOH$) appears relatively insensitive to uncouplers. Thus to the extent that uncouplers dissipate transmembrane protonmotive force, it is unlikely that such a force is used to drive ATP formation by direct protonations of P_i oxygens.

When only P_i and ADP are added and formation of ATP from added ADP by adenylate kinase and subsequent ATP hydrolysis are adequately blocked, no $P_i \rightleftharpoons HOH$ exchange can be observed, demonstrating a requirement of energization by ATP binding and cleavage for such an exchange. This uncoupler-insensitive energization is suggested to represent a conformationally energized state that can be used reversibly to develop a transmembrane protonmotive force accompanying ADP and P_i release.

Rates of various exchanges as estimated by improved procedures are compatible with all oxygen exchanges occurring by dynamic reversal of ATP hydrolysis at the catalytic site.

For the understanding of the present status of oxidative phosphorylation, it is instructive to consider the three components of the overall process, namely how energy is captured in

* This work was supported in part by Grant GM 11094 of the Institute of General Medical Science, United States Public Health Service, and Contract AT(04-3)-34 of the Energy Research and Development Administration.

‡ Recipient of a NATO Fellowship awarded by the Netherlands Organization for Advancement of Pure Research (Z. W. O.).

§ Recipient of a Science Fellowship awarded by the Scientific and Technical Research Council of Turkey.

the oxidation enzyme complexes, how energy is transmitted from oxidation complexes to phosphorylation complexes, and how energy is used in phosphorylation complexes to drive ATP synthesis (1, 2). A decade ago the suggestion was made that all three steps or stages might depend upon energy-linked changes in protein conformation (3). Subsequently stimulated principally by the experimental work and suggestions of P. Mitchell, considerable evidence has accumulated consistent with or favoring the transmission of energy by a transmembrane electrochemical potential or pH gradient (4). Convincing evidence for energy transmission by an interlocking protein network has not developed. But irrespective of how energy is transmitted, the formidable problem remains of how energy is used to cause phosphorylation of ADP by P_i.

Experimental observations in Slater's laboratory on the presence of ATPase-bound nucleotides (5, 6) and in Boyer's laboratory on the uncoupler sensitivity of exchange reactions (7) have led to the suggestion that ATP synthesis may involve conformationally induced changes in ATP affinity. Attention has been focused recently on this possibility (8) and on a contrasting suggestion, developed earlier by P. Mitchell as part of his chemiosmotic hypothesis, that ATP synthesis occurs by effective removal of an "O^{2-}" group from P_i accomplished by protonations at the catalytic site of the coupling factor ATPase, F_1 (9). The principal purpose of this paper is to present additional measurements of exchange reactions that expand and clarify the concept of energy-linked conformational changes in substrate binding sites as key components of the phosphorylation reaction sequence, and that point to an energized membrane state that can exist in presence of relatively high concentrations of uncouplers.

The present experiments were prompted in part by the observation that the ADP-dependent $P_i \rightleftharpoons HOH$ exchange catalyzed by submitochondrial particles was inhibited by additions of hexokinase and glucose. This result suggested that energy may also affect one or more of the steps leading to the formation of ATP at the catalytic site (10). A prominent portion of the clarifications and extensions presented in the present paper depend upon the separation of the overall $P_i \rightleftharpoons HOH$ exchange into two components, the "medium" exchange and the "intermediate" exchange.[1] In addition to reporting meas-

[1] Both intermediate and medium exchanges of P_i have been ob-

urements of these oxygen exchanges, the present paper also includes improved procedures for estimation of various exchanges and their uncoupler sensitivity. Such procedures may be of value because of the growing evidence that the relative uncoupler sensitivity of the exchange reactions can give basic information about how energy is used in ATP formation.

EXPERIMENTAL PROCEDURES

Materials – Water of approximately 9.49 or 26.11 atom % excess ^{18}O was purchased from Yeda Research and Development Co., Rehovoth, Israel. $KH_2P^{18}O_4$ with about 33 atom % excess ^{18}O was prepared as described by Cohn and Drysdale (13). $^{32}P_i$ was obtained from ICN Pharmaceuticals, Inc. 2,4-Dinitrophenol was purified by recrystallization from chloroform. S-13[2] was the gift of Monsanto Chemical Co. Hexokinase, pyruvate kinase, and lactate dehydrogenase were purchased from Boehringer Mannheim Co. and dialyzed before use. Activated charcoal (Matheson, Coleman and Bell) was treated as follows. Ten grams of charcoal was suspended in 1 liter of 1 N HCl and stirred for 30 min. The charcoal was filtered off by suction and washed with 1 M KCl until the filtrate was neutral. The acid-treated charcoal was suspended in 100 ml of a solution containing 0.3 M perchloric acid, 50 mM sodium pyrophosphate, 100 mM phosphoric acid, and 2 mM AMP and was stirred for 15 min. The charcoal was filtered off by suction, suspended in 1 liter of H_2O, and suspended in 200 ml of 95% ethanol:1 M NH_4OH (40:60 v/v). The suspension was stirred for 15 min at 30° and filtered again. The charcoal was suspended in 100 ml of H_2O and used for isolation of adenine nucleotides from perchlorate extracts.

Mitochondrial Preparations – Rat liver mitochondria were prepared by the method of Johnson and Lardy (14). Heavy beef heart mitochondria were prepared by a modification of the method of Smith (15) and used for preparation of submitochondrial particles (ETPH/Mg^{2+}/Mn^{2+}) essentially as described by Beyer (16). Protein was estimated by the method of Lowry *et al.* (17) with bovine serum albumin as a standard.

Preparation of [β-^{32}P]ADP – Rat liver mitochondria (3 mg of protein) were incubated at room temperature for 30 min in a 2-ml reaction mixture containing 75 mM sucrose, 50 mM Tris/Cl, 20 mM KCl, 2.5 mM EDTA, 0.5 mM $^{32}P_i$ (~10⁷ cpm/nmol), 5 mM $MgCl_2$, 5 mM succinate, 0.3 mM AMP, and 50 μM ATP at pH 7.5. Under these conditions, AMP is phosphorylated to a mixture of [β-^{32}P]ADP and [β,γ-^{32}P]ATP because of the combined adenylate kinase and phosphorylation activities present in the mitochondria. The mitochondria were removed by centrifugation and the [β,γ-^{32}P]ATP was converted to [β-^{32}P]ADP with hexokinase and glucose. The reaction was stopped with 1 ml of 1 M perchloric acid and the adenine nucleotides were adsorbed to 40 mg of acid-treated charcoal. The charcoal was filtered off by suction and washed with 2.5 ml of a solution containing 25 mM sodium pyrophosphate, 0.1 M H_3PO_4, and 0.3 M perchloric acid and rinsed with 10 ml of H_2O. The nucleotides were eluted from the charcoal with 6 ml of ethanol: 1 M ammonia (40:60 v/v) and applied to a column (0.5 × 3 cm) of anion exchange resin (Bio-Rad, AG 1-X4, 200 to 400 mesh) in order to separate the [β^{32}P]ADP from traces of $^{32}P_i$ and [β,γ-^{32}P]ATP. The P_i was eluted with 5 ml of 0.2 M Tris/Cl at pH 7.5, and the ADP with 3 ml of 60 mM HCl. ATP can be eluted from this type of column with 1 M HCl.

Measurement of ATPase Activity and Isotope Incorporation – Experiments were conducted under conditions given in the legends to the tables and figures. After stopping the reactions with 1 M perchloric acid the protein was removed by centrifugation. Measurement of P_i was performed by the method of Sumner (18). ATP was determined with hexokinase and glucose-6-phosphate dehydrogenase, and ADP with pyruvate kinase and lactate dehydrogenase essentially as described by Bergmeyer (19).

The ATPase activity was calculated either from the change in P_i concentration or the change in adenine nucleotide concentrations dependent on the accuracy of the determinations. ATP hydrolysis was determined by measurement of $^{32}P_i$ formation in the experiments described in Fig. 2 and Table I.

For determination of the amount of $P_i \rightleftharpoons$ ATP exchange concen-

trated HCl and 50 mM aqueous ammonium molybdate were added to final concentrations of 1 M and 12 mM, respectively, and the phosphomolybdate complex was removed by repeated extraction with cold isobutyl alcohol:benzene (1:1 v/v). An 0.5-ml aliquot of the lower layer was counted in 10 ml of water using Cerenkov light (20).

P_i was isolated from the perchlorate extract and analyzed for its ^{18}O content as described elsewhere (21) to determine the $P_i \rightleftharpoons$ HOH exchange. Calculations of ^{18}O content were based on recoveries of ^{18}O from standard [^{18}O]P_i added to reaction mixtures.

For measurement of the ^{18}O present in ATP, the adenine nucleotides present in the perchlorate extract were adsorbed to acid washed charcoal (14 mg of charcoal/μmol of adenine nucleotide). The charcoal was filtered off by suction and washed with 5 ml of a solution containing 0.3 N perchloric acid, 25 mM sodium pyrophosphate, and 0.1 M H_3PO_4. The charcoal was rinsed with 20 ml of H_2O, suspended in 2 ml of 2 M HCl, and boiled for 30 min to release the β- and γ-phosphoryl groups of ADP and ATP. Phosphate was isolated from the filtrate and analyzed for its ^{18}O content.

For measurement of conversion of [^3H]ADP or [β-^{32}P]ADP into ATP, the adenine nucleotides present in the perchlorate extracts were adsorbed to charcoal and the incorporation of radioactive label from ADP into ATP was measured after separation of the nucleotides as described for the preparation of [β-^{32}P]ADP. Radioactivity was measured in a scintillation liquid containing 3 g of 2,5-diphenyloxazole and 0.2 g of 1,4-bis[2-(5-phenyloxazolyl)]benzene per liter of xylene:Triton X-114 (3:1 v/v).

Estimation of Exchange Rates – For calculation of the $P_i \rightleftharpoons$ ATP exchange, the total counts of ^{32}P found in the ATP + ADP fractions were divided by the counts per nmol of P_i present to give the nanomoles of exchange (^{32}P appears in both ADP and ATP because of adenylate kinase action).

The rate of ATP $\rightleftharpoons$ ADP exchange was calculated from the rate of incorporation of ^{32}P and ^3H from, respectively, [β-^{32}P]ADP and [^3H]ADP into ATP. The rate of ^{32}P incorporation into ATP represents the rate of ATP $\rightleftharpoons$ ADP exchange plus twice the rate of the adenylate kinase reaction. The rate of ^3H incorporation into ATP is the sum of the adenylate kinase rate and ATP $\rightleftharpoons$ ADP exchange rate. From this it follows that the rate of ATP $\rightleftharpoons$ ADP exchange = (2 × rate of ^3H exchange) − (rate of ^{32}P exchange).

Estimations were made of total, intermediate and medium oxygen exchanges, as defined and explained under "Results," by measurements of the incorporation of water oxygens from $H^{18}OH$ into P_i and of loss of ^{18}O from [^{18}O]P_i to water. Such separation of oxygen exchanges of oxidative phosphorylation has not been made in previous studies.

A number of factors need to be considered for calculation of exchanges of oxidative phosphorylation from primary data. Estimations might be made under conditions where net ATP hydrolysis occurs, as in the present paper, or under conditions where net ATP synthesis may result. For estimation of the intermediate and medium oxygen exchange of P_i, as measured by gain of ^{18}O from $H^{18}OH$ into P_i, reactions that change the ^{18}O content of P_i, in addition to intermediate and medium exchange, are as follows: (*a*) Gain of ^{18}O from the total hydrolytic cleavage of ATP, equal to the sum of the P_i formed by any net hydrolysis and the $P_i \rightleftharpoons$ ATP exchange. This gives incorporation of 1 oxygen from $H^{18}OH$ into each P_i formed. (*b*) Gain of ^{18}O from that which is incorporated into ATP by $P_i \rightleftharpoons$ HOH exchange, then appears in P_i through ATP cleavage. (*c*) Gain of ^{18}O from that which is incorporated into ATP through the $P_i \rightleftharpoons$ ATP exchange, then reappears in P_i through ATP cleavage. (*d*) Loss of ^{18}O from that which appears in medium P_i, but is then transferred to ATP and to HOH by the total amount of ATP formation, equal to the sum of the $P_i \rightleftharpoons$ ATP exchange and of any ATP formed by net synthesis. This causes 1 P_i oxygen to appear in water and 3 in ATP. For the present data, corrections were made for Items *a* and *d* only as estimations of *b* and *c* indicated that they were negligible.

For estimation of the medium exchange from measurement of loss of ^{18}O from P_i, those reactions that can change the ^{18}O content of P_i, in addition to medium exchange, are as follows: (*a*) Loss of ^{18}O by disappearance of medium P_i through the $P_i \rightleftharpoons$ ATP exchange and any net ATP synthesis. Corrections for this can be appreciable; each molecule of P_i forming ATP removes 4 atoms of P_i-bound oxygen; more than one goes to water and the balance to ATP. (*b*) Gain of ^{18}O by transfer to ATP and reappearance in P_i through ATP cleavage. For the present data correction for Item *b* was estimated to be negligible.

Estimation of the total incorporation of water oxygens into P_i when $H^{18}OH$ was present was made as follows. The fraction of

---

served to accompany hydrolysis of ATP by myosin (11, 12), and the definitions of such exchanges adopted here follows that as given for myosin hydrolysis of ATP.

[2] The abbreviation used is: S-13, 5-chloro-3-*t*-butyl-2'-chloro-4'-nitrosalicylanilide.

isotopic equilibrium, F, was calculated by dividing the observed atom per cent excess ^{18}O in the isolated P_i by that in the water; the total nanoatoms of oxygen in P_i that had been replaced by water oxygens was calculated by correcting for the approach to isotopic equilibrium (21) and multiplying by the total nanoatoms of phosphate oxygen present, that is $4 \times$ nanomoles of $P_i \times \ln(1 - F)^{-1}$; subtraction of the nanomoles of ATP hydrolyzed gives the total atoms of water oxygen incorporated by exchange.

For calculation of the total oxygens incorporated from $H^{18}OH$ into ATP, the observed atom per cent excess in the P_i formed by acid hydrolysis of the ATP + ADP fraction was multiplied by $(^4/_3)$ $(2 \times$ nanomoles of ATP + nanomoles of ADP)/nanomoles of ATP to give the expected atom per cent excess in the γ-phosphoryl group of ATP, assuming that all ^{18}O in the P_i formed from ADP + ATP fraction comes from this group. The total nanoatoms of exchange is estimated by correction for approach to isotopic equilibrium as given above for the $P_i \rightleftharpoons HOH$ exchange. This probably gives a slight overcorrection because not all the ^{18}O will be present in the γ-phosphoryl group of ATP.

Calculation of exchanges by the above procedures can be regarded as estimations only because several complicating factors introduce uncertainty. This does not modify the conclusions made in this paper, as these are based on very large differences in relative effects on various exchanges. Nonetheless, it was felt preferable to make appropriate correction and to outline procedures here as they may be useful in future studies.

One factor that may introduce appreciable error is the lack of correction for approach to isotopic equilibrium of P_i bound at the catalytic site. For example, although medium P_i may contain little ^{18}O, each bound P_i might contain appreciably more than 1 oxygen from water, so that additional exchange with $H^{18}OH$ may not always increase the ^{18}O content of P_i. For example, if all 4 oxygens of bound P_i participate equally in exchange and if we assume that each P_i that leaves the site contains 2 oxygens from water, the fraction of isotopic equilibrium of bound P_i would equal 0.5 and $1/\ln(1 - F)$ would equal about 1.4. Calculated oxygen exchange rates would then need to be multiplied by 1.4. Such corrections were not attempted for these studies, but may be appropriate in later studies if necessary data become available.

Other uncertainty is introduced by changes in reactant concentrations that may occur during the assay period. In the present studies in absence of uncouplers such corrections are relatively small. But if considerable net ATP hydrolysis occurs, attempted corrections can be somewhat complicated. Specific activities of the labeled P_i and ADP will decrease with time of incubation. Thus a better estimation is made if the specific activities are taken as (original specific activity + final specific activity)/2; such a correction was made in the present experiments. Similarly, for estimation of total amount of exchanges, the average concentration of reactants present was used. A further correction could be made for both the $P_i \rightleftharpoons ATP$ and ATP $\rightleftharpoons$ $H^{18}OH$ exchanges by estimation of the loss of ^{18}O and ^{32}P previously incorporated into ATP by hydrolysis of the ATP. Such loss would cause some underestimation of the $P_i \rightleftharpoons ATP$ and ATP $\rightleftharpoons H^{18}OH$ exchanges and some overestimation of the $P_i \rightleftharpoons HOH$ exchange. Such corrections were not made for the data presented in this paper; calculations were based on the final ATP and ADP concentrations. If corrections are made, exchange values in presence of uncoupler where ATP cleavage was appreciable would be somewhat higher, but as noted earlier, this would not modify conclusions from the data.

When both medium and intermediate exchanges were measured, a second identical incubation was performed with ^{18}O in the P_i instead of the HOH. The fraction of total phosphate oxygens that had exchanged was estimated from the fraction of isotope exchange as given above. The fraction of total phosphate oxygens that had exchanged times the average nanomoles of P_i present gave the total nanomoles of oxygen lost from P_i. This was corrected for oxygen loss by $P_i \rightleftharpoons ATP$ exchange as mentioned above, to give the nanoatoms of oxygen lost by medium exchange.

The amount of total $P_i \rightleftharpoons HOH$ exchange (from $H^{18}OH$ experiments) minus the amount of medium exchange (from $[^{18}O]P_i$ experiments) gives the amount of intermediate exchange. This value divided by the total amount of ATP hydrolytic cleavage (net cleavage + $P_i \rightleftharpoons ATP$ exchange) gives the value for water oxygens incorporated by intermediate exchange for each ATP cleaved.

Exchange rates per mg of protein present were calculated on the assumption that rates were linear over the time period used. This was verified experimentally for exchanges in the absence of added uncoupler. It should be noted, however, that incubation of particles

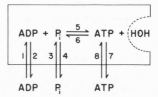

FIG. 1. A schematic representation of the minimal steps of substrate binding and release and ATP formation and cleavage. Enzyme bound components are indicated within the *rectangle*; whether a specific binding site exists for H_2O is uncertain, as indicated by the *dashed indentation*.

with ATP for about 2 min prior to adding isotopes was necessary to obtain linear exchange rates.

RESULTS

Experimental Rationale and Exchange Mechanisms – For presentation of our results it is important for the reader to understand the potential significance of the exchanges associated with oxidative phosphorylation. For this purpose it is helpful to consider the diagram of Fig. 1 depicting binding, release and interconversion steps during steady state ATP hydrolysis or oxidative phosphorylation.[3] In this figure reactants at the catalytic phosphorylation site in the membrane are depicted in the rectangle. Because the oxygen exchanges are more rapid than other exchanges (23–25) and because no localization of water has been detected (26), either no specific binding site for water exists or the water binding and dissociation is more rapid than other steps involved.

The total oxygen exchange reactions observed with substrates such as P_i and ATP can usefully be separated into two components, the medium and intermediate exchanges. Medium exchange occurs when a reactant binds to a catalytic site, undergoes exchange, and is released as the same reactant. Intermediate exchange occurs when a reactant binds, undergoes exchanges and conversion to a product, and the product containing atoms incorporated by exchange is released. Intermediate exchange is defined as an exchange of the product released. For example, if ATP that binds and is subsequently released as ATP contains water oxygens, a medium ATP $\rightleftharpoons HOH$ exchange has occurred. If ATP binds and the P_i formed from ATP and released to the medium contains more than the 1 oxygen required for ATP cleavage, an intermediate $P_i \rightleftharpoons HOH$ exchange has occurred. Such definitions of exchange are independent of the mechanism of exchange.

In accord with Fig. 1, oxygen exchanges of ATP and P_i and the $P_i \rightleftharpoons ATP$ and ADP $\rightleftharpoons ATP$ exchanges require reaction steps as summarized in Table I.

In Fig. 1 and Table I, only one bound species of each reactant is indicated. More than one species may exist, for example a loosely bound form not capable of undergoing covalent change, and a more tightly or competently bound form that undergoes substrate interconversion. The single binding steps of Fig. 1 and Table I include any intermediate species between free reactants and bound reactants that are catalytically competent.

---

[3] We assume that the oxygen exchanges associated with oxidative phosphorylation reflect occurrence of dynamic reversal of ATP synthesis at the catalytic site. It must be noted, however, that an alternate mechanism for oxygen exchange has been proposed (22). This mechanism is regarded as unlikely by us, but has not been disproved.

TABLE I

Required reaction steps for oxygen exchanges and the $P_i \rightleftharpoons ATP$ exchange of oxidative phosphorylation

Exchange reaction	Minimal required steps						
	ADP binding (Step 1)	ADP release (Step 2)	P_i binding (Step 3)	P_i release (Step 4)	Substrate interconversion (Steps 5 & 6)	ATP release (Step 7)	ATP binding (Step 8)
ADP ⇌ ATP[a]	+	+			+	+	+
P_i ⇌ ATP[b]			+	+	+	+	+
Medium P_i ⇌ HOH			+	+	+		
Intermediate P_i ⇌ HOH				+	+		+
Medium ATP ⇌ HOH					+	+	+
Intermediate[b] ATP ⇌ HOH			+		+	+	

[a] Requires presence of bound P_i derived either from medium P_i or from ATP cleavage.
[b] Requires presence of bound ADP derived either from medium ADP or from ATP cleavage.

Table I illustrates well the power of the exchange measurements, as they require different steps of the overall reaction sequence and may thus reveal changes in those steps not measurable by other approaches. Modifiers of the different steps of the reaction sequence given in Fig. 1 may have different effects on the rates of the exchange reactions (*cf.* Ref. 27). This offers the possibility of demonstrating the steps affected by energy in ATP formation by measuring the effect of uncouplers on the exchange reactions in which case uncouplers are used to change the energy level in the submitochondrial particles.

Apparent Requirement of ATP Hydrolysis for $P_i \rightleftharpoons HOH$ Exchange – Cross and Boyer (10) noted that the rapid $P_i \rightleftharpoons$ HOH exchange catalyzed by submitochondrial particles in the presence of added ADP and P_i, and in the absence of an added energy donor, was inhibited considerably by addition of glucose and hexokinase. This raised the possibility that the exchange might be stimulated by ATP formed by adenylate kinase present in submitochondrial particle preparations. It was thus desirable to ascertain if any ATP formed by adenylate kinase escaped removal by hexokinase and was hydrolyzed by the mitochondrial ATPase. To test this, we repeated experiments similar to these of Cross and Boyer but in the presence of [β-^{32}P]ADP. The ATP formed by adenylate kinase will be labeled with ^{32}P in both the β and γ positions. Any hydrolysis of this ATP can be measured as a release of [^{32}P]P_i.

Fig. 2 shows the effect of hexokinase and glucose on the $P_i \rightleftharpoons$ HOH exchange measured in the presence of ADP and P_i and the hydrolysis of ATP formed from this ADP by adenylate kinase. It is clear that the $P_i \rightleftharpoons$ HOH exchange is accompanied by a considerable ATP hydrolysis and that the exchange and the ATP hydrolysis are inhibited to the same extent when glucose and varying amounts of hexokinase are present. The fact that the number of oxygen atoms incorporated into P_i per mol of ATP hydrolyzed is essentially constant suggests that ATP hydrolysis is necessary for the $P_i \rightleftharpoons$ HOH exchange.

That the $P_i \rightleftharpoons$ HOH exchange is indeed driven by hydrolysis of ATP formed by adenylate kinase is shown by data in Table II. A 90% inhibition of the $P_i \rightleftharpoons$ HOH exchange was observed in the absence of added energy donor but in the presence of an amount of AMP that nearly completely inhibited ATP formation via adenylate kinase. Complete abolishment of the $P_i \rightleftharpoons$ HOH exchange, within experimental error, was obtained by addition of uncoupler, AMP, and hexokinase plus glucose. The

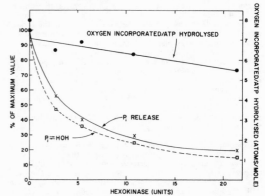

FIG. 2. Effect of hexokinase plus glucose on $P_i \rightleftharpoons$ HOH exchange and ATP hydrolysis in the absence of added energy donor. The reactions were carried out in a 1.0-ml volume at 30° in a reaction mixture containing 5 mM [β-^{32}P]ADP (208 cpm/nmol), 10 mM MgCl₂, 40 mM Tris/HCl, 10 mM P_i, 40 mM glucose, 0.76 atom % excess H^{18}OH at pH 7.4 and amounts of hexokinase as indicated. The reactions were started by addition of 1.9 mg of beef heart submitochondrial particles and stopped after 5 min by addition of 0.45 ml of cold 1 M perchloric acid. The samples were analyzed for ^{18}O incorporation into P_i and [^{32}P]P_i liberation as described under "Experimental Procedures." For $P_i \rightleftharpoons$ HOH exchange, 100% is 720 nmol min^{-1} mg^{-1}; 100% for ATP hydrolysis is 90 nmol min^{-1} mg^{-1}.

$P_i \rightleftharpoons$ HOH exchange thus does not take place in the complete absence of an energy donor. These results demonstrate that net ATP hydrolysis is required for the $P_i \rightleftharpoons$ HOH exchange, implying an energy requirement for one of the steps leading to the formation of ATP at the catalytic site.

Effect of Uncouplers on Exchange Reactions – The above findings prompted further investigation of the effects of uncouplers on the exchange reactions. The basis of our approach is that uncouplers collapse an energized state of the mitochondria, probably the transmembrane electrochemical potential or pH gradient, that can serve to drive both oxidative phosphorylation and the exchange reactions. Fig. 3 shows that, as anticipated, oxidative phosphorylation and $P_i \rightleftharpoons$ ATP exchange catalyzed by submitochondrial particles are equally sensitive to the uncoupler 2,4-dinitrophenol and that the inhi-

TABLE II

Effect of AMP, hexokinase and glucose, and 2,4-dinitrophenol on the total $P_i \rightleftharpoons HOH$ exchange and ATP hydrolysis

The reactions were carried out in a 1-ml final volume at 30° in a reaction mixture at pH 7.4 containing 1 mM $[\beta\text{-}^{32}P]ADP$ (1250 cpm/nmol), 10 mM $MgCl_2$, 40 mM Tris/Cl, 10 mM P_i, 40 mM glucose, $H^{18}OH$ (0.75 atoms % excess) and hexokinase, AMP, and 2,4-dinitrophenol as indicated. The reaction was started by addition of 2 mg of beef heart submitochondrial particles and stopped after 5 min by addition of 0.45 ml of cold 1 M perchloric acid. The samples were analyzed for the ^{18}O content in P_i and the $^{32}P_i$ release as described under "Experimental Procedures."

Additions	ATP hydrolysis		Total $P_i \rightleftharpoons HOH$ exchange	
	$nmol$ min^{-1} mg^{-1}	% inhibition	$nanoatoms$ min^{-1} mg^{-1}	% inhibition
None, control	54		735	
21.5 units of hexokinase	10	81	73	90
10 mM AMP	4.9	91	59	92
21.5 units of hexokinase, 10 mM AMP	2.1	96	15	98
100 μM 2,4-dinitrophenol	58		161	78
100 μM 2,4-dinitrophenol, 10 mM AMP, 21.5 units of hexokinase	0.6	99	11	99

bition parallels the increase in the ATPase activity. Such equal sensitivity gives more credence to the differential sensitivity of other exchanges as noted later.

Fig. 4 shows effects of 2,4-dinitrophenol on the ATP $\rightleftharpoons$ ADP exchange carried out in the presence of AMP to inhibit ATP formation from ADP via adenylate kinase. The low rate of P_i $\rightleftharpoons$ ATP exchange under these conditions might result from AMP inhibition of this exchange reaction. The important point of Fig. 4 is that the inhibition of the ADP $\rightleftharpoons$ ATP exchange by uncoupler is quite similar to the inhibition of the $P_i \rightleftharpoons$ ATP exchange.

To gain information about the additional sites of energy input we evaluated the uncoupler effects on the medium and intermediate exchange components of the $P_i \rightleftharpoons$ HOH exchange. Data from experiments with 2,4-dinitrophenol, similar to those reported for Figs. 3 and 4, suggested that the apparent insensitivity of the total $P_i \rightleftharpoons$ HOH exchange to uncouplers resulted from the fact that intermediate $P_i \rightleftharpoons$ HOH exchange was uncoupler-insensitive but the medium exchange was uncoupler sensitive. At 0.5 mM 2,4-dinitrophenol, within experimental error, the $P_i \rightleftharpoons$ ATP exchange was completely inhibited, the intermediate exchange was not inhibited, and the medium exchange was 85% inhibited. To test the relative sensitivities of the medium and intermediate exchanges further, we titrated the exchange reactions with the potent uncoupler S-13. Results of such a titration are given in Fig. 5; they demonstrate the lack of appreciable inhibition of the intermediate $P_i \rightleftharpoons$ HOH exchange and the apparently complete inhibition of the medium exchange by this uncoupler.

It is evident from the data of Fig. 5 that at higher uncoupler

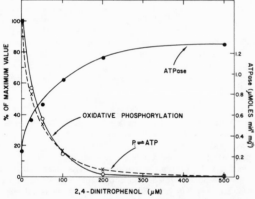

FIG. 3. Effect of the uncoupler 2,4-dinitrophenol on oxidative phosphorylation, $P_i \rightleftharpoons$ ATP exchange, and ATPase catalyzed by beef heart submitochondrial particles. For measurement of oxidative phosphorylation, beef heart submitochondrial particles (0.5 mg) were incubated at 30° in 0.8 ml of a reaction mixture containing 188 mM sucrose, 63 mM glucose, 63 mM Tris/Cl, 8 mM P_i, 3.8 mM $MgCl_2$, 50 units of dialyzed hexokinase, and 10 mM succinate. After 2 min 50 s, DNP was added to give final concentrations as given in the figure, and 10 s later a mixture of ADP and carrier-free ^{32}P was added to give a final ADP of 2.5 mM and a final volume of 1 ml. The reactions were stopped 2 min later by addition of 1 ml of 1 M perchloric acid. For measurement of the $P_i \rightleftharpoons$ ATP exchange and ATPase, 0.5 mg of beef heart submitochondrial particles were incubated at 30° in 0.8 ml of a reaction mixture containing 188 mM sucrose, 25 mM Tris/Cl, 12.5 mM P_i, 18.8 mM $MgCl_2$, 3.75 mM ADP, and 18.8 mM ATP at pH 7.5. After 2 min 50 s, a 2,4-dinitrophenol solution was added to give final concentrations as given in the figure, and 10 s later carrier-free ^{32}P was added to give a final volume of 1 ml. The reactions were stopped 2 min later by addition of 1 ml of 1 M perchloric acid. In both cases the amount of esterified ^{32}P was determined as described under "Experimental Procedures." For phosphorylation, 100% is 250 nmol min^{-1} mg^{-1}; 100% for ATP $\rightleftharpoons$ P_i is 330 nmol min^{-1} mg^{-1}.

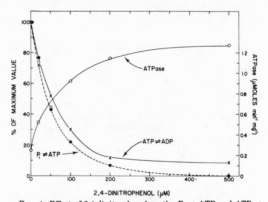

FIG. 4. Effect of 2,4-dinitrophenol on the $P_i \rightleftharpoons$ ATP and ATP $\rightleftharpoons$ ADP exchange and ATP hydrolysis catalyzed by beef heart submitochondrial particles. Beef heart submitochondrial particles were incubated at 30° in 0.9 ml of a reaction mixture containing 75 mM sucrose, 40 mM Tris/Cl, 15 mM $MgCl_2$, 10 mM P_i, 15 mM AMP, 15 mM ADP, and 15 mM ATP at pH 7.5. After 1 min 50 s, 2,4-dinitrophenol was added to give final concentrations as given in the figure, and 10 s later $^{32}P_i$ was added to give a specific activity of 2750 cpm/nmol. The total volume after these additions was 1 ml. The reactions were stopped 4 min later by addition of 1 ml of cold 1 M perchloric acid. An analogous incubation was carried out for the measurement of the ATP $\rightleftharpoons$ ADP exchange. In this case the exchange reaction was started by addition of a mixture of $[^3H]ADP$ and $[\beta\text{-}^{32}P]ADP$ to give specific activities of 400 and 552 cpm/nmol, respectively. Addition of the $[^{32}P]P_i$, $[^3H]ADP$, and $[\beta\text{-}^{32}P]ADP$ gave a negligible change in the corresponding concentrations. The perchlorate extracts were analyzed as given under "Experimental Procedures." For $P_i \rightleftharpoons$ ATP exchange, 100% is 120 nmol min^{-1} mg^{-1}; 100% for ATP $\rightleftharpoons$ ADP exchange is 180 nmol min^{-1} mg^{-1}.

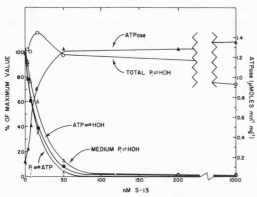

FIG. 5. Effect of S-13 on exchange reactions and ATP hydrolysis catalyzed by beef heart submitochondrial particles. Beef heart submitochondrial particles (2 mg) were incubated at 30° in a reaction mixture containing 150 mM sucrose, 20 mM Tris/Cl, 15 mM MgCl$_2$, 7.5 mM P$_i$, 3 mM ADP, and 15 mM ATP at pH 7.5. After 1 min 50 s, S-13 was added to give final concentrations as indicated in the figure, and 10 s later a mixture of [^{32}P]P$_i$ and H^{18}OH was added to give a final concentration of 10 mM P$_i$ and a final 1.96 atom % excess H^{18}OH. The total volume was 1.0 ml. The reactions were stopped 5 min later by addition of 1 ml of cold 1 M percholoric acid and analyzed as described under "Experimental Procedures." An analogous incubation was carried out for the measurement of the [^{18}O]P$_i$ $\rightleftharpoons$ HOH exchange. In this case the exchange reaction was started after 2 min by addition of [^{18}O]P$_i$ to give a final concentration of P$_i$ of 10 mM containing 8.3 atom % excess ^{18}O. For total P$_i$ $\rightleftharpoons$ HOH exchange, 100% is 1700 nanoatoms min^{-1} mg^{-1}; 100% for medium P$_i$ $\rightleftharpoons$ HOH exchange is 972 nanoatoms min^{-1} mg^{-1}; 100% for total ATP $\rightleftharpoons$ HOH exchange is 690 nanoatoms min^{-1} mg^{-1}; 100% for P$_i$ $\rightleftharpoons$ ATP exchange is 280 nmol min^{-1} mg^{-1}.

concentrations there is still considerable oxygen incorporated by exchange into each P$_i$ formed from ATP; the amount decreased with increase in the S-13 concentration from about 1.7 to 1.0 atoms of water oxygen incorporated into each P$_i$ formed. Such continued exchange can readily be explained if the reversible formation of bound ATP from bound ADP and P$_i$ continues in presence of relatively high uncoupler concentrations. A continued exchange with each P$_i$ released can also explain the observed increase of the total amount of intermediate exchange at low uncoupler concentration because uncouplers increase considerably the total amount of ATP hydrolyzed. In agreement with Cross and Boyer (10), we found that the uncoupler insensitive P$_i$ $\rightleftharpoons$ HOH exchange, now demonstrated to be the intermediate exchange, is sensitive to the inhibitor oligomycin.

It is important to note that the purified ATPase from mitochondria shows little or no capacity to catalyze either the prominent intermediate exchange or the medium exchange characteristic of the competent membrane-bound ATPase.[4]

Effect of 2,4-Dinitrophenol on Intermediate P$_i$ $\rightleftharpoons$ HOH Exchange Measured in Presence of ATP Regenerating System — Because measurements of the intermediate P$_i$ $\rightleftharpoons$ HOH exchange may be subject to comparatively large error resulting from high medium exchange, it would be advantageous if uncoupler effects could be measured when medium exchange was low or absent. The effect of uncouplers on the intermediate P$_i$ $\rightleftharpoons$ HOH exchange can be checked more directly when the oxygen incorporation from H^{18}OH into P$_i$ arising from ATP

[4] G. L. Choate and P. D. Boyer, unpublished observations.

TABLE III

Effect of 2,4-dinitrophenol on intermediate P$_i$ $\rightleftharpoons$ HOH exchange and ATP hydrolysis measured in presence of ATP regenerating system

The reactions were carried out at 30° in a medium containg 5 mM ATP, 10 mM MgCl$_2$, 40 mM Tris/Cl, 150 mM sucrose, 5 mM phosphoenol pyruvate, 0.35 mM NADH, 0.2 mg of rotenone, 100 units of pyruvate kinase, 200 units of lactate dehydrogenase, 3.9 atom % excess H^{18}OH at pH 7.5, and amounts of 2,4-dinitrophenol as given in the table. Reactions were started by addition of beef heart submitochondrial particles to give a final concentration of 0.15 mg/ml and stopped after 7 min by addition of 1 ml of cold 1 M perchloric acid. The ATPase was calculated from the rate of NADH disappearance and P$_i$ was analyzed for its ^{18}O content as described under "Experimental Procedures."

2,4-Dinitro-phenol	ATPase	Intermediate P$_i$ $\rightleftharpoons$ HOH exchange	
		Exchange rate	Oxygens exchanged per ATP cleaved
μM	*nmol min^{-1} mg^{-1}*	*nanoatoms min^{-1} mg^{-1}*	
	750	350	0.46
25	960	550	0.57
50	1100	410	0.37
100	1200	490	0.41
250	1200	630	0.53

is measured in the presence of an ATP regenerating system (Table II). Medium P$_i$ $\rightleftharpoons$ HOH exchange does not occur under these conditions due to lack of free ADP and the low concentrations of medium P$_i$ present. The ^{18}O incorporation into P$_i$ results exclusively from intermediate P$_i$ $\rightleftharpoons$ HOH exchange. The results given in Table III show continuation of prominent intermediate exchange in the presence of uncoupler. This supports the above mentioned suggestion that uncouplers do not effect the reversible formation of bound ATP from bound ADP and P$_i$.

DISCUSSION

Measurements of the effects of energy depletion on the various exchange and net reactions catalyzed by submitochondrial particles appear to deserve recognition as a powerful approach to the understanding of how energy is used for ATP synthesis. Applications of this approach presented in this paper have demonstrated some important new points, one of which is that depletion of the energized state of the mitochondrial membrane results in a loss of the ability of P$_i$ to be bound at the catalytic site so as to participate in the oxygen exchange reactions characteristic of oxidative phosphorylation.

It deserves emphasis that the above conclusion about P$_i$ binding and participation is independent from the mechanism of oxygen exchanges (*cf.* Ref. 22). The continuation of the intermediate P$_i$ $\rightleftharpoons$ HOH exchange and the ATPase in the presence of uncouplers means that P$_i$ bound to the catalytic site is still undergoing oxygen exchange and is still capable of being rapidly released to the medium. What is lost in the presence of uncoupler is the ability for medium P$_i$ to be bound in the manner necessary for participation in the exchange reaction.

An important conclusion from our present data about the exchange of P$_i$ oxygens with water is that the presence of Mg^{2+}, ADP, and P$_i$ alone with submitochondrial particles but without oxidizable substrates does not allow the medium P$_i$ $\rightleftharpoons$ HOH exchange to occur. No P$_i$ $\rightleftharpoons$ HOH exchange was detected when the availability of ATP formed from added ADP by adenylate kinase action was blocked (Fig. 2 and Table II). Net ATP cleavage is necessary for the exchange. Thus the apparent absolute requirement of added ADP for the $P_i \rightleftharpoons HOH$ exchange reported earlier (25) reflects not only the presence of ADP but also formation and net hydrolysis of ATP. We can explain this only by the requirement of energization by ATP binding and cleavage to drive this $P_i \rightleftharpoons HOH$ exchange.

The experimental findings are also of interest because they indicate that this energization of the mitochondrial membrane is distinct from the presence of a transmembrane potential or proton gradient. The continuation of a prominent intermediate exchange in the presence of the uncoupler S-13 at a 10-fold higher concentration than necessary to stop net oxidative phosphorylation indicates a remarkable insensitivity of the covalent bond forming and breaking step $(ADP + P_i \rightleftharpoons ATP + HOH)$ to uncouplers. That this continued exchange does not result from some transmembrane potential that might remain in presence of high uncoupler levels is made unlikely by the observation that presence of valinomycin and K^+ in addition to S-13 did not further reduce intermediate exchange.[4] We interpret these results to mean the energized state of the enzyme complex derived from ATP binding and cleavage is separate and distinct from that primarily dissipated by uncouplers, and is present even when the protonmotive force is dissipated. We hypothesize that the enzyme complex capable of reversible ATP cleavage is in a conformationally energized state. Such an energized state could be converted to transmembrane potential or pH gradient by movement of protons concurrent with changes favoring ADP and P_i release.

If uncouplers abolish protonmotive force (4), then present findings are not compatible with the suggestions of Mitchell about how an effective proton gradient may drive ATP synthesis (9). The reactions leading to P—O bond cleavage and reformation, as required for the exchanges, can obviously continue under conditions where the protonmotive force is largely or entirely dissipated. Mitchell's mechanism requires the use of a potentially activated proton for cleavage of the P—O bond of P_i leading to ATP formation. Our results thus add to chemical objections (8, 28) to Mitchell's mechanism. A suggestion of the type of mechanism by which a potential or proton gradient might drive conformational changes for ATP formation has been presented elsewhere (29).

The existence of a conformationally energized state in the presence or absence of a membrane potential or proton gradient is in harmony with the concept of conformational coupling in biological energy transductions (3, 30). Other conformationally energized states might exist in the enzymes of the electron transport chain. A conformationally energized state might be responsible for the light-induced exchange of water protons with the chloroplast CF_1-ATPase noted in the important paper of Ryrie and Jagendorf (31). Some characteristics of the exchange reactions are not readily rationalized by a conformationally energized state as depicted here and a single catalytic site for ATP formation. They can be explained by a multisite mechanism; such explanations and the role of bound nucleotides are presented elsewhere (32, 33).

The evidence from our data that energization is necessary for medium P_i to undergo transformations at the catalytic site should not be interpreted as suggesting that binding alone is sufficient for the overall reaction. The sequence of events may involve steps such as the following.

$$E + P_i + ADP \leftrightarrow E \cdot {}^{P_i}_{ADP} \xrightarrow[\text{transition}]{\text{energy-coupled}} *E \cdot {}^{P_i}_{ADP} \xrightarrow{HOH} E \cdot ATP$$

where $*E$ represents an energized form of the phosphorylation complex. Energy input might not change the initial binding steps, but the conversion of the initial complex to the productive complex. In the productive complex, the environment of the bound P_i and ADP is such as to promote bound ATP formation. We further suggest that the energized state is capable of promoting ATP dissociation with return of the enzyme to the nonenergized form. There appear to be two ways of achieving the energized form, $E * \cdot {}^{ADP}_{P_i}$: one is by binding and cleavage of ATP and the other is by use of energy as transmitted from oxidations.

If energy promotes formation of a productive complex from ADP and P_i, the apparent Michaelis constants of ADP and P_i for net oxidative phosphorylation would be expected to be increased by uncoupler. This prediction recently has been confirmed (34).

An interesting analogy may be made between energization events in muscle contraction and oxidative phosphorylation (30, 35, 36). In muscle, binding of ATP to actomyosin causes actin dissociation accompanied by conformational changes in myosin. An intermediate oxygen exchange occurs associated with reversal of the cleavage of bound ATP and the myosin molecule with the bound ADP and P_i may be regarded as being in an energized state. Upon recombination with actin, ADP and P_i dissociate and the energized state is used to slide the filaments. Hypothetically, one could energize myosin by dissociation of actin from actomyosin, thus promoting binding of ADP and P_i and formation of ATP at the catalytic site of myosin, then allow actin to recombine when bound ATP is present causing release of ATP to the medium.

Previous results from this laboratory localized the uncoupler-insensitive portion of the scheme as depicted in Fig. 1 to the chemical interconversion and P_i binding steps. The present results now further localize the insensitive portion solely to the interconversion step. In independent studies, Mitchell *et al.* have also demonstrated that the intermediate oxygen exchange is insensitive to uncouplers (37).

Consideration is also necessary of the observations of Eisenhardt and Rosenthal (38) and of Cross and Boyer (10) on the rapid incorporation of ${}^{32}P_i$ into a small amount of ATP in the presence of sufficient 2,4-dinitrophenol to nearly stop net oxidative phosphorylation. Such incorporation is considerably more sensitive to uncouplers than the intermediate $P_i \rightleftharpoons HOH$ exchange accompanying ATP hydrolysis as noted in this paper. In the experiments of Cross and Boyer, added ADP would have been rapidly converted to ATP by adenylate kinase and both conformational and transmembrane potential or proton gradient energization may have resulted. The amount of uncoupler present (for example, 100 μM 2,4-dinitrophenol) may have been insufficient to cause rapid dissipation of all energized states, thus allowing some binding of $[{}^{32}P]P_i$ and formation of $[{}^{32}P]ATP$. The $[{}^{32}P]ATP$ present could represent that at the catalytic site in addition to a small, steady state amount present in the medium.

The simplest mechanism for the oxygen exchanges remains as that suggested earlier, namely that the exchanges result from dynamic reversal of the cleavage of ATP at the catalytic site. As noted by Mitchell *et al.* (24), for such a simple mechanism the rates of the total $P_i \rightleftharpoons HOH$ exchange and the ATP $\rightleftharpoons$ HOH exchange cannot both be much greater than the $P_i \rightleftharpoons ATP$ exchange, although the ratio of the $P_i \rightleftharpoons HOH$ to the $P_i \rightleftharpoons ATP$ exchange can approach high values if the ratio of the ATP $\rightleftharpoons$ HOH to $P_i \rightleftharpoons ATP$ exchange is only slightly greater than 3. The exchange ratios reported in this paper using the improved methodology fall within the available limits of the simple mechanism. Also, the derivations given by Mitchell *et al.* (24) only apply to a system without net ATP hydrolysis. ATP hydrolysis can under some conditions give rise to disparity of exchange rates much larger than expected on basis of equilibrium considerations alone. Such conditions are met in experiments in the presence of phosphoenolpyruvate and pyruvate kinase in which the $P_i \rightleftharpoons$ ATP exchange can be inhibited completely (Kayalar *et al.* (31)) while the intermediate $P_i \rightleftharpoons$ HOH exchange is not affected (Table II). Both ATP and P_i at the catalytic site could be labeled with ^{18}O from $H^{18}OH$, and their release could give considerable $P_i \rightleftharpoons$ HOH and ATP $\rightleftharpoons$ HOH exchange with little or no $P_i \rightleftharpoons$ ATP exchange. Thus the disparity of the exchange rates under these conditions should not be taken as requiring alternate exchange mechanisms (22).

The fact that oxygen exchanges on the basis of present information for both mitochondrial and myosin ATPase can be explained by dynamic reversal of ATP formation at the catalytic site does not eliminate the possible detection of additional intermediates in the sequence. For example, a transient formation of a bound metaphosphate at the catalytic site remains as a possibility that is difficult to assess experimentally.

Acknowledgments – We wish to thank Donna Bryan and Jeanette Yamamoto for their excellent technical assistance in performing ^{18}O analyses for these researches.

REFERENCES

1. Rosing, J., Kayalar, C., and Boyer, P. D. (1975) in *The Structural Basis of Membrane Function* (Hatefi, Y., and Ojavadi-Ohaniance, L., eds) pp. 189-204, Academic Press, New York
2. Boyer, P. D., Smith, D. J., Rosing, J., and Kayalar, C. (1975) in *Electron Transfer Chains and Oxidative Phosphorylation* (Quagliariello, E., Papa, S., Palmieri, E., Slater, E. C., and Siliprandi, N., eds) pp. 361-372, North Holland Publishing Company, Amsterdam
3. Boyer, P. D. (1965) in *Oxidases and Related Redox Systems* (T. E. King, H. S. Mason, and M. Morrison, eds) pp. 994-1008, John Wiley & Sons, New York
4. Mitchell, P. (1966) *Chemiosmotic Coupling in Oxidative and Photosynthetic Phosphorylation*, Glynn Research, Bodmin, Cornwall, England
5. Slater, E. C. (1974) in *Dynamics of Energy Transducing Membranes* (Ernster L., Estabrook, R. W., and Slater, E. C., eds) Vol. 13, BBA Library, pp. 1-20, Elsevier, Amsterdam
6. Harris, D. A., and Slater, E. C. (1975) *Biochim. Biophys. Acta* 387, 335-348
7. Boyer, P. D., Cross, R. L., and Momsen, W. (1973) *Proc. Natl. Acad. Sci. U. S. A.* 70, 2837-2839
8. Boyer, P. D. (1975) *FEBS Lett.* 50, 91-94
9. Mitchell, P. (1974) *FEBS Lett.* 43, 189-194
10. Cross, R. L., and Boyer, P. D. (1975) *Biochemistry* 14, 392-398
11. Levy, H. M., and Koshland, D. E., Jr. (1959) *J. Biol. Chem.* 234, 1102-1107
12. Dempsey, M. E., Boyer, P. D., and Benson, E. S. (1963) *J. Biol. Chem.* 238, 2708-2715
13. Cohn, M., and Drysdale, G. R. (1955) *J. Biol. Chem.* 216, 831-846
14. Johnson, D., and Lardy, H. (1967) *Methods Enzymol.* 10, 94-96
15. Smith, A. L. (1967) *Methods Enzymol.* 10, 81-86
16. Beyer, R. E. (1967) *Methods Enzymol.* 10, 186-194
17. Lowry, O. H., Rosebrough, N. J., Farr, A. L., and Randall, R. J. (1951) *J. Biol. Chem.* 193, 265-275
18. Sumner, J. B. (1944) *Science* 100, 413-414
19. Bergmeyer, H. U. (1970) *Methoden der Enzymatischen Analyse*, Verlag Chemie, Weinheim
20. Clausen, T. (1968) *Anal. Biochem.* 22, 70-73
21. Boyer, P. D., and Bryan, D. M. (1967) *Methods Enzymol.* 10, 60-71
22. Young, J. H., Korman, E. F., and McLick, J. (1974) *Bioorg. Chem.* 3, 1-15
23. Boyer, P. D., Luchsinger, W. W., and Falcone, A. B. (1956) *J. Biol. Chem.* 223, 405-421
24. Mitchell, R. A., Hill, R. D., and Boyer, P. D. (1967) *J. Biol. Chem.* 242, 1793-1801
25. Jones, D. H., and Boyer, P. D. (1969) *J. Biol. Chem.* 244, 5767-5772
26. Kaplan, A., and Boyer, P. D. (1969) *J. Biol. Chem.* 244, 4659-4663
27. Wedler, F., and Boyer, P. D. (1973) *J. Theor. Biol.* 38, 539-558
28. Williams, R. J. P. (1975) *FEBS Lett.* 53, 123-125
29. Boyer, P. D. (1975) *FEBS Lett.* 58, 1-7
30. Boyer, P. D. (1974) in *Dynamics of Energy Transducing Membranes* (Ernster, L., Estabrook, R. W., and Slater, E. C., eds) Vol. 13, BBA Library, pp. 289-301, Elsevier, Amsterdam
31. Ryrie, I. J., and Jagendorf, A. T. (1972) *J. Biol. Chem.* 247, 4453-4459
32. Kayalar, C., Rosing, J., and Boyer, P. D. (1977) *J. Biol. Chem.* 252, 2486-2491
33. Kayalar, C., Rosing, J., and Boyer, P. D. (1976) *Fed. Proc.* 35, 1601
34. Kayalar, C., Rosing, J., and Boyer, P. D. (1976) *Biochem. Biophys. Res. Commun.* 72, 1153-1159
35. Wolcott, R. G., and Boyer, P. D. (1974) *Biochem. Biophys. Res. Commun.* 57, 709-716
36. Bagshaw, C. R., Trentham, D. R., Wolcott, R. G., and Boyer, P. D. (1975) *Proc. Natl. Acad. Sci. U. S. A.* 72, 2592-2596
37. Mitchell, R. A., Lamos, C. M., and Russo, J. A. (1975) *170th American Chemical Society Meeting, Chicago* Abstr. 108
38. Eisenhardt, R. H., and Rosenthal, O. (1968) *Biochemistry* 7, 1327-1333

Editor's Comments
on Papers 25 and 26

THE MEMBRANE ADENOSINE TRIPHOSPHATASE

Increasing attention has been directed toward the molecular configuration and enzymatic activities of the membrane ATPase in procaryotes. The manifold functions of this enzyme suggest that its structure and dynamic interactions with cellular constituents ought to be complex, and the two selections presented here confirm that suspicion.

25

Reprinted from Arch. Biochem. Biophys. **159**:664–670 (1973)

Effect of Removal or Modification of Subunit Polypeptides on the Coupling Factor and Hydrolytic Activities of the Ca^{2+} and Mg^{2+}-Activated Adenosine Triphosphatase of *Escherichia coli*

P. D. BRAGG, P. L. DAVIES, AND C. HOU

Department of Biochemistry, University of British Columbia, Vancouver 8, B. C., Canada

Received August 23, 1973

The effect of removal or modification of the polypeptide subunits (α, β, γ, δ, and ϵ) of the Ca^{2+} and Mg^{2+}-activated ATPase of *Escherichia coli* was investigated. Removal of the δ-polypeptide, although giving some decrease in ATPase activity, resulted in complete loss of coupling activity, where coupling activity was measured by the restoration of the energy-dependent transhydrogenase activity of ATPase-stripped respiratory particles. Modification of the γ-polypeptide, as found in the ATPase of an energy transfer coupling mutant (*etc-15*), resulted in diminution of the ATPase and coupling activities. The diminished coupling activity could be overcome by using more of the enzyme which suggested that this enzyme may not be able to bind to the membrane as firmly as the enzyme from the wild type.

Calcium or magnesium ion-activated adenosine triphosphatase (ATPase) has been implicated in the coupling of electron transport to the formation or use of ATP in mitochondria (1), chloroplasts (1), and bacteria (2, 3). The molecular weight of the membrane-bound, Ca^{2+} or Mg^{2+}-activated ATPase solubilized from different organisms is remarkably similar. Thus, the molecular weight of the enzyme from rat liver and beef heart mitochondria is 360,000 (4), from yeast mitochondria, 340,000 (5), from spinach chloroplasts, 325,000 (6), from *Escherichia coli*, 365,000–390,000 (7), from *Bacillus megaterium*, 379,000–410,000 (8), and from *Streptococcus faecalis*, 385,000 (9). It is likely that the enzyme from *Micrococcus lysodeikticus* has a molecular weight in the same range since it has a sedimentation constant of 14–15 s (10). With the exception of the enzyme from *S. faecalis* (9) which is made up of two nonidentical polypeptides of MW 33,000, the other enzymes show a similar polypeptide composition. The mitochondrial ATPase from beef heart contains poly-

peptides of MW 53,000, 50,000, 25,000, 12,500, and 7,500 (4), while that from chloroplasts has subunits of MW 59,000, 56,000, 37,000, 17,500, and 13,000 (11). The enzyme from *E. coli* also contains five polypeptides (av MW: 56,800; 51,800; 30,500; 21,000; 11,500) (12). Fewer polypeptides have been found in the ATPases of *M. lysodeikticus* (13) and *B. megaterium* (8). This is probably due to insufficient protein having been applied to the gels to detect the smaller polypeptides since it is the two subunits of highest molecular weight which stain most strongly with coomassie blue. However, the major polypeptides of the enzyme from *B. megaterium* had molecular weights of 68,000 and 65,000 (8), while those of the *M. lysodeikticus* ATPase were 62,000, 60,000, and 35,000 (13).

Recently Nelson *et al.* (11, 14) have reported on the function of the polypeptides of the chloroplast enzymes, but much still remains unknown. The similarity in function and polypeptide composition of the ATPase from the various sources raises the problem of whether the polypeptides also have an analogous function in the different enzymes. The availability of a number of mutants of *E. coli* in which the ATPase activity has been altered (2, 15, 16) prompted us to study the functions of the polypeptide subunits of the ATPase from this organism. The initial results are given in this paper. For convenience of identification of the five subunit polypeptides of the *E. coli* ATPase we follow the procedure of Nelson *et al.* (11) and refer to them as the α, β, γ, δ, and ϵ polypeptides in order of decreasing molecular weights.

METHODS

Escherichia coli strains NRC-482, ML308-225 (wild type) and its electron transfer coupling mutant *etc-15* (17), were grown with vigorous aeration on a minimal salts–glucose (0.4%) medium containing 12 μM ferric citrate. The cells were harvested in the late exponential phase and converted to washed respiratory particles as described previously (18). ATPase was stripped from these particles by dialysis against 0.5 mM EDTA at low ionic strength, and purified to homogeneity by a combination of chromatography on DEAE-cellulose and Sepharose 6B, followed by sucrose density gradient centrifugation. The procedure followed the method used before (12). The stripped particles were suspended in 50 mM Tris–H_2SO_4 buffer, pH 7.8, containing 10 mM $MgCl_2$, and 1% bovine serum albumin, at a concentration of 10–20 mg protein/ml.

Protein, Ca²⁺-activated ATPase, aerobic- and ATP-driven energy-dependent transhydrogenase activities were measured exactly as described previously (18) except that the final concentration of sucrose in the transhydrogenase assays was 0.133 M. ATPase activity was determined in the presence of 5 mM $CaCl_2$. The activities of the energy-dependent transhydrogenases were corrected for that of the energy-independent transhydrogenase. Enzyme activities were measured at 37°C.

For reconstitution of transhydrogenase activity the stripped particles (50 μl) in a cuvette with 1 ml Tris–H_2SO_4 buffer, pH 7.8, containing 10 mM $MgCl_2$, 0.1% bovine serum albumin, 0.1 mM dithiothreitol, and 0.16 M sucrose, were preincubated for 5 min at 37°C with various amounts of ATPase. Following preincubation, the transhydrogenase assay was carried out directly on the contents of the cuvette (18). The final volume of the complete assay mixture was 1.2 ml.

Analytical disc gel electrophoresis was performed either on 5% polyacrylamide gels prepared and run in 0.05 M Tris–glycine buffer, pH 8.7, or on 7.5% polyacrylamide gels containing 0.1% sodium dodecyl sulfate (SDS). For the latter system the protein sample was depolymerized at 37°C for 1 hr, and then at 100°C for 3 min, in 4 M urea–1% SDS–1% mercaptoethanol, and run in system 1 as described previously (19). Protein bands were stained with Coomassie blue.

When the ATPase was purified on polyacrylamide gels a slab gel vertical electrophoresis apparatus (E-C Apparatus Corp.) was used. Partially purified ATPase of *E. coli* NRC-482 (1.2 mg protein) obtained following chromatography on Sepharose 6B (12) was applied to a 4 × 100 mm slot in a 5% polyacrylamide gel made in 0.05 M Tris–glycine buffer, pH 8.7, which had been prerun to remove charged compounds. The buffer compartments contained the same buffer. Electrophoresis was carried out at 300 V for 90 min at which time the bromophenol blue marker dye had migrated ca. 13 cm through the gel. During electrophoresis the gel was cooled by circulating water at 10°C. Guide strips were cut from the gel slab after electrophoresis and were stained for ATPase activity using the assay reagents normally used to quantitate the enzyme. The area containing the ATPase was cut out from the remainder of the gel and extracted with 0.05 M Tris–HCl buffer, pH 7.5, containing 0.5 mM EDTA, 0.1 mM dithiothreitol, and 10% glycerol. The enzyme solution was concentrated immediately to about 0.7 mg protein/ml by ultrafiltration through a PM 10 membrane (Amico Corp.). The recovery of ATPase activity from the gel was about 35%.

RESULTS

Effect of gel electrophoresis on ATPase of E. coli NCR-482. In experiments designed to purify ATPase the almost homogeneous enzyme was separated on polyacrylamide gels at pH 8.7. Although the enzyme could be reextracted from the gels there was a considerable loss of enzyme units. Furthermore, there was some decline in the specific activity of the enzyme (Table I) even though the enzyme appeared to migrate as a single protein band on the gel. When the extracted enzyme was disaggregated into its constituent polypeptides by heating with 1% SDS in the presence of 4 M urea and 1% mercaptoethanol and examined by electrophoresis in SDS-containing gels, the δ-polypeptide of the ATPase was found to be missing (Fig. 1). Since these gels were overloaded with sample to show the minor bands, the α- and β-polypeptides have not resolved

BRAGG, DAVIES, AND HOU

Strain	Final purification step	Specific activity[a]
NRC-482	Sucrose gradient	38.9
NRC-482	Gel electrophoresis	26.9
ML308-225	Sucrose gradient	31.3
etc-15	Sucrose gradient	18.6

[a] μmoles/min/mg protein.

from one another on these gels. In other gels (not shown) where less sample was applied to the gel the α- and β-polypeptides were found to be identical in the two preparations. In the gel shown in Fig. 1 there is a trace of another polypeptide band migrating more slowly than the γ-subunit of the ATPase obtained from the gel. It is not clear if this represents an impurity or whether this is derived from the missing polypeptide. Although the increased molecular size of this band over the δ-polypeptide could be explained by the formation of disulfide bridges between two molecules of the δ-polypeptide, it seems unlikely that these bridges would not have been cleaved by the disaggregation technique used to prepare the sample for analysis on the SDS-containing gels.

Removal of ATPase from membrane particles of *E. coli* results in loss of both aerobic- and ATP-driven transhydrogenase activities. These activities can be restored to the stripped particles by incubating them in the presence of the purified ATPase and magnesium ions or salts (12). Figure 2 shows the restoration of these activities to stripped particles by an electrophoretically homogeneous ATPase purified on a sucrose gradient. In contrast to this ATPase, the ATPase extracted from the polyacrylamide gel had no ability to restore either of the energy-dependent transhydrogenase activities even after preincubation with mercaptoethanol or dithiothreitol.

ATPase of electron transfer coupling mutant. Preliminary experiments with *E. coli etc-15* showed that membrane particles prepared from this strain had lower energy-

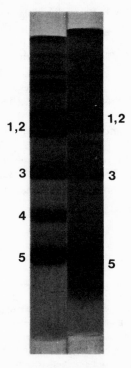

FIG. 1. Electrophoresis of purified preparations of the ATPase of *E. coli* NRC-482 purified in the final step either by sucrose density gradient centrifugation (left gel) or by gel electrophoresis at pH 8.7 (right gel). The samples were depolymerized as described in Methods and electrophoresis was carried out in the presence of 0.1% SDS. Bands 1–5 indicate polypeptides α–ϵ.

dependent transhydrogenase activities than the parent strain, ML308-225, while the nonenergy dependent transhydrogenase, as measured by the reduction of 3-acetylpyridine-NAD⁺ by NADPH, was much less affected. Moreover the specific activity of the membrane-bound Ca²⁺-activated ATPase of the mutant was about half that of the parent (Table II). In mitochondria the energy-dependent transhydrogenase enzyme appears to be the same enzyme that functions in the nonenergy-dependent reaction (20). Thus, the lower activity of the energy-dependent reactions suggested that the supply of energy to the transhydrogenase enzyme was impaired. This would agree with the results of Hong and Kaback (17) who found that energy-dependent transport of amino acids was much reduced in this strain

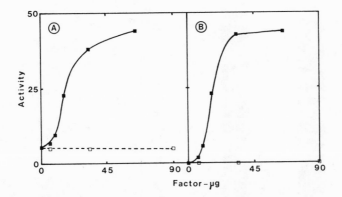

F ɪ ɢ. 2. Effect of purified ATPase ("factor") on the aerobic-driven (A) and ATP-driven (B) transhydrogenase activities of stripped particles of *E. coli* NRC-482. The final step in the purification of the ATPase of *E. coli* NRC-482 was either sucrose density gradient centrifugation (solid points) or gel electrophoresis (open points). Activity is expressed as nmoles NADPH formed/min. Stripped particles, 0.94 mg protein.

TABLE II

Sᴘᴇᴄɪꜰɪᴄ Aᴄᴛɪᴠɪᴛɪᴇs[a] ᴏꜰ ATPₐₛₑ, ᴀᴇʀᴏʙɪᴄ-
ᴀɴᴅ ATP-Dʀɪᴠᴇɴ Tʀᴀɴsʜʏᴅʀᴏɢᴇɴᴀsᴇ, ᴀɴᴅ
Eɴᴇʀɢʏ-Nᴏɴᴅᴇᴘᴇɴᴅᴇɴᴛ[b] Tʀᴀɴsʜʏᴅʀᴏɢᴇɴᴀsᴇ
ᴏꜰ Wᴀsʜᴇᴅ ᴀɴᴅ Sᴛʀɪᴘᴘᴇᴅ Pᴀʀᴛɪᴄʟᴇs ᴏꜰ *E. ᴄᴏʟɪ*
ML308-225 ᴀɴᴅ *ᴇᴛᴄ-15*

Particles	ATPase	Aerobic-TH	ATP-TH	Nonde-pendent-TH
Washed				
ML308-225	100	74	38	424
etc-15	48	24	14	345
Stripped				
ML308-225		35	0	922
etc-15		14	0	646

[a] nmoles/min/mg protein.

[b] Assayed as in Ref. 23 as reduction of 3-acetyl-pyridine-NAD⁺ by NADPH.

when compared to the wild type. In order to see if the energy defect was related to the lower specific activity of the ATPase we purified this enzyme to homogeneity. The homogeneous enzyme had a lower specific activity than that from ML308-225 (Table I) although the two enzymes comigrated on polyacrylamide gels at pH 8.7 (Fig. 3; left gel). Examination of the subunit structure of the two enzymes on polyacrylamide gels in the presence of SDS revealed a distinct difference in the rate of migration of the γ-polypeptide of the ATPase (Fig. 3; middle and right gels). The increased rate of migra-

tion of this polypeptide, although small, has been verified numerous times and appears to be a real difference between the two enzymes. No difference in the rate of migration of the α, β, δ, and ε-polypeptides between the mutant and the parent could be detected. The increased rate of migration of the γ-subunit in the enzyme from the mutant would be consistent with the deletion of a small part of the polypeptide chain.

The ability of the electrophoretically homogeneous ATPases from ML308-225 and *etc-15* to restore aerobic- and ATP-dependent transhydrogenation to stripped particles of both strains is shown in Fig. 4. On a weight basis the mutant ATPase appeared to be less efficient in restoring energy-dependent transhydrogenation than the enzyme from the parent strain. However, the final activity achieved with both enzymes was similar. These results suggest that the mutant ATPase may bind less efficiently to the stripped particles such that larger amounts are required for saturation of the binding sites.

It is also clear from Fig. 4 that an additional defect to that present in the ATPase must occur in the mutant strain. Even at saturating levels of the ATPase the energy-dependent transhydrogenase activities were lower than in the parent strain. It is probably this defect, and not that in the ATPase, which accounts for the drastic lowering

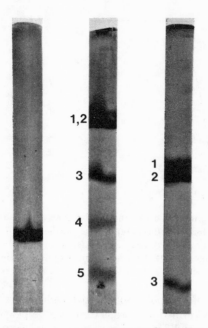

FIG. 3. Electrophoresis of purified preparations of the ATPases of *E. coli* ML308-225 and *etc-15*. The gels were run using the split gel technique (24) with the enzyme from strain ML308-225 applied to the left half of the top of each gel and with that of *etc-15* to the right half. The middle and right-hand gels were run in the presence of 0.1% SDS following depolymerization of the enzymes as described in Methods. Smaller amounts of the two enzymes were applied to the right-hand gel to obtain resolution of the α- and β-polypeptides. The durations of electrophoresis for the middle and right-hand gels were 2 and 3.5 h, respectively. Bands 1–5 indicate polypeptides α–ε. The enzymes on the left-hand gel were not depolymerized and were run in Tris–glycine buffer, pH 8.7.

of energy-dependent transhydrogenase and transport activities which initially prompted examination of the ATPase of *etc-15*.

DISCUSSION

Much remains to be discovered about the function of the individual subunit polypeptides of the coupling factor ATPases of mitochondria, chloroplasts, and the bacterial cytoplasmic membrane. The most extensive studies have been carried out with the ATPase from chloroplasts by Nelson *et al.* (11, 14). These workers observed that a preparation having α, β, and γ polypeptides

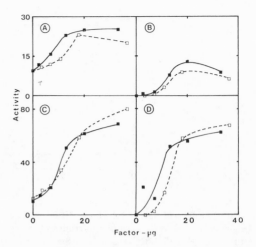

FIG. 4. Effect of purified ATPases ("factor") of *E. coli* ML308–225 (solid points) or *etc-15* (open points) on the aerobic-drive (A, C) and ATP-driven (B, D) transhydrogenase activities of stripped particles from ML308-225 (C, D) or *etc-15* (A, B). Activity is expressed as nmoles NADPH formed/min. The amounts of stripped particles of ML308–225 and *etc-15* were 0.73 and 0.89 mg protein, respectively.

was still active as a coupling factor for photophosphorylation, and retained its ATPase activity (14). The precise function of the α, β, and γ subunits was not determined. However, antibodies against both α and γ polypeptides were required to inhibit the ATPase activity of the complete coupling factor. Antibodies against β or δ polypeptides were ineffective. This suggested that the α and γ subunits might have the active site for ATP hydrolysis (11). The ε polypeptide appeared to have a regulatory function since it would inhibit the ATPase activity of the complete coupling factor (14). It seems to be analogous in function to the ATPase inhibitor of mammalian mitochondria which is believed to control the back flow of energy from ATP to the mitochondrial electron- and ion-transport systems (21). No function for the δ subunit was determined.

The only previous information regarding the role of the subunits of ATPase in bacterial systems has been provided by Salton and Schor (13). These workers solubilized the ATPase from the membranes of *Micrococcus lysodeikticus* by butanol treatment.

It differed from another form of ATPase which was released by a washing procedure in that it had only the α and β polypeptides, that it would not rebind to ATPase-depleted membranes, and that it was not stimulated by trypsin. Thus, for ATPase activity the α and β subunits had to be present, whereas one (or more) of the other subunits was required for binding of the enzyme to the membrane and for the masking of the ATPase activity. It is possible that one of these other polypeptides might correspond to nectin. Nectin is a protein (MW 37,000) which is not found as a subunit of the ATPase of *Streptococcus faecalis*, as isolated, but is required for the binding of the enzyme to the cytoplasmic membrane (22). The ATPases of *M. lysodeikticus* (13) and of *E. coli* (12) prepared by washing procedures do not require a dissociable binding protein like nectin for attachment to the membrane, but a protein with this function is presumably a subunit of these ATPases as isolated.

The results described in the present paper extend the information given above particularly with regard to the coupling factor activity of the ATPase in bacterial systems. Modification of the γ-polypeptide as occurs in the ATPase of *etc-15* is associated with a somewhat lower ATPase activity. This agrees with the results for chloroplast ATPase where the γ-subunit has some involvement in ATPase activity. The coupling factor activity is partly affected in that more of the enzyme from the mutant than from the parent is required to obtain full stimulation of the energy-dependent transhydrogenase. This might be due to impairment of binding of the ATPase to the membrane but we have no clear evidence for this yet.

Removal, or possibly modification, of the δ-subunit of the ATPase by alkaline gel electrophoresis has a much greater effect on coupling factor activity than on ATPase activity. Thus, although this result agrees with those of Salton and Schor (13) and of Nelson *et al.* (14) which indicate this subunit is not directly involved in ATP hydrolysis, it differs from the findings of the latter workers with the chloroplast ATPase in that it appears to be essential for energy coupling in *E. coli*. If this difference is substantiated,

it will show that, regardless of the apparently similar polypeptide subunit structure of ATPases from various sources, the function of the individual polypeptides in these enzymes may not be the same.

The reason why gel electrophoresis appears to remove the δ-subunit from the ATPase of *E. coli* has not been completely determined. If the process simply involved dissociation of the subunit at the alkaline pH of the gel then the liberated subunit should be detectable on alkaline gels heavily loaded with the enzyme. However, we have not been able to detect the released subunit under these conditions. The reason for this is unclear, but this result may indicate that the δ-subunit has undergone some modification on the gels. It is possible that the other subunits of the ATPase may have been modified also, but we have no evidence for this. Attempts to duplicate the results of gel electrophoresis by taking the enzyme to pH 9 during the purification step on the sucrose gradient have at present been only partially successful in causing removal of the δ-subunit.

ACKNOWLEDGMENTS

We are pleased to acknowledge the generosity of Dr. H. R. Kaback in providing us with cultures of *E. coli* ML308–225 and *etc-15*. This work was supported by a Grant from the Medical Research Council of Canada and by the award of a Medical Research Council Studentship to P. L. Davies.

REFERENCES

1. RACKER, E. (1970) *in* Membranes of mitochondria and chloroplasts (Racker, E., ed.), p. 127, Van Nostrand Reinhold Co., New York.
2. BUTLIN, J. D., COX, G. B., AND GIBSON, F. (1971) *Biochem. J.* **124,** 75.
3. ISHIKAWA, S. (1970) *J. Biochem.* **67,** 297.
4. SENIOR, A. E. AND BROOKS, J. C. (1971) *FEBS Lett.* **17,** 327.
5. TZAGOLOFF, A., AND MEAGHER, P. (1971) *J. Biol. Chem.* **246,** 7328.
6. FARRON, F. (1970) *Biochemistry* **9,** 3823.
7. DAVIES, P. L., AND BRAGG, P. D. (1972) *Biochim. Biophys. Acta* **266,** 273.
8. MIRSKY, R., AND BARLOW, V. (1973) *Biochim. Biophys. Acta* **291,** 480.
9. SCHNEBLI, H. P., VATTER, A. E., AND ABRAMS, A. (1970) *J. Biol. Chem.* **245,** 1122.
10. MUNOZ, E., SALTON, M. R. J., NG, M. H.,

AND SCHOR, M. T. (1969) *Eur. J. Biochem.* **7**, 490.

11. NELSON, N., DETERS, D. W., NELSON, H., AND RACKER, E., (1973) *J. Biol. Chem.* **248**, 2049.

12. BRAGG, P. D. AND HOU, C. (1972). *FEBS Lett.* **28**, 309.

13. SALTON, M. R. J., AND SCHOR, M. T. (1972) *Biochem. Biophys. Res. Commun.* **49**, 350.

14. NELSON, N., NELSON, H., AND RACKER, E. (1972). *J. Biol. Chem.* **247**, 7657.

15. KANNER, B. I., AND GUTNICK, D L. (1972) *FEBS* Lett. **22**, 197.

16. SIMONI, R. D., AND SCHALLENBERGER, M. K. (1972) *Proc. Nat. Acad. Sci. USA* **69**, 2663.

17. HONG, J. S., AND KABACK, H. R. (1972) *Proc. Nat. Acad. Sci. USA* **69**, 3336.

18. BRAGG, P. D., DAVIES, P. L., AND HOU, C.

(1972) *Biochem. Biophys. Res. Commun.* **47**, 1248.

19. BRAGG, P. D. AND HOU, C. (1972) *Biochim, Biophys. Acta* **274**, 478.

20. KAWASAKI, T., SATOH, K., AND KAPLAN, N. O. (1964) *Biochem. Biophys. Res. Commun.* **17**, 648.

21. VAN DE STADT, R. J., DE BOER, B. L., AND VAN DAM, K. (1973) *Biochim. Biophys. Acta* **292**, 338.

22. BARON, C., AND ABRAMS, A. (1971) *J. Biol. Chem.* **246**, 1542.

23. KAPLAN, N. O. (1967) *in* Methods in enzymology (Estabrook, R. W., and Pullman, M. E., eds.), Vol. 10, p. 317, Academic Press, New York.

24. DUNKER, A K., AND RUECKERT, R. R. (1969) *J. Biol. Chem.* **244**, 5074.

Reprinted from *Biochemistry* **15**:4163–4170 (1976)

Molecular Polymorphism and Mechanisms of Activation and Deactivation of the Hydrolytic Function of the Coupling Factor of Oxidative Phosphorylation[†]

Robert Adolfsen and Evangelos N. Moudrianakis*

ABSTRACT: The 13S coupling factor of oxidative phosphorylation from *Alcaligenes faecalis* has a latent adenosine triphosphatase (ATPase) function that can be activated by heating at 55 °C for 10 min at pH 8.5 in 50% glycerol. The specific activity increases from 0.1 to 20–30 μmol min^{-1} mg^{-1}. Adenosine 5'-triphosphate (ATP) is not required for stabilization at 55 °C when glycerol is present. Activation involves displacement of the endogenous ATPase inhibitor subunit (ϵ subunit), and readdition of this subunit results in deactivation. In the deactivation process the ATPase inhibitor subunit can be replaced by other cationic proteins such as protamine, histones, or poly(lysine). Mg^{2+} and H^+ also are effective deactivators. The fact that every positively charged substance tested deactivated the enzyme suggests that the inhibitor subunit is complexed with the enzyme at a site containing a surplus of negative charges. The activated enzyme is not cold labile, but it is salt labile, having a half-life of 2–3 min in 0.1 M KI at either 25 or 0 °C. The activated ATPase is also inhibited by aurovertin, 7-chloro-4-nitrobenzo-2-oxa-1,3-diazole (NBD), and by the cross-linking agent dimethyl suberimidate. Evidence for polymorphism comes from finding that the properties of the unactivated enzyme (intrinsic ATPase) are different in many ways from the properties of activated ATPase. With respect to the coupling factor's ability to hydrolyze ATP, the data in this study suggest that there are at least four distinct functional allomorphs of this enzyme: (1) the latent enzyme, which has no kinetically measurable ATPase activity, (2) intrinsic ATPase, which is catalyzed by a small percentage of the molecular population that has been activated by some natural mechanism, (3) activated ATPase, which has properties different from those of intrinsic ATPase, and (4) aged activated ATPase, in which some of the properties (K_m for substrate, sensitivity to deactivation by Mg^{2+} and H^+) spontaneously change within 30 min.

The coupling factor of oxidative phosphorylation is a polymorphic enzyme (Moudrianakis and Adolfsen, 1975). *Structural polymorphism* of HLF[1] (and also of F_1 and CF_1) was the subject of a previous publication (Adolfsen et al., 1975). Five electrophoretically distinct species of HLF were found. Since polyacrylamide gel electrophoresis resolves proteins on the basis of their size and charge, each of these species must be slightly different in terms of its size and/or charge. Sodium dodecyl sulfate gel electrophoresis showed that each species contained four classes of subunits (α, β, γ, and ϵ). This suggested that all of the allomorphs had the same molecular weight. Therefore, the differences between them could be due to differences either in the three dimensional arrangement of subunits or in the tertiary structure of the individual subunits. Conceptually, such differences could easily give rise to species having different surface charge distributions and/or different molecular volumes. The allomorphs were also *interconvertible* by treatment with ATP, by aging, or by exposure to phosphate buffer during the isolation procedure. The interconvertibility of species is referred to as *polymorphic flux*.

HLF also exhibits *functional polymorphism* (Adolfsen and Moudrianakis, 1976). By this we mean that the enzyme population consists of a number of different allomorphs, the presence of which can be detected by some functional assay—for example, nucleotide binding. One species of HLF did not bind any nucleotide (ADP or ATP), another bound nucleotide very slowly (turnover time 1–2 h), and a third had sites available for very rapid interaction with nucleotide. This last species is responsible for the very low level of ATPase activity (about 0.1 μmol min^{-1} mg^{-1}) that is catalyzed by an enzyme preparation that hs not been subjected to any treatment that would "activate" the hydrolytic function. Since the enzyme preparations did not exhibit a rapidly equilibrating site, even during equilibrium nucleotide binding studies, we concluded that the allomorph responsible for the low ATPase activity was present in very small amounts in the enzyme population. As in the case of structural polymorphism, there was also some indication that these functionally different species were interconvertible.

The low level of ATPase activity catalyzed by the enzyme preparation was termed "intrinsic" ATPase, since it was manifest without any special treatment that would result in activation. Most investigators in this field of research prefer to study the properties of an enzyme that has been activated either by heat treatment, treatment with a reducing agent, or trypsinization. We felt that it was important to study the indigenous or intrinsic level of activity because of the possibility that the harsh treatments used to activate the enzyme might alter basic catalytic properties and give rise to kinetic anomalies (Adolfsen and Moudrianakis, 1973). The data in the present paper demonstrate that this is no longer a speculative possibility: heat activation does indeed give rise to changes in the kinetic properties of the enzyme. This means that any

[†] From the Department of Biology, The Johns Hopkins University, Baltimore, Maryland 21218. *Received April 15, 1976.* Contribution No. 868. This work was supported by National Institutes of Health Grant AI-02443.

[1] Abbreviations used are: HLF, heat-labile factor, the 13S coupling factor from *Alcaligenes faecalis;* F_1, the 13S coupling factor from beef heart mitochondria; CF_1, the 13S coupling factor from spinach chloroplasts; NBD-Cl, 7-chloro-4-nitrobenzo-2-oxa-1,3-diazole chloride; Mes, 2-(*N*-morpholino)ethanesulfonic acid; EDTA, ethylenediaminetetraacetic acid; Tris, 2-amino-2-hydroxymethyl-1,3-propanediol; Hepes, 4-(2-hydroxyethyl)-1-piperazineethanesulfonic acid; AMP, ADP, ATP, adenosine mono-, di-, and triphosphate; ATPase, adenosine triphosphatase; P_i, inorganic phosphate; $HClO_4$, perchloric acid.

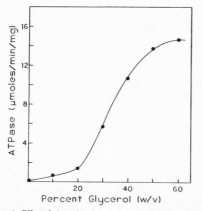

FIGURE 1: Effect of glycerol on heat activation of ATPase. HLF was incubated at 0.1 mg/ml in 10 mM Tris (pH 8.5) plus the indicated concentration of glycerol for 5 min at 60°C, after which ATPase activity was measured as described under Methods.

studies that are performed on activated ATPase are subject to restrictive interpretations, and that generalizations as to how the enzyme functions when it is membrane-bound and in vivo should not be made. The value of studies on the activated HLF is, at this point, solely to learn about the protein chemistry of the active site and the details of the chemical mechanism by which ATP is hydrolyzed. Subsequent experiments on intrinsic ATPase or the ATpase activity of the membrane-bound enzyme may yield the information necessary to deduce how ATP is utilized as a source of energy for various cellular processes in vivo.

This paper has four themes: the first is mechanisms of activation and deactivation of the hydrolytic function; the second is comparison of the properties of intrinsic ATPase and activated ATPase; the third is functional polymorphism of the activated ATPase; the fourth is comparison of the properties of HLF ATPase to those of other ATPases, especially F_1, to further demonstrate how similar these types of enzymes are.

A note on terminology: we will use the term "heat activation" or simply "activation" to refer to the effect of incubating the enzyme at high temperature prior to commencing the assay. This is distinct and separate from "kinetic activation", which refers to the essentially instantaneous activation by ions and/or other effectors that occurs in the reaction mixture in the course of the assay. The term "deactivation" will be used to describe a reduction in the ATPase function (either intrinsic or activated) that occurs when the enzyme is preincubated under specified conditions. This term will be applied only when the loss of activity occurs without dissociation of the enzye into subunits. Loss of activity due to dissociation into subunits is simply "lability." The term "inhibition" will be used to refer to a decrease in the kinetic parameters of the enzyme caused by changes in the composition of the assay medium.

Methods and Materials

HLF was isolated by the previously described procedure (Adolfsen et al., 1975), which gave type IB HLF (the most native electrophoretic species) with small amounts of type IA enzyme. Occasionally, small amounts of type IIB also were present.

The hydrolytic function was activated by incubating HLF at a concentration of 0.10 mg/ml in 10 mM Tris or trietha-

nolamine buffer at pH 8.5, containing 50% glycerol (w/v), at 55 °C for 10 min (or 60 °C for 5 min), after which the enzyme was placed on ice.

ATPase activity was assayed by incubating 2 μg of enzyme for 1 min at 37 °C in 0.50 ml of reaction mixture containing 1 mM ATP, about 50 000 cpm of [γ-^{32}P]ATP, 0.3 mM KCl, and 10 mM Tris (pH 8.5). Substrate hydrolysis was between 5 and 10%. The reaction was terminated by adding 0.5 ml of 10% HClO$_4$, which was followed by 1 ml of 5% HClO$_4$ containing 25 mg/ml of Norit A to adsorb nucleotide. The charcoal was removed by suction filtration through a glass fiber filter, and the filtrate (containing the product [^{32}P]P$_i$) was collected in a scintillation vial. The reaction vessel was washed with two successive 2-ml volumes of 1% HClO$_4$ to ensure quantitative transfer of radioactivity, and Čerenkov radiation was measured in a Packard Model 2002 liquid scintillation spectrometer at 65% gain.

Intrinsic ATPase was measured by incubating 2 μg of HLF for 20 min at 37 °C in 0.50 ml of reaction mixture containing 0.10 mM ATP, about 50 000 cpm of [γ-^{32}P]ATP, 0.10 mM MgCl$_2$, 30 mM KCl, and 10 mM Tris (pH 8.5). The rest of the procedure was the same as described above.

Electrophoresis in 5% polyacrylamide in the Hepes–imidazole buffer system was carried out as previously described (Adolfsen et al., 1975). Sodium dodecyl sulfate gel electrophoresis was carried out according to Weber and Osborn (1969).

Materials. Aurovertin was isolated by Dr. John Barnes of this laboratory, using the method described by Chang and Penefsky (1974). Reagent [γ-^{32}P]ATP was synthesized by the method of Weiss et al. (1968), using [^{32}P]P$_i$ obtained from New England Nuclear Corp. Dimethyl suberimidate was from Pierce Chemical Co. Buffers and other reagents were obtained from Sigma Chemical Co.

Results

Heat Activation of HLF ATPase. Heat activation of coupling factor ATPase is usually optimized by having a high concentration of ATP present to prevent heat denaturation. About 30 mM was optimal for CF$_1$ (Farron and Racker, 1970). However, this procedure brought the activity of HLF up to only about 1 μmol min^{-1} mg^{-1} (Adolfsen and Moudrianakis, 1971b). During attempts to improve the activation, we found that glycerol was an effective stabilizing agent for HLF (Figure 1) with a maximal activity evident at 50–60% (w/v). Glycerol had no effect on activity unless the enzyme was incubated at high temperatures. Since glycerol can bind to proteins (Detrich et al., 1976), and since higher concentrations of glycerol can induce conformational changes in a variety of proteins (Myers and Jakoby, 1975), it was important to determine whether the glycerol in the reaction mixture (carried over with the enzyme from the preincubation step) had any effect on initial velocity. We found that the initial velocity of ATP hydrolysis by heat-activated HLF was not affected by glycerol when the concentration of glycerol in the assay medium did not exceed 25%; higher glycerol concentrations were inhibitory. In all the assays reported in the present study the only glycerol present was that carried together with the enzyme from the heat-activation pretreatment; this amounted to a final glycerol concentration of 2–4% in the assay mixture. Thus, it is clear that the effect shown in Figure 1 is due entirely to the stabilizing effect of glycerol on the enzyme at elevated temperature and cannot be attributed to any kinetic effects of glycerol on the assay.

Time courses of activation at various temperatures are

TABLE I: Polymorphic Flux of Activated ATPase.[a]

Preincubation at Room Temp (min)	Sp Act. (μmol min^{-1} mg^{-1})	% Decrease	Apparent V_m	Apparent K_m
0	18.4	0	29	0.41
30	13.4	27	19	0.35
90	9.0	51	13	0.29

[a] The enzyme was heat activated for 5 min at 60 °C as described under Methods, after which substrate saturations were performed with 0, 30, or 90 min of preincubation at room temperature. MgCl$_2$ and ATP were varied at a constant ratio of 1:3, which was the optimal ratio. The kinetic constants were determined from double-reciprocal plots.

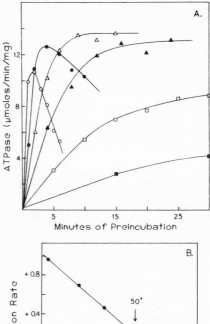

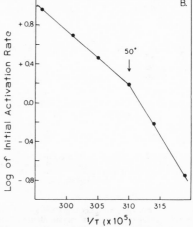

FIGURE 2: Effect of temperature on heat activation of ATPase. (A) Time courses of activation were carried out with HLF at 0.1 mg/ml in 10 mM Tris (pH 8.5) and 50% (w/v) glycerol at the indicated temperatures: (■) 40 °C; (□) 45 °C; (▲) 50 °C; (△) 55 °C; (●) 60 °C; (○) 65 °C. (B) Arrhenius plot of initial velocity of heat activation.

shown in Figure 2A. The highest level of activation was reached after 10 min at 55 °C, and there was no significant heat denaturation for at least 15 min at this temperature. Figure 2B is an Arrhenius plot of the initial velocity of heat activation. A discontinuity occurred at 50 °C. Below 50 °C the activation energy was 47 kcal, while above this temperature it decreased to 25 kcal.

Attempts to further optimize activation resulted in the following findings: maximal activation occurred between pH 8 and 9 (measured at 25 °C), and it declined sharply below pH 7.5 and above pH 9.0. Activation was greatest at 0.10 mg/ml of enzyme protein; specific activities were about 50% lower when the enzyme was 1.0 or 0.01 mg/ml. Supplementing the incubation mixture with 1 mM ATP had no effect, 1 mM ADP inhibited activation by 40%, 1 mM AMP had no effect, and 1 mM P$_i$ inhibited activation by 40%. Inclusion of 1 mM MgCl$_2$ inhibited activation by 50%, while 1 mM EDTA gave a small and variable stimulation (usually about 10%). Increasing the ionic strength by adding KCl to 0.1 M resulted in a 40% inhibition of activation. Dithiothreitol (1 or 10 mM) had no effect, 0.1% Triton X-100 had no effect, 0.5 M urea inhibited by 50%, and 2% ethanol inhibited 100%. Polyacrylamide gel electrophoresis showed that ethanol caused a very rapid dissociation of the enzyme into subunits at elevated temperatures.

Stability of Activated ATPase. The activated enzyme exhibited a partial lability that was dependent upon the temperature to which it was exposed subsequent to its activation. When kept at 0 °C, there was no significant change in activity for at least 1 h. At 25 °C (room temperature), the activity decreased by about 30% in the first 30 min and by about 50% within 2 h. The remaining activity was stabe for at least 2 days longer at room temperature. The partial lability was accelerated by incubation at 37 °C, with about 50% loss of activity in 30 min.

This partial lability was not due simply to denaturation of the activated enzyme. If it were, the apparent V_m would decrease while the apparent K_m remained constant. The data in Table I show that the K_m decreased by 15% after 30 min and by 30% after 90 min. These data indicate that there are at least two forms of activated ATPase, which may be distinguished by their K_m values. Their interconversion is another instance of polymorphic flux. Other properties of the activated enzyme also change during aging (see below).

As part of a search for further evidence of polymorphism of activated ATPase, the kinetic parameters K_m and V_m were determined during a time course of activation at 60 °C similar

to the one illustrated in Figure 2A. The K_m was constant from 1 to 10 min of incubation at 60 °C, with the only variation being in the V_m. The K_m was also constant when the enzyme was activated for 30 min at 45 °C, for 20 min at 50 °C or for 10 min at 55 °C. Thus, the process of activation can be described as a simple two-state conversion—unactivated to activated.

The activated enzyme is *not* cold labile as long as the incubation medium does not contain significant amounts of salt. This may also be true of F$_1$ to some extent, although the importance of salts is not usually stressed. Figure 3 shows the lability of heat-activated HLF in 0.1 M KI. The half-life was 2–3 min, and temperature did not have a significant effect on it. Because of these results, we will refer to this property as "salt lability" instead of cold lability.

The mechanism of salt lability is the same as that usually described for cold lability. Polyacrylamide gel electrophoresis

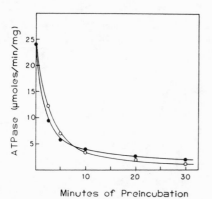

FIGURE 3: Salt lability of activated ATPase. The activated enzyme was incubated for the indicated length of time in 0.1 M KI and assayed. The protein concentration was 0.01 mg/ml and glycerol was 5%. (O) 0 °C; (●) 25 °C.

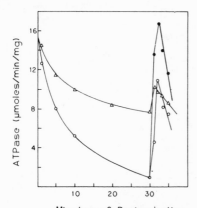

FIGURE 4: Reversibility of deactivation of ATPase by Mg^{2+}. Freshly activated enzyme was incubated at 37 °C with or without 1 mM $MgCl_2$. At 30 min, the temperature was changed to 60 °C. (△) control system without $MgCl_2$; (O) system with $MgCl_2$; (●) system with $MgCl_2$ that was made 1 mM in EDTA just before changing the incubation temperature. ATPase activity was measured as described under Methods.

showed that KI acted by promoting dissociation of the enzyme into subunits. KI also promoted dissociation of the unactivated enzyme into subunits, though at a much slower rate than for the activated enzyme.

Salt lability is also important when ATPase activity is measured in reaction mixtures containing 30 mM KCl (or higher). The half-life of activated enzyme preincubated in unlabeled reaction mixture and then sampled for subsequent assay in labeled reaction mixture was about 7 min. This is quite different from the results obtained with intrinsic ATPase, where preincubation in 30 mM KCl had no significant effect on activity and where time courses were linear for at least 20 min of incubation at 37 °C (10% hydrolysis of substrate).

In addition to its role during heat activation, glycerol also plays a role in stabilizing the activated enzyme. When the activated enzyme was diluted tenfold in 10 mM Tris (pH 8.5) the partial lability that occurred at room temperature more than doubled. However, this additional lability did not occur

TABLE II: ATPase Inhibitor Subunit of HLF.[a]

Preincubation (min)	% Deactivation by a Given Molar Excess of Inhibitor		
	2.5×	5×	10×
3	16	76	91
10	35	83	91
20	55	81	85

[a] Freshly activated HLF was mixed with the supernatant fraction of heat-denatured HLF (prepared as described in text) and incubated for the indicated length of time at room temperature before being assayed for ATPase activity. The percent deactivation was computed with respect to a system incubated with the same solvent that the ATPase inhibitor preparation contained. This compensated for lability of ATPase activity due to addition of some KCl to the activated ATPase along with the inhibitor. The molar excess of ATPase inhibitor was computed assuming complete release during heat treatment.

when the dilution was performed in buffer containing 50% glycerol. Glycerol also reduced the salt lability, increasing the half-life in 0.1 M KI from 2 min to more than 10 min.

ATPase Inhibitor Subunit of HLF. The ATPase inhibitor subunit of F_1 can be released from the enzyme by heat treatment (Warshaw et al., 1968). To determine if HLF contained an inhibitor subunit, the enzyme was incubated for 2 min at 100 °C at 1 mg/ml in the presence of 0.1 M KCl. KCl promoted coagulation of the denatured large polypeptides, which facilitated their removal by centrifugation. The supernatant fraction contained less than 10% of the total enzyme protein. Sodium dodecyl sulfate gel electrophoresis showed only one polypeptide present in large amounts. This was the small one having a molecular weight of about 12 000 (ϵ subunit). The experiment shown in Table II demonstrates that this supernatant fraction also contained an ATPase inhibitor. If we assume complete release and recovery of the inhibitor by this procedure, then the system containing undiluted extract had a tenfold molar excess of inhibitor over activated ATPase. The results show that the more dilute inhibitor solution was effective if longer preincubation was permitted before assay. The ATPase inhibitor in the heat extract was also excluded from a Bio-Gel P-6 column, which indicated that it is a macromolecule. Taken together, these facts indicate that the small polypeptide subunit of HLF is the ATPase inhibitor subunit and that it is similar to those reported in F_1 and CF_1 (Pullman and Monroy, 1963; Horstman and Racker, 1970; Brooks and Senior, 1971; Nelson et al., 1972). An interesting question (which we cannot answer at present) is whether there is 1 or more than 1 ATPase inhibitor subunit/molecule of HLF.

Deactivation of ATPase. When F_1 is incubated with Mg^{2+}, ATPase activity is rapidly lost (Caterall and Pedersen, 1972). When HLF was incubated with 1 mM Mg^{2+} for 10 min at 37 °C, a 60% decrease in activity was observed. Similar degrees of deactivation were found with 1 mM Ca^{2+}, Mn^{2+}, Zn^{2+}, Cd^{2+}, Cu^{2+}, Fe^{2+}, Co^{2+}, Ba^{2+}, or Sr^{2+}. The deactivation by Mg^{2+} was completely prevented by having equimolar amounts of ATP present to chelate the cation. Polyacrylamide gels showed that this deactivation did not involve dissociation of the enzyme into subunits.

Mg^{2+} deactivation is reversible (Figure 4). A second heat treatment step resulted in recovery of all of the lost activity. The extent of reactivation was higher when EDTA was added before heating. A control system incubated with EDTA at 37

TABLE III: Deactivation of ATPase by Polycationic Substances.[a]

System	Sp Act.	% Deactivation
Control	14.0	
Spermine	6.7	53
Spermidine	10.4	26
Histones	12.4	12
Cytochrome c	11.4	18
Protamine	3.9	73
Polylysine:		
mol wt 2 000	6.5	54
15 000	6.1	57
30 000	4.9	65
85 000	3.8	74

[a] HLF (100 μg/ml) was activated for 10 min at 55 °C, cooled to room temperature, and incubated with each of the indicated cationic materials (50 μg/ml) for 10 min, after which specific activity (μmoles min^{-1} mg^{-1}) was determined as described under Methods.

°C showed only a threefold increase of activity in 60 min (not shown). This result suggests that temperature is more important than EDTA with respect to reactivation. In another experiment, the free Mg^{2+} was removed by passing the enzyme through a Bio-Gel A 0.5 column. The ATPase activity did not increase significantly, but full reactivation was obtained by heating at 60 °C for 2 min. EDTA had no significant effct on this reactivation, indicating that the stimulation by EDTA in the experiment shown in Figure 4 was due to removal of free Mg^{2+} and not due to interaction of EDTA with the enzyme. This conclusion is supported by the finding (reported above) that 1 mM $MgCl_2$ inhibited heat activation of ATPase by nearly 50%.

Another method of deactivation was incubation at a lower pH. When Mes buffer at pH 6.0 was added to a final concentration of 20 mM to give a final pH of 7.0, ATPase activity decayed with a half-life of about 3 min, with about 90% deactivation being attained after 15 min of incubation at 37 °C. Polyacrylamide gel electrophoresis showed once again that the deactivation did not involve dissociation of the enzyme into subunits. Partial reactivation was obtained by raising the pH back up to 8 and heating for 2 min at 60 °C.

The three types of deactivation have different characteristics. Mg^{2+} deactivation was prevented by chelating agents such as EDTA or ATP, whereas deactivation by adding H^+ or ATPase inhibitor subunit was not affected. Also, freshly activated enzyme was almost totally deactivated by adding Mg^{2+} or H^+, but after aging for 1 h at room temperature Mg^{2+} deactivated only about 50%, and adding H^+ gave only about 40% deactivation. In contrast, aging had no effect at all on the ability of the enzyme to be deactivated by the ATPase inhibitor. This deactivation was nearly complete, even after aging for 1 day at 25 °C.

The properties of intrinsic ATPase were significantly different from those of activated ATPase. With intrinsic ATPase, incubation with 2 mM $MgCl_2$ gave about 20% deactivation. Lowering the pH to neutrality resulted in no reduction of activity at all. And the equivalent of a tenfold molar excess of ATPase inhibitor gave only 15% deactivation.

Mechanism of Deactivation. All three ways of obtaining deactivation of ATPase involve adding a positively charged material—Mg^{2+}, H^+, or the ATPase inhibitor subunit. (Knowles and Penefsky (1972) have reported that the inhibitor subunit of F_1 has an isoelectric pH of about 10.) This raised the possibility that any cationic substance could cause deac-

tivation. The results in Table III show that all of the cationic substances tested were indeed effective in promoting deactivation. The least effective were cytochrome c and histones. When the length of the preincubation was increased from 10 to 60 min, the deactivation by histones increased to 42% and the deactivation by cytochrome c increased to 43%. Polyanions, such as poly(glutamate) and poly(ethylene sulfonate) (also at 50 μg/ml), had no effect at all when preincubated with the ATPase for up to 60 min. These results suggest that deactivation involves covering up important negative charges on the surface of the activated enzyme.

Partial reactivation of ATPase was obtained as follows: first, deactivation was effected by incubating the ATPase for 10 min at 25 °C with poly(lysine) at 50 μg/m; then poly(glutamat) was added to 50 μg/ml to remove the excess poly(lysine) by complexing with it. There was no reversal of deactivation. However, when the system was incubated for 5 min at 55 °C, the activity increased from 1.5 to 5.5 μmol min^{-1} mg^{-1}. This may be compared to the activity of the untreated control, which was 10 μmol min^{-1} mg^{-1}.

Poly(glutamate) also protected the enzyme against poly(lysine)-induced activation. There was no detectable deactivation when poly(glutamate) was added to the enzyme before the poly(lysine) or when the two polyions were mixed first and then added to the enzyme.

Aurovertin. As part of a continuing effort to determine whether intrinsic and activated ATPase are similar or different, we tested their sensitivity to a number of substances that are known to have potent effects on other coupling factor ATPases. Thus, the kinetic effect of aurovertin on both the intrinsic and activated ATPase functions of HLF was examined. Intrinsic ATPase was inhibited 80% by 1 μM aurovertin, and activated ATPase was inhibited 60%. Increasing the concentration up to 20 μM had no further effect. Even preincubating the enzyme with 10 μM aurovertin for 10 min at 25 °C gave the same amount of inhibition as that observed by simply having 1 μM aurovertin present in the assay mixture. This ruled out the possibility that the inhibition was partial because binding of aurovertin to the enzyme was slow, and it demonstrated that there is no preincubation effect of aurovertin on purified HLF.

Aurovertin was also a very potent inhibitor of ATP synthesis by the membrane-bound coupling factor. Using the previously described assay (Adolfsen and Moudrianakis, 1971a), oxidative phosphorylation was 95% inhibited by 1 μM aurovertin. Half-maximal inhibition occurred at 0.05 μM aurovertin.

NBD-Cl. Ferguson et al. (1975) reported that NBD-Cl deactivates the ATPase function of F_1 by reacting with tyrosine at the active site. Time courses of deactivation of the ATPase function of HLF were performed in 0.1 mM NBD at 25 °C. Semilog plots of the remaining activity were linear with time, indicating that the decay was first order. The half-life of intrinsic ATPase was about 2 min, while that of activated ATPase was about 3 min (not significantly different). Aging the activated ATPase for 1 h at room temperature did not affect the half-life.

It was also of interest to determine whether the unactivated enzyme was sensitive to NBD. The unactivated enzyme was incubated for 20 min at 25 °C with 0.1 mM NBD, passed through a Sephadex G-50 M column to remove excess NBD, and then heat activated. The specific activity was 0.7 μmol min^{-1} mg^{-1}, compared to 11.2 for another sample of enzyme treated in exactly the same manner but with no NBD present. Thus, the target residues are accessible to NBD even before heat activation.

Suberimidate. Bragg and Hou (1975) reported that the *E. coli* membrane ATPase is sensitive to a cross-linking agent called dithiobis(succinyl propionate). The ATPase activity of HLF is sensitive to another cross-linking agent, dimethyl suberimidate. When activated ATPase was incubated with 0.01% suberimidate in 20 mM triethanolamine buffer (pH 8.5), a first-order decay of activity was found, which had a half-life of 6 min. After aging for 1 h at 25 °C, the half-life was about 4 min (not significantly different). Under these same conditions, suberimidate had no effect on intrinsic ATPase activity. Increasing the concentration by tenfold gave 30% deactivation of intrinsic ATPase activity after 10 min at 25 °C. These results suggested that the groups that were cross-linked to result in deactivation of the activated ATPase did not have the same spatial geometry as those in the intrinsic ATPase.

It was also of interest to determine whether the unactivated enzyme could be influenced by suberimidate. The unactivated enzyme was incubated with 0.1% suberimidate for 30 min at 25 °C, passed through a Sephadex G-50 M column to remove excess reagent, and then heat activated. The specific activity was 12.3 μmol min^{-1} mg^{-1}, which was about the same as that of the untreated control. Thus, the groups in the activated ATPase that are sensitive to the cross-linking agent have a different spatial orientation in the unactivated enzyme.

Kinetic Activation by Ions. Further differences between intrinsic and activated ATPases were found in studies on effects of ionic activators. First, the enzyme hydrolyzes free ATP at a slow rate in the complete absence of any added divalent cation activators. We previously suggested that this might be due to the presence of a tightly bound metal in the enzyme—i.e., that the enzyme was a metalloprotein (Adolfsen and Moudrianakis, 1973). The specific activity of intrinsic Mg^{2+}-independent ATPase was about 0.1 μmol min^{-1} mg^{-1}. After heat activation it was about 1.0 μmol min^{-1} mg^{-1}. The K_m of both intrinsic and activated enzyme was approximately 0.1 mM. Both activities were inhibited by a variety of metal-complexing agents, such as EDTA, azide, and citrate. However, the enzyme changed its response to hydroxyquinoline as a consequence of heat activation. There was very little inhibition (about 15%) by 2 mM hydroxyquinoline before heat treatment, but after heat treatment the inhibition was 85%. A similar effect was seen with *o*-phenanthroline (also 2 mM). The enzyme behaved in the same manner toward the more hydrophobic chelator bathophenanthroline, except that 85% inhibition occurred at a concentration of 5 μM instead of 2 mM. These data suggest that the site with which the chelators interact is more accessible in the activated ATPase than it is in the intrinsic ATPase and also that it is hydrophobic.

Further differences were found with respect to activation by divalent cations. Mg^{2+} stimulated intrinsic ATPase by about 1.5-fold. Activated ATPase was stimulated more than 20-fold. Also, monovalent cations controlled the selectivity of intrinsic ATPase for the divalent cation activator. Almost any divalent cation could stimulate intrinsic ATPase if the reaction mixture did not contain monovalent cations, but only Mg^{2+} and Fe^{2+} were stimulatory when monovalent cations were present (Adolfsen and Moudrianakis, 1973). This interesting regulatory property was absent from the activated ATPase. The order of effectiveness of stimulation for activated ATPase was $Mg^{2+} > Mn^{2+} > Co^{2+} > Cd^{2+} > Zn^{2+}$, and monovalent cations did not change it.

Discussion

We propose the following hypothesis for the mechanism of activation and deactivation of ATPase: The ATPase inhibitor subunit is cationic and is electrostatically complexed with the enzyme at a region containing a number of negative charges; heat activation involves displacement of the inhibitor subunit and a conformational change in the protein; negative charges that become exposed during heat activation are instrumental in holding the protein in the proper conformational state for ATP hydrolysis; deactivation involves covering these negative charges, which permits a return to an inactive conformational state. Support for the individual aspects of this hypothesis is given below.

The presence of negative charges in the bonding domain between the enzyme and the inhibitor subunit can be inferred from the deactivation studies. Preincubating the activated ATPase with every cationic substance tested here promoted deactivation (Tables II, III, Figure 4). Preincubating the activated enzyme with anions either had no effect, as in the case of poly(glutamate) and poly(ethylene sulfonate), or it prevented deactivation by a cationic substance, as in prevention of Mg^{2+} deactivation by EDTA or ATP, or as in prevention of poly(lysine) deactivation by poly(glutamate). These effects can be explained in terms of the formation of complexes between the anionic substances and the appropriate cationic substances, which makes the cationic substances unavailable for complexing with the enzyme.

The data presented here underscore the potential for the appearance of serious artifacts during attempts to isolate an inhibitor for the ATPase function of the 13S coupling factor. All the polycationic peptides tested in Table III could erroneously qualify for this, thus raising the possibility that many more cellular basic polypeptides could fit in this category. It appears to us then, that before deciding that a certain polypeptide is indeed a specific inhibitor of the ATPase function of the 13S coupling factor, it must be demonstrated that this polypeptide normally exists in a molecular complex with the coupling factor.

The two most important conditions for obtaining high levels of activation were alkaline pH and high temperature. Since the ATPase inhibitor protein is cationic, it is reasonable to expect that negative charges in solution (OH^-) would stabilize the inhibitor and thereby promote its solubility. The temperature requirement for activation (Figure 2A) suggests that high temperature increases the rate constant for the approach to the new equilibrium. Figure 2A also shows that the maximal level of activation was higher at higher temperatures. This suggests that temperature may also affect the absolute magnitude of the equilibrium constant.

The occurrence of a conformational change during heat activation is suggested by the discontinuity in the Arrhenius plot in Figure 2B. Warshaw et al. (1968) also report a conformational change during heat activation of F_1, which they detected by optical rotatory dispersion measurements. The fact that deactivation of HLF was not reversible simply by removing the deactivation agent—by gel filtration, by increasing pH, by adding EDTA to remove Mg^{2+}, or by adding poly(glutamate) to remove poly(lysine)—but required a second exposure to high temperature, suggests that the deactivation process involves a second conformational change. The deactivation is presumably a return to a state resembling the original, unactivated enzyme. The events occurring during reactivation may be a repeat of the changes that occurred during the first heat activation. Moyle and Mitchell (1975) have also reported on reversible active/inactive state transitions in mitochondrial F_1, which may be similar to those mentioned here for HLF.

The involvement of negative charges, in general, in holding

TABLE IV: Comparison of Properties of HLF Allomorphs.

Property	E_1 (Latent)	E_2 (Intrinsic)	E_3 (Activated)	E_4 (Aged)
Salt lability	Low	Low	High	
Deactivation by $MgCl_2$		20%	90%	50%
Deactivation by lowering pH		0%	90%	40%
Deactivation by ATPase inhibitor subunit		15%	95%	95%
Aurovertin inhibition		80%	60%	
Inhibition by NBd)0.1 mM)	Sensitive	$t_{1/2}$ 2 min	$t_{1/2}$ 3 min	$t_{1/2}$ 3 min
Inhibition by suberimidate (0.01%)	Not sensitive	Not sensitive	$t_{1/2}$ 6 min	$t_{1/2}$ 4 min
Inhibition by bathophenanthroline (10 μM)		15%	85%	
Stimulation by $MgCl_2$		2×	20×	
Regulation by KCl		Yes	No	
K_m for ATP		0.1 mM	0.4 mM	0.3 mM

the protein in the activated state is suggested by the lack of specificity for the deactivating agent that was observed during the deactivation studies. Any substance that can neutralize these charges promotes deactivation. Lowering the pH may actually play a dual role. First, addition of H^+ can result in neutralization of the negative charges on the enzyme. Second, the equilibrium of the ATPase inhibitor subunit may be shifted back toward association with the enzyme due to a reduction in the number of stabilizing charges in solution. It is interesting to note that the effectiveness of the inhibitor subunit of F_1 in deactivating the ATPase function of this enzyme was found to be greater at lower pH values (Pullman and Monroy, 1963; Horstman and Racker, 1970).

The reason for the partial lability of the activated enzyme is not understood. One possibility that has been ruled out is dissociation of some of the molecules into subunits, since this would not explain changes in the properties of the enzyme (lower K_m and decreased sensitivity to Mg^{2+} and H^+). It is possible that a partial deactivation could be effected by the very dilute inhibitor subunit (5 μg/ml at most) that is still present in the solution. The inhibitor may not complex in the same way as it was originally complexed, so that deactivation is only partial and other properties also change. An alternative explanation is that the activated enzyme is metastable and spontaneously relaxes into a different conformational state that does not have inhibitor bound to it but which is sufficiently different to result in changes in some of its properties.

Differences in the properties of intrinsic, activated, and aged activated ATPase indicated that there was functional polymorphism in the enzyme preparation. This polymorphism may be explained by the simple scheme in Figure 5. The previously reported finding that the enzyme did not have a detectable rapidly equilibrating nucleotide binding site led to the conclusion that only a small portion of the molecules are responsible for the intrinsic ATPase activity of the preparation (Adolfsen and Moudrianakis, 1976). Thus, the unactivated preparation is mostly E_1 with a small amount of E_2. E_2 may be molecules that have undergone activation by some other, natural mechanism, since the preparation was not treated in any manner that would cause activation. Heat activation converts E_1 into E_3, and extended exposure to high temperature leads to denaturation (Figure 2A). The properties of E_3 are different from those of E_2; these differences are summarized in Table IV. The properties of activated ATPase are stable for at least 1 h if the enzyme is kept at 0 °C. (There is no significant lability at 0 °C unless salt is added.) However, the K_m for substrate decreases and the ability of the enzyme to be deactivated by Mg^{2+} and H^+ drops by approximately 50% when

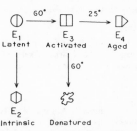

FIGURE 5: Proposed scheme to explain polymorphism of ATPase. The symbols represent different overall conformations of the enzyme functioning as an ATPase (not an ATP synthetase), and the bilateral symmetry is consistent with current views on the subunit stoichiometry of the enzyme. The arrows indicate the observed sequence of events and are not meant to imply irreversibility of conversions.

the enzyme is incubated at higher temperatures. This is a case of polymorphic flux, in which E_3 converts into E_4 with a half-time of about 30 min. It is important to prevent this from happening if careful studies are to be done on the enzyme kinetics of ATP hydrolysis. To study the properties of E_3, the enzyme is placed on ice immediately after heat activation and used within 10 min. To study E_4, the enzyme is aged for 2 h at 25 °C prior to being assayed.

The polymorphism observed in this system so far is quite extensive. There are five separate and distinct electrophoretic forms of HLF (Adolfsen et al., 1975). In addition to this structural polymorphism, we now have evidence for five functional allomorphs. There are the four described in the present paper (Figure 5) plus an additional form, which was detected in nucleotide binding studies as being incapable of binding any nucleotide (Adolfsen and Moudrianakis, 1976). This form would be a subpopulation of E_1 in the scheme in Figure 5. Thus far, we have found no evidence for any direct or one-to-one correspondence between the structural and functional allomorphs. If each functional allomorph can exist in each of the five structural states (or vice versa), then there may be a total of 25 different states in which this enzyme may exist in vitro. This is a theoretical maximum. If, on the other hand, a direct one-to-one correlation could be established between each structural allomorph and one and only one functional allomorph, then the theoretical minimum of five states could be reached. However, we have not yet been able to demonstrate such one-to-one correspondence, and our experimental obervations suggest that this number could be closer to ten. The question arises as to whether these different states are all just in vitro artifacts or whether they have some significance in vivo. Undoubtedly, some of them exist only under special in vitro conditions. However, previous studies showed that the native slow and fast electrophoretic species (types IA and IB) were present on the membrane and could undergo interconversions while bound to the membrane. If we also concede that the enzyme can exist in either a latent or an activated state on the membrane, there are a minimum of four species which may have in vivo significance. One may ask what is the use of having all of these different species on the membrane. The answer to this question may be that the 13S coupling factor is a multienzyme system that in the cell is required to perform a number of different functions (not only ATP synthesis, but also several other energy-linked functions, including various forms of transport), and plasticity of structure is advantageous for adapting the multienzyme system to these various functions. In short, the enzyme may need to be polymorphic simply because it is polyfunctional.

Acknowledgments

We thank Dr. Morris Burke for a gift of dimethyl suberimidate. We also thank Mr. Mark McDonnell for his excellent technical assistance in isolating the enzyme used in most of these studies.

References

Adolfsen, R., McClung, J. A., and Moudrianakis, E. N. (1975), *Biochemistry 14*, 1727.

Adolfsen, R., and Moudrianakis, E. N. (1971a), *Biochemistry 10*, 434.

Adolfsen, R., and Moudrianakis, E. N. (1971b), *Biochemistry 10*, 2247.

Adolfsen, R., and Moudrianakis, E. N. (1973), *Biochemistry 12*, 2926.

Adolfsen, R., and Moudrianakis, E. N. (1976), *Arch. Biochem.* *Biophys. 172*, 425.

Bragg, P. D., and Hou, C. (1975), *Arch. Biochem. Biophys. 167*, 311.

Brooks, J. C., and Senior, A. E. (1971), *Arch. Biochem. Biophys. 147*, 467.

Caterall, W. A., and Pedersen, P. L. (1972), *J. Biol. Chem. 247*, 7969.

Chang, T., and Penefsky, H. S. (1974), *J. Biol. Chem. 249*, 1090.

Detrich, H. W., Berkowitz, S. A., Kim, H., and Williams, R. C. (1976), *Biochem. Biophys. Res. Commun. 68*, 961.

Farron, F., and Racker, E. (1970), *Biochemistry 9*, 3829.

Ferguson, S. J., Lloyd, W. J., Lyons, M. H., and Radda, G. K. (1975), *Eur. J. Biochem. 54*, 117.

Horstman, L. L., and Racker, E. (1970), *J. Biol. Chem. 245*, 1336.

Knowles, A. F., and Penefsky, H. S. (1972), *J. Biol. Chem. 247*, 6624.

Moudrianakis, E. N., and Adolfsen, R. (1975), in Electron Transfer Chains and Oxidative Phosphorylation, Quagliariello, E., et al., Ed., Amsterdam, North Holland Publishing Co., pp 373–378.

Moyle, J., and Mitchell, P. (1975), *FEBS Lett. 56*, 55.

Myers, J. S., and Jakoby, W. B. (1975), *J. Biol. Chem. 250*, 3785.

Nelson, N., Nelson, H., and Racker, E. (1972), *J. Biol. Chem. 238*, 3762.

Pullman, M. E., and Monroy, G. C. (1963), *J. Biol. Chem. 238*, 3762.

Warshaw, J. B., Lam, K. W., Nagy, B., and Sanadi, D. R. (1968), *Arch. Biochem. Biophys. 123*, 385.

Weber, K., and Osborn, M. (1969), *J. Biol. Chem. 244*, 4406.

Weiss, B., Live, T. R., and Richardson, C. C. (1968), *J. Biol. Chem. 243*, 4530.

Editor's Comments
on Papers 27 and 28

27   **BUTLIN, COX, and GIBSON**
Oxidative Phosphorylation in Escherichia coli *K12: Mutations Affecting Magnesium Ion- or Calcium Ion-Stimulated Adenosine Triphosphatase*

28   **KANNER and GUTNICK**
Use of Neomycin in the Isolation of Mutants Blocked in Energy Conservation in Escherichia coli

THE GENETIC APPROACH

Butlin, Cox, and Gibson had earlier carried out a careful study of ubiquinone function in the respiration of *Escherichia coli* using the mutant approach.[1] (Contrast the conclusions reached by that group with those obtained by Kashket and Brodie,[2] who employed classical biochemical techniques in their investigation of the role of quinones in terminal electron transport.) The isolation of ATPase-deficient mutants incapable of oxidative phosphorylation, described in Paper 27, initiated a most fruitful series of experiments, by several investigators, which have combined searches for mutants deficient in energy conservation with biochemical characterization of the ATPase as in Papers 27 and 28. Gibson and Cox reviewed their progress in 1973.[3]

Enrichment for a desired mutant is frequently a difficult and time-consuming task. Kanner and Gutnick in Paper 28 provide an imaginative selection procedure for mutants deficient in energy conservation. The relationship of neomycin sensitivity to energy-conserving mechanisms is still unclear.

The discovery of plasmid-borne genes encoding for respiratory enzymes, especially in the pseudomonads, has furnished a further experimental technique for modifying the ability of procaryotes to attach substrates oxidatively. An outstanding example of such work is found in reference 4.

REFERENCES

1. Cox, G. B., N. A. Newton, F. Gibson, A. M. Snoswell, and J. A. Hamilton. *Biochem. J.*, **117**, 551–562, 1970.
2. Kashket, E. R., and A. F. Brodie. *Biochim. Biophys. Acta,* **78**, 52–65, 1963.
3. Gibson, F., and G. B. Cox. *Essays in Biochemistry,* **9**, 1–31, 1973.
4. Chakrabarty, A. M. *J. Bacteriol.,* **112**, 815–823, 1972.

27

Reprinted from *Biochem. J.* **124**:75–81 (1971)

Oxidative Phosphorylation in *Escherichia coli* K12

MUTATIONS AFFECTING MAGNESIUM ION- OR CALCIUM ION-STIMULATED ADENOSINE TRIPHOSPHATASE

By J. D. BUTLIN, G. B. COX AND F. GIBSON

Department of Biochemistry, John Curtin School of Medical Research, Institute of Advanced Studies, Australian National University, Canberra, A.C.T. 2601, Australia

(*Received* 18 *March* 1971)

1. Two mutants of *Escherichia coli* K12 were isolated which, although able to grow on glucose, are unable to grow with succinate or D-lactate as the sole source of carbon. 2. Genetic mapping of these mutants showed that they both contain a mutation in a gene (designated *uncA*) mapping at about minute 73.5 on the *E. coli* chromosome. 3. The *uncA*⁻ alleles were transferred by bacteriophage-mediated transduction into another strain of *E. coli* and the transductants compared with the parent strain to determine the nature of the biochemical lesion in the mutants. 4. The mutants gave low aerobic growth yields when grown on limiting concentrations of glucose, but oxidase activities in membranes from both the mutants and the normal strain were similar. 5. Measurement of P/O ratios with D-lactate as substrate indicated that a mutation in the *uncA* gene causes uncoupling of phosphorylation associated with electron transport. 6. Determination of the Mg^{2+},Ca^{2+}-stimulated adenosine triphosphatase activities in the mutant and normal strains indicated that the *uncA* gene is probably the structural gene for Mg^{2+},Ca^{2+}-stimulated adenosine triphosphatase. 7. Mg^{2+},Ca^{2+}-stimulated adenosine triphosphatase therefore appears to be essential for oxidative phosphorylation in *E. coli*.

Oxidative phosphorylation coupled to electron transport, in both fractionated mitochondrial (Linnane & Titchener, 1960) and bacterial (Pinchot, 1953) systems, has been shown to require, in addition to a respiring membrane fraction, a number of soluble coupling factors. These factors have been classified as phosphoryltransferases, energy-transfer factors or oligomycin-sensitizing factors (see Lardy & Ferguson, 1969). Purification of the various coupling factors has been attempted but, with the exception of the Mg^{2+}-stimulated adenosine triphosphatase activity from mitochondria (Penefsky & Warner, 1965), most preparations seem to consist of mixtures of coupling factors or mixtures of coupling factors and other membrane components (Lam, Warshaw & Sanadi, 1968; Racker, 1964).

It is a difficult practical problem to damage membrane preparations specifically and reproducibly in such a way as to obtain a system lacking only the one factor under consideration (see Lehninger, 1964). The methods used generally involve sonication followed by treatment with trypsin, trypsin–urea, or phosphatides (Racker,

1963). In theory, the study of microbial mutants that lack specific enzymic activities concerned in the coupling reactions could be used to overcome the problem of lack of specificity inherent in other approaches. A mutant of *Saccharomyces cerevisiae* that had the phenotype expected for an 'uncoupled' mutant, i.e. lack of growth on oxidizable non-fermentable carbon sources, normal amounts of cytochromes and apparently normal respiration, has been described (Kovac, Lachowicz & Slonimsky, 1967). However, a detailed biochemical investigation (Somlo, 1970) seems to indicate that strains carrying this mutation cannot be considered as uncoupled. The use of bacteria with their simpler cellular organization than eucaryotic cells, and of *Escherichia coli* in particular, with its amenability to genetic manipulations, seems a promising experimental system for a combined genetic and biochemical approach to the problem of coupling of phosphorylation to electron transport. The present paper describes an investigation of two mutant strains of *E. coli* which have the phenotypic characteristics expected for mutants in which phosphorylation is uncoupled from electron transport.

MATERIALS AND METHODS

Chemicals and enzymes. Piericidin A was kindly provided by Professor S. Tamura, Department of Agricultural Chemistry, University of Tokyo, Japan. Chemicals generally were of the highest purity available commercially and were not further purified. Glucose 6-phosphate dehydrogenase and hexokinase were obtained from Boehringer G.m.b.H., Mannheim, Germany.

Organisms. All the bacterial strains used in this work were derived from *E. coli* K12 and are shown in Table 1.

Media. The mineral-salts minimal medium 56 described by Monod, Cohen-Bazire & Cohn (1951) was used. Sterile solutions of various carbon sources to give a final concentration of 30 mM were added to the sterilized mineral-salts base. Additional amino acid supplements (0.2 mM) and thiamin (0.2 μM) were added as required. The cells used for genetic experiments were grown on a tryptone–yeast extract broth (Luria & Burrous, 1957). The nutrient broth was solidified with 2% (w/v) Difco agar as required.

Streptomycin-resistant mutants. Spontaneous streptomycin-resistant mutants were obtained by the method of Cox, Gibson & Pittard (1968).

Transduction techniques. The generalized transducing bacteriophage P1kc was used for transduction experiments as described by Pittard (1965).

Conditions for conjugation experiments. The conditions under which mating was carried out were similar to those described by Taylor & Thoman (1964), with the modifications used by Cox et al. (1968).

Growth conditions. Growth yields of various strains were obtained as described by Cox, Newton, Gibson, Snoswell & Hamilton (1970), by using a medium containing limiting glucose. The turbidities were measured at intervals until growth was complete, i.e. when two successive readings taken at 60 min intervals on a Klett–Summerson colorimeter were similar.

For growth under anaerobic conditions, the cultures were incubated at 37°C in tubes with loosely fitting tops in an atmosphere of H_2, in a Gallenkamp anaerobic culture jar fitted with a platinum catalyst.

For the preparation of cell extracts (from strains AN120 and AN180) the growth from a nutrient agar slope was suspended in medium 56 and added to 1 litre of medium 56 supplemented with glucose, arginine and thiamin. This culture was shaken overnight at 37°C, and then used to inoculate 9 litres of medium in a 14 litre New Brunswick fermenter. The fermenter was kept at 37°C, aerated at 12 litres/min, stirred at 600 rev./min and the culture harvested at about 0.6 mg dry wt. of cells/ml.

Preparation and fractionation of cell extracts. The cells were washed, a cell extract was prepared with a Sorvall Ribi Cell Fractionator at 20000 lb/in² and the membranes were separated by $(NH_4)_2SO_4$ precipitation as described by Cox et al. (1970). The procedure was modified slightly for the preparation of membranes for adenosine triphosphatase determinations. In this case, the cells were washed in 0.05 M-imidazole buffer (pH 7.2), resuspended in fresh imidazole buffer (4 ml of buffer/1.0 g wet wt. of cells) and then fractionated as described above. The precipitate obtained after $(NH_4)_2SO_4$ fractionation was resuspended in 4 ml of imidazole buffer per original 1.0 g wet wt. of cells. All operations on the harvested cells were conducted at 0–4°C. Proteins were determined with Folin's phenol reagent (Lowry, Rosebrough, Farr & Randall, 1951) with bovine serum albumin (fraction V; Sigma Chemical Co., St Louis, Mo., U.S.A.) as standard.

Determination of fermentation products. The supernatants obtained after centrifuging cultures grown in the

---

Table 1. *Strains of* E. coli *K12 used*

Genes coding for enzymes in various biosynthetic pathways are denoted as follows: *thi*, thiamin; *ilv*, isoleucine–valine; *arg*, arginine; *met*, methionine; *leu*, leucine; *pro*, proline; *pur*, purine; *trp*, tryptophan; *thr*, threonine; *ubi*, ubiquinone. Streptomycin resistance is denoted by *str^R*. The two mutant alleles *uncA401* and *uncA402* are described in this paper. Abbreviation: MNNG, *N*-methyl-*N*′-nitro-*N*-nitrosoguanidine.

Strain	Sex	Relevant genetic loci	Other information
AB259	Hfr	*thi⁻*	Hfr Hayes. Obtained from J. Pittard
AN118	♀	*thi⁻, uncA401*	Derived from strain AB259 after MNNG treatment
AN119	♀	*thi⁻, uncA401, str^R*	Derived from strain AN118 by spontaneous mutation
JP58	♀	*ilvC7, argE3, thi-1, str^R*	Obtained from J. Pittard
AN120	♀	*argE3, thi-1, str^R, uncA401*	Isolated after transduction with strain AN119 as donor and strain JP58 as recipient
AN180	♀	*argE3, thi-1, str^R*	Isolated after transduction with strain AN119 as donor and strain JP58 as recipient
AB3311	Hfr	*metB⁻, thi⁻*	Hfr Reeves, Hfr1 (Echols et al. 1961). Obtained from J. Pittard
AN181	Hfr	*metB⁻, thi⁻, uncA402*	Derived from strain AB3311 after MNNG treatment
AB1515	♀	*leu⁻, proC⁻, purE⁻, trp⁻, str^R*	Obtained from J. Pittard
AN182	♀	*proC⁻, purE⁻, trp⁻, thi⁻, uncA402*	Recombinant obtained after conjugation between strains AN181 and AB1515
AN183	♀	*argE3, thi-1, str^R, uncA402*	Isolated after transduction with strains AN182 as donor and strain JP58 as recipient
AN59	Hfr	*thr-1, leu-6, ubiB⁻*	See Cox, Young, McCann & Gibson (1969)
AB2154	Hfr	*metE⁻, thr-1, leu-6*	Obtained from J. Pittard
AB2826	♀	*aroB351*	Obtained from J. Pittard

New Brunswick fermenters were examined by g.l.c. for volatile and non-volatile fermentation products (Doelle, 1969). Volatile fermentation products were determined by g.l.c. on a Porapak Q column at 180°C with N_2 as carrier gas. Trimethylsilyl derivatives of the non-volatile fermentation products were determined on a 10% SE-30 Chromosorb W(60–80) column with N_2 as carrier gas, the temperature being raised from 100°C to 250°C at 4°C/min.

Measurement of oxygen uptake. Measurements of oxidase activity were made by using an oxygen electrode as described by Cox *et al.* (1970). The reaction mixture contained (final concentrations): 1.3mg of protein, 15mM-sodium–potassium phosphate buffer (pH 7.4), 1.9mM-$MgCl_2$, in a final volume of 2.5ml. The substrates, succinate (8mM), lactate (4mM) or NADH (1.2mM), were added as indicated. Buffer solutions were calibrated for oxygen content by the method of Chappell (1964).

Difference spectra. Difference spectra for the determination of cytochromes b_1, a_1, a_2 and o and the flavoproteins in the membrane preparations were recorded as described by Cox *et al.* (1970) except that an Aminco Chance spectrophotometer was used.

Determination of quinones. The ubiquinone and menaquinone contents of 5g samples of whole cells were determined as described by Cox *et al.* (1968).

Assay of adenosine triphosphatase. Membrane fractions prepared in imidazole buffer were assayed for Mg,Ca-ATPase* activity as described by Evans (1969). The reaction mixture contained, in a final volume of 1ml, 0.1M-tris–HCl buffer (pH 9), 5mM-ATP and other additions as described in the text. The reaction was initiated by the addition of 50µl of membrane preparation containing about 250µg of protein. The tubes were shaken at 37°C in a water bath for 30min and the reaction was terminated by the addition of 1.0ml of 5% (v/v) $HClO_4$. Phosphate was determined by the method of King (1932) on 0.5ml samples of the reaction mixture, with correction for acid hydrolysis of ATP.

P/O ratios. Oxygen uptake was measured in constant-volume Warburg manometers at 30°C (Umbreit, Burris & Stauffer, 1951). CO_2 was removed by 0.2ml of 10% (w/v) KOH in the centre well of the manometer flasks. The flasks were incubated for 10min before being sealed, after which membrane preparations (150µl) containing 3.9mg of protein were tipped from the side arm into the main section of the flasks, which contained, in a total volume of 3.0ml, 20mM-glucose, 13mM-KF, 5mM-sodium–potassium phosphate buffer (pH 7), 5mM-$MgCl_2$, 16.7mM-AMP, 4.2mM-ADP, hexokinase and other additions as indicated in the text. Lactate (20mM, pH 7) was used as substrate. The reactions were terminated after 30min by the addition of 0.3ml of 35% (v/v) $HClO_4$, the precipitated protein was removed by centrifugation and the supernatants were neutralized with 10% KOH. The precipitated $KClO_4$ was removed by centrifugation and the glucose 6-phosphate contents of samples of the supernatants were determined fluorimetrically (Greengard, 1963). The reaction mixture contained 0.8mM-$NADP^+$, 17mM-$MgCl_2$, 3mM-EDTA (pH 7.4) and 17mM-triethanolamine buffer (pH 7) in a total volume of 1.5ml. The formation of NADPH after the addition of glucose 6-phosphate dehydrogenase (0.5 Kornberg unit) was determined fluori-

* Abbreviation: Mg,Ca-ATPase, Mg^{2+},Ca^{2+}-stimulated adenosine triphosphatase activity.

metrically with an Aminco–Bowman spectrophotofluorimeter (excitation wavelength, 360nm; emission wavelength, 460nm, uncorrected). The estimated amount of glucose 6-phosphate formed was corrected for the amount formed in the absence of lactate, which amounted to about 25% of the total glucose 6-phosphate formed by membranes from the normal strain.

RESULTS

During the examination of a number of mutants able to grow with glucose but not succinate as the sole source of carbon (Suc⁻ mutants), two strains were found which gave low aerobic growth yields in a glucose medium, but appeared to possess normal activities of the NADH oxidase and D-lactate oxidase systems. The mutant strains (AN118 and AN181) were therefore examined in detail.

Genetic mapping. Strain AN118, although derived from an Hfr male, was found to be a female and therefore the mutation causing the Suc⁻ phenotype could be mapped by using interrupted-mating experiments. A spontaneous streptomycin-resistant derivative of strain AN118 was obtained and designated AN119. The latter strain was then used in an interrupted mating experiment with the Hfr strain AB3311, and Suc⁺ recombinants selected on a medium containing succinate as sole carbon source together with streptomycin to kill the ex-conjugant

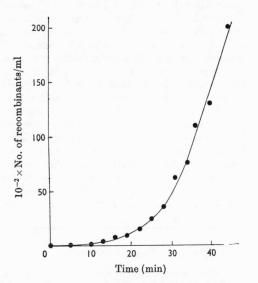

Fig. 1. Kinetics of zygote formation when the female strain AN119 was mated with the Hfr strain AB3311. The ordinate scale shows the interval between the time when the parental cultures were mixed together (zero time) and the time at which the sample was vortexed to interrupt mating.

males. A time of entry of about 10 min for the wild-type allele was obtained (Fig. 1) indicating that the mutation causing the Suc⁻ phenotype was in a gene transferred early by the Hfr strain AB3311. The marker (*phoS*) nearest to the origin of transfer of this Hfr strain maps at about minute 73.5 on the *E. coli* genome (Echols, Garen, Garen & Torriani, 1961; Taylor, 1970). The mutation causing the Suc⁻ phenotype was located more precisely by tests for co-transduction with two genes, namely *metE* at minute 74.5 and *ilvC* at minute 74. The generalized transducing bacteriophage Plkc was grown on strain AN119 and used for co-transduction experiments with strains AB2154 (*metE⁻*) and JP58 (*ilv⁻*). All the 200 *metE⁺* transductants examined were able to grow with succinate as sole carbon source, whereas only 50 out of 84 *ilv⁺* transductants were able to grow on succinate. The mutation affecting growth on succinate and the *ilvC* gene were therefore co-transducible at a frequency of about 40%. The co-transduction results are consistent with the mutation present in strain AN119 being located at about minute 73.5 on the *E. coli* genome, and the gene carrying this mutation was designated *uncA401*. An *ilv⁺*, *unc⁻* transductant (strain AN120) and an *ilv⁺*, *unc⁺* transductant (strain AN180) were retained for further study.

The mutation in the second strain (AN181), in which oxidative phosphorylation was possibly uncoupled, was also mapped. Strain AN181 was an Hfr male, and a mating was carried out with the female AB1515 (*leu⁻*, *proC⁻*, *purE⁻*, *trp⁻*) selecting for either Leu⁺, Pro⁺, Pur⁺ or Trp⁺ recombinants. Ex-conjugant males were killed by the inclusion of streptomycin in the selective media. The recombinants were then examined for the Suc⁻ phenotype. Aerobic growth yields of the Suc⁻ recombinants showed that a Leu⁺, Suc⁻ strain (AN182) had the same low growth yield as strain AN120 (*unc⁻*). Strain AN182 was then used as a recipient in an interrupted mating experiment with the Hfr male AB3311. A time of entry which was similar to that described above for the mating with strain AN119 was obtained for the wild-type allele. Co-transduction tests were carried out with strain AN182 as donor and strain JP58 as recipient. Transductants that were Ilv⁺ were then screened

for their ability to grow on succinate as sole source of carbon, and 45% of the Ilv⁺ recombinants (27 out of 60 tested) were found to be of the Suc⁻ phenotype. One of the Suc⁻ transductants (strain AN183) was retained for further investigation.

The mutation in strain AN183 affecting growth on succinate was apparently in the same region of the chromosome as the *unc* mutation in strain AN120. A bacteriophage lysate prepared on strain AN120 (*uncA401*) was used as donor and strain AN182 as recipient, selecting for Suc⁺ transductants. The numbers of Suc⁺ transductants obtained were normalized with respect to the numbers of Pro⁺ transductants obtained by using the same bacteriophage lysates. The Suc⁺ transductants were detected at frequencies of about 2% of the frequencies obtained by using a bacteriophage lysate prepared on a wild-type strain (AB2826) (Table 2). The mutations in strains AN182 and AN120 affecting growth on succinate were probably in the same gene and the mutation in strains AN182 and AN183 was therefore designated *uncA402*.

A study of the biochemical effects of mutations in the *uncA* gene was made by a comparison of three of the strains referred to above. These were strain AN120 carrying the *uncA401* allele, strain AN183 carrying the *uncA402* allele and, as a control, the Ilv⁺, Unc⁺ transductant (strain AN180). The latter strain will be referred to as the normal strain. The results obtained with both mutant strains were identical within experimental error, and therefore only the results with one of them (strain AN120) are described in detail.

Growth characteristics and the metabolic products of normal and mutant strains. Apart from the inability of the mutant strains to grow on a medium with succinate or D-lactate as sole source of carbon, the mean generation time in glucose–mineral salts medium was longer for the mutants, being 1.5 h compared with 1 h for the normal strain. Examination by g.l.c. of the products of glucose metabolism by the mutant and the normal strains grown under aerobic conditions showed that the concentrations of succinate, lactate and ethanol in the culture supernatants were the same for the normal and mutant strains. However, the concentrations of acetate in the culture supernatants of the normal

---

Table 2. *Transduction crosses involving strains AN120 (uncA401) and AN182 (uncA402)*

The transducing bacteriophage Plkc was grown on either strain AB2826 (Pro⁺, Suc⁺) or on strain AN120 (Pro⁺, Suc⁻) and used as donor with strain AN182 (Pro⁻, Suc⁻) as recipient. Either Pro⁺ or Suc⁺ transductants were selected.

Donor	Recipient	Number of Pro⁺ transductants	Number of Suc⁺ transductants
AB2826	AN182 (*uncA402*)	125	290
AN120 (*uncA401*)	AN182 (*uncA402*)	370	10

and mutant strains differed, and were 9mM and 14mM respectively.

Determination of the growth yields, measured as turbidities, of the strains growing on media containing limiting concentrations of glucose showed (Fig. 2) that the aerobic growth yield of strain AN120 (*unc⁻*) was lower than that of the normal strain. However, the aerobic growth yield of strain AN120 (*unc⁻*) was higher than the anaerobic growth yield of the normal strain.

Concentrations of membrane components in strains AN180 and AN120 (unc⁻). Concentrations of total flavin and cytochromes in the membrane fractions from strain AN120 (*unc⁻*) and strain AN180 were determined from the reduced-minus-oxidized difference spectra. It was found (Table 3) that the concentrations in the normal and mutant strains did not differ significantly. Similarly the concentrations of ubiquinone and vitamin K in the normal and mutant strains, determined after extraction and partial purification, were not significantly different (Table 3). Examination of the membranes by electron-spin-resonance spectroscopy showed that the signal attributed to ubisemiquinone (Hamilton, Cox, Looney & Gibson, 1970) and the signal attributed to 'non-haem iron' could be demonstrated in both the normal and the mutant strains (J. A. Hamilton, personal communication).

Oxidase systems in strains AN180 and AN120 (unc⁻). The NADH oxidase and lactate oxidase systems have been shown to be quantitatively the most significant in membranes from *E. coli* K12 grown with glucose as carbon source (Cox *et al.* 1970). Comparison of these two oxidase systems in strains AN180 and AN120 showed that there was no significant difference in NADH oxidase activity between the normal and mutant strains (about 1000ng-atoms of O/min per mg of protein), whereas the lactate oxidase activity in membranes from the mutant (340ng-atoms of O/min per mg of protein) was 35% higher than that in membranes from the normal strain. It was found that there was considerable variation in the succinoxidase activities of different batches of membranes, although a similar range of activities was found in both the normal and mutant strains.

Oxidative phosphorylation by membranes from strains AN180 and AN120 (unc⁻). Oxidative phosphorylation was examined by using lactate rather than NADH as the oxidizable substrate, since the presence of the reduced nicotinamide nucleotide interfered with the assay system used. A mixture of AMP and ADP was used for the determination of oxidative phosphorylation to inhibit adenylate kinase activity (Slater, 1953) present in the membrane preparations. The P/O ratio of 0.12 found for the normal strain (Table 4) is low but consistent with the values found for most

bacterial systems (see Gel'man, Lukoyanova & Ostrovskii, 1967).

2,4-Dinitrophenol (0.3 mM) uncoupled oxidative phosphorylation by 75% whereas piericidin A (0.13mM) completly prevented phosphorylation. This concentration inhibited lactate oxidase activity by only 41% (Table 4).

There was no detectable phosphorylation by strain AN120 (*unc⁻*) and it therefore appears that

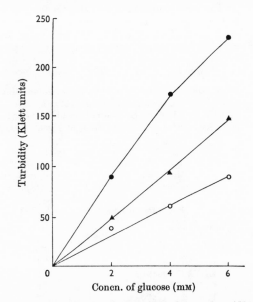

Fig. 2. Growth yields (turbidity) for strains AN180 and AN120 (*unc⁻*) grown on limiting concentrations of glucose. Cultures were aerated by shaking at 37°C and anaerobic cultures were incubated in an anaerobic jar. ●, Strain AN180, aerobic; ○, strain AN180, anaerobic; ▲, strain AN120 (*unc⁻*), aerobic.

Table 3. *Concentrations of some membrane components in strains AN180 and AN120* (unc⁻)

Experimental methods are described in the Materials and Methods section.

Membrane component	Conc. of component (nmol/mg of protein)	
	Strain AN180	Strain AN120 (*unc⁻*)
Total flavin	1.3	1.0
Cytochrome b_1	0.54	0.65
Cytochrome a_2	0.02	0.02
Cytochrome o	0.24	0.28
Cytochrome a_1*	+	+
Ubiquinone	6.1	6.7
Menaquinone	2.0	2.3

* Cytochrome a_1 was present but the quantities were too low for determination.

Table 4. *Oxidative phosphorylation by membranes from strains AN180 and AN120 (unc⁻)*

Experimental details are given in the Materials and Methods section.

Membrane from strain	Alteration to basal systems in Warburg flask	Oxygen uptake* (ng-atoms/min per mg of protein)	Glucose 6-phosphate formed (nmol/min per mg of protein)	P/O ratio
AN180	—	103	12.4	0.12
AN180	Flask gassed with oxygen-free nitrogen	0	<0.1	0
AN180	2,4-Dinitrophenol (300 μM) included	84	2.3	0.03
AN180	Piericidin A (130 μM) included	58	<0.1	<0.001
AN120 (*unc⁻*)	—	121	<0.1	<0.001

* The presence of AMP and ADP in the reaction mixture used for the determination of P/O ratios inhibits the lactate oxidase system.

Table 5. *Mg,Ca-ATPase activity of membranes from strains AN180 and AN120 (unc⁻)*

Adenosine triphosphatase activity was determined by the method of Evans (1969) except that P_i was determined by the method of King (1932). Membranes were incubated with ATP (5mM) for 30min at 37°C in 0.1M-tris–HCl buffer, pH9, with other additions as indicated, in a final volume of 1ml. $MgCl_2$ was added at a final concentration of 2mM or $CaCl_2$ at 1mM.

Additions and final concn.	P_i released (μmol/mg of protein in 30 min)		Stimulation of adenosine triphosphatase activity by metal ions (μmol of P_i released/mg of protein in 30 min)	
Membranes from strain ...	AN180	AN120 (*unc⁻*)	AN180	AN120 (*unc⁻*)
None	12	6	—	—
Mg^{2+}	45	7.5	33	1.5
Ca^{2+}	30	6	18	0
EDTA (7.5μM)	1.6	0.5	—	—
EDTA (7.5μM)+Mg^{2+}	38	1.3	36	0.8
EDTA (7.5μM)+Ca^{2+}	18	1.3	16	0.8
Piericidin A (400μM)	12	—	—	—
Piericidin A (400μM)+Mg^{2+}	40	—	28	—
Piericidin A (400μM)+Ca^{2+}	30	—	18	—

a consequence of a mutation in the *uncA* gene is uncoupling of phosphorylation from electron transport.

Mg,Ca-ATPase activity of membranes from strains AN180 and AN120 (unc⁻). Evans (1969) studied adenosine triphosphatase activity in membranes from *E. coli* and suggested that there may be a single adenosine triphosphatase present activated by either Mg^{2+} or Ca^{2+}. Preliminary experiments with the membrane preparations used in the present study indicated that they possessed about the same amount of Mg^{2+}- or Ca^{2+}-stimulated adenosine triphosphatase activity as found by Evans (1969) and that Na^+ or K^+ inhibited the activity in the presence of Ca^{2+}. The stimulation by Ca^{2+} was less than that reported by Evans (1969) and the reason for this is not known. The addition of EDTA to the assay system in the absence of added Mg^{2+} or Ca^{2+} decreased the endogenous adenosine triphosphatase activity (Table 5), but the stimulation by

the bivalent metal ions remained about the same. Piericidin A had no effect on the adenosine triphosphatase activity (Table 5) and, as found by Evans (1969), 2,4-dinitrophenol did not stimulate, and azide and *p*-chloromercuribenzoate inhibited adenosine triphosphatase.

Comparison of the Mg,Ca-ATPase activity from strains AN180 and AN120 (*unc⁻*) shows that the mutation in the *uncA* gene resulted in a virtually complete (>95%) loss of activity.

DISCUSSION

The *uncA* gene mapping near minute 73.5 on the *E. coli* genome is probably the structural gene for the membrane-bound Mg,Ca-ATPase. Mutations in this gene resulted in loss of Mg^{2+},Ca^{2+}-activated adenosine triphosphatase activity, prevented growth on succinate or D-lactate as carbon source and decreased the growth rate with glucose as carbon source. Aerobic growth yields of the mutant strain grown on limiting glucose were less than those from the normal strain but not as low as the anaerobic growth yield of the normal strain. Unlike membrane preparations from the normal strain, those from the mutant strain lacked the ability to couple phosphorylation to electron transport with D-lactate as substrate. The oxidase activities in the membranes and the concentrations of a number of membrane components were not altered by lack of Mg,Ca-ATPase.

The P/O ratio of 0.12 for the normal strain *in vitro* with D-lactate as substrate makes it difficult to decide whether phosphorylation at more than one site is being measured. However, the mutants, although possessing derepressed values for D-lactate oxidase activity, are unable to grow with D-lactate as sole source of carbon, indicating that the Mg,Ca-ATPase is required for phosphorylation at both the sites coupled to lactate oxidation.

The aerobic growth yield of the Mg,Ca-ATPase-deficient strain was higher than the anaerobic growth yield of the normal strain. If it is assumed that Mg,Ca-ATPase is required for ATP production at each of the three postulated sites for NADH oxidation in the electron-transport system it would appear that some oxidative energy may be conserved via the 'energy-linked' reactions. These reactions, such as the NAD(P) transhydrogenase, utilize high-energy intermediates rather than ATP (Snoswell, 1962).

Recent work on the function of ubiquinone in *E. coli* K12, using mutants unable to form ubiquinone, has led to the proposal of a scheme for electron transport in this organism (Cox *et al.* 1970). It was suggested (Cox *et al.* 1970) that piericidin A separated ubiquinone from the remainder of the electron-transport chain. In the present experiments it has been shown that piericidin A completely uncouples oxidative phosphorylation when used at a concentration that inhibited lactate oxidation by only 41%. Piericidin A may have two points of action, the more sensitive reaction lying between the proposed iron–ubisemiquinone complex and the Mg,Ca-ATPase. Vallin & Löw (1968) have found, using mitochondria, that piericidin A has an uncoupler-like action when used at concentrations that do not affect NADH oxidase activity.

We thank Mrs R. McDowall, Mrs J. Tetley and Miss B. Humphrey for technical assistance, Mr D. Abigail for growing cultures and preparing cell extracts, and Mr L. B. James for g.l.c. determinations. We are grateful to our colleagues, Dr N. A. Newton and Dr I. G. Young, for helpful discussions.

REFERENCES

Chappell, J. B. (1964). *Biochem. J.* **90**, 225.
Cox, G. B., Gibson, F. & Pittard, J. (1968). *J. Bact.* **95**, 1591.
Cox, G. B., Newton, N. A., Gibson, F., Snoswell, A. M. & Hamilton, J. A. (1970). *Biochem. J.* **117**, 551.
Cox, G. B., Young, I. G., McCann, L. M. & Gibson, F. (1969). *J. Bact.* **99**, 450.
Doelle, H. W. (1969). *J. Chromat.* **39**, 398.
Echols, H., Garen, A., Garen, S. & Torriani, A. (1961). *J. molec. Biol.* **3**, 425.
Evans, D. J. (1969). *J. Bact.* **100**, 914.
Gel'man, N. S., Lukoyanova, M. A. & Ostrovskii, D. N. (1967). In *Respiration and Phosphorylation of Bacteria*, pp. 182–189. Ed. by Pinchot, G. B. New York: Plenum Press.
Greengard, P. (1963). In *Methods of Enzymatic Analysis*, p. 551. Ed. by Bergmeyer, H. V. New York: Academic Press Inc.
Hamilton, J. A., Cox, G. B., Looney, F. D. & Gibson, F. (1970). *Biochem. J.* **116**, 319.
King, E. J. (1932). *Biochem. J.* **26**, 292.
Kovac, L., Lachowicz, T. M. & Slonimsky, P. P. (1967). *Science, N.Y.*, **158**, 1564.
Lam, K. W., Warshaw, J. B. & Sanadi, D. R. (1968). *Archs Biochem. Biophys.* **119**, 477.
Lardy, H. A. & Ferguson, S. M. (1969). *A. Rev. Biochem.* **38**, 991.
Lehninger, A. L. (1964). In *The Mitochondrion*, p. 98. New York and Amsterdam: W. A. Benjamin Inc.
Linnane, A. W. & Titchener, E. B. (1960). *Biochim. biophys. Acta*, **39**, 469.
Lowry, O. H., Rosebrough, N. J., Farr, A. L. & Randall, R. J. (1951). *J. biol. Chem.* **193**, 265.
Luria, S. E. & Burrous, J. W. (1957). *J. Bact.* **74**, 461.
Monod, J., Cohen-Bazire, G. & Cohn, M. (1951). *Biochim. biophys. Acta*, **7**, 585.
Penefsky, H. S. & Warner, R. C. (1965). *J. biol. Chem.* **240**, 4694.
Pinchot, G. (1953). *J. biol. Chem.* **205**, 65.
Pittard, J. (1965). *J. Bact.* **89**, 680.
Racker, E. (1963). In *Energy-Linked Functions in the Mitochondrion*, p. 75. Ed. by Chance, B. New York and London: Academic Press.
Racker, E. (1964). *Biochem. biophys. Res. Commun.* **14**, 75.
Slater, E. C. (1953). *Biochem. J.* **53**, 521.
Snoswell, A. M. (1962). *Biochim. biophys. Acta*, **60**, 143.
Somlo, M. (1970). *Archs Biochem. Biophys.* **136**, 122.
Taylor, A. L. (1970). *Bact. Rev.* **34**, 155.
Taylor, A. L. & Thoman, M. S. (1964). *Genetics*, **50**, 659.
Umbreit, W. W., Burris, R. H. & Stauffer, J. F. (1951). In *Manometric Techniques and Tissue Metabolism*, 2nd ed., p. 1. Minneapolis: Burgess Publishing Co.
Vallin, I. & Löw, H. (1968). *Eur. J. Biochem.* **5**, 402.

28

Reprinted from *J. Bacteriol.* **111**:287–289 (1972)

Use of Neomycin in the Isolation of Mutants Blocked in Energy Conservation in *Escherichia coli*

BARUCH I. KANNER AND DAVID L. GUTNICK

Department of Microbiology, Tel Aviv University, Tel Aviv, Israel

Received for publication 22 November 1971

A neomycin-resistant mutant of *Escherichia coli* K-12 unable to grow on Krebs cycle intermediates has been isolated. The mutant retained its respiratory capacity, but lacked membrane Mg^{2+}-Ca^{2+}-stimulated adenosine triphosphatase activity (EC 3.6.1.3).

Selection for neomycin resistance has been used in the isolation of hemin-deficient mutants of *Escherichia coli* K-12 (13) and *Salmonella typhimurium* (12). It was postulated that respiratory-deficient cells incorporated less neomycin than normal cells (12). One explanation for this may be the inability of these mutants to generate sufficient energy to concentrate the antibiotic. It appeared possible, therefore, to employ neomycin in the positive selection of mutants rendered resistant by virtue of a defect in the ability to couple respiration to the synthesis of adenosine triphosphate (ATP). This report describes the isolation and partial characterization of one such neomycin-resistant mutant of *E. coli* K-12.

Strain A428 (F⁻, Pro⁻, Lac₁⁻, T6ᴿ, Gal₂⁻, Ara⁻, His⁻, Xyl⁻, Man⁻, B₁⁻, Strᴿ) was used as a parent organism and grown in nutrient broth to a cell density of 1.5×10^9 bacteria/ml. The cell suspension was diluted 10-fold into Davis minimal medium (4) and 4-ml portions were irradiated in petri dishes with a Phillips germicidal lamp (30 w) at a distance of 57.5 cm for 90 sec. Under these conditions the viable count was reduced about 1,000-fold. After irradiation, cells were diluted into nutrient broth containing glucose (0.5%) and yeast extract (0.5%) and incubated for 2 hr at 37 C. Samples containing between 10^4 and 10^6 cells were passed through membrane filters (Sartorius; pore size, 0.45 µm; diameter, 50 mm). The filters were washed with saline and placed on agar plates containing supplemented Davis medium (see legend to Fig. 1), glucose (0.5%), and neomycin sulfate (50 µg/ml, Sigma Chemical Co.). The plates were incubated for 3 days at 37 C, and small colonies were picked and transferred to minimal plates supplemented as above but without neomycin, and incubated at 37 C. They were then replicaplated onto supplemented minimal plates containing either succinate, malate, α-ketoglutarate, or glucose (all at 0.5%) as sole source of carbon. Out of 500 neomycin-resistant colonies examined, 14 were able to grow on glucose but were unable to utilize these Krebs cycle intermediates as sole sources of carbon and energy. Respiration was then examined in washed whole cells of these 14 mutants by using either glucose or the tricarboxylic acid cycle intermediates as substrates. A mutant blocked in coupled ATP synthesis would be expected to grow on glucose but not on Krebs cycle intermediates, yet it should retain its ability to oxidize these compounds. Three mutants were found which respired on each of the substrates to the same extent as the parent. One of these, N₁₄₄, was retained for further study.

A mutant unable to couple respiration to the synthesis of ATP might be expected to exhibit much lower growth yield under aerobic conditions than the corresponding parent strain in the presence of limiting concentrations of a carbon source (1–3, 8). A comparison of the growth yields of mutant N₁₄₄ with those of the parent A428 on limiting glucose concentrations is illustrated in Fig. 1. Under aerobic conditions the growth yield of the mutant was much lower than that of the parent. Anaerobically, the yield of mutant and parent differed slightly. Nitrate has been shown to serve as a terminal electron acceptor in place of oxygen under anaerobic conditions, and its reduction is coupled to the synthesis of ATP (11). It is of interest that, whereas the anaerobic growth yield of the parent was stimulated by the presence of nitrate, no effect of nitrate was observed in the case of the mutant (Fig. 1).

Butlin et al. (2) recently described a mutant of *E. coli* K-12, *uncA*, with similar growth characteristics (although the effect of nitrate was not reported). Evidence from cell-free studies was presented indicating that *uncA* was defective in oxidative phosphorylation and that this defect was due to an impaired Mg^{2+}-Ca^{2+}-stimulated adenosine triphosphatase (EC 3.6.1.3). The Mg^{2+}-Ca^{2+}-stimulated adenosine triphosphatase activity was therefore examined in preparations of A428 and N_{144} (Table 1). Membrane ghosts were prepared, and the adenosine triphosphatase was assayed by the procedure of Evans (5). Virtually no membrane-bound adenosine triphosphatase activity could be detected in the mutant. Evans has shown that treatment of *E. coli* membrane ghosts with sodium dodecyl sulfate (SDS) results in the solubilization and stimulation of cation-dependent adenosine triphosphatase (6). The data in Table 1 demonstrate that the

TABLE 1. *Membrane-bound and solubilized Mg^{2+}-Ca^{2+}-activated adenosine triphosphatase activity in strains A428 and N_{144}[a]*

Addition	Specific activity[b]			
	Membrane-bound		Solubilized	
	A428	N_{144}	A428	N_{144}
None	5.4	0	19.0	1.0
Mg^{2+}	29.4	0	66.0	3.6
Ca^{2+}	18.1	0	74.4	0.6

[a] Bacteria were grown to late exponential phase on supplemented Davis minimal medium (see legend to Fig. 1) containing 0.5% glucose. Membrane ghosts were prepared as described by Evans (5).

[b] The enzyme was assayed and solubilized with sodium dodecyl sulfate according to the procedures of Evans (5, 6). Magnesium chloride and calcium chloride were added where indicated at 2 mM and 1 mM, respectively. Protein was determined by the method of Lowry et al. (9) with bovine serum albumin (Sigma Chemical Co.) as a standard. Specific activity is recorded as micromoles of orthophosphate (7) released per milligram of protein per hour.

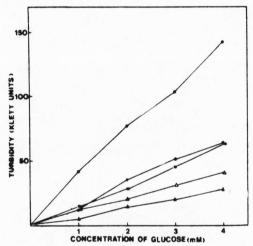

FIG. 1. *Growth yields of strains A428 and N_{144} grown on limiting concentrations of glucose. The measurement of aerobic growth yields was carried out as described by Cox et al. (3) except that Davis minimal medium (4) supplemented with citrate, histidine (50 µg/ml), proline (50 µg/ml), and vitamin B_1 (1 µg/ml) was used. Anaerobic experiments were performed in glass-stoppered Thunberg tubes, especially adapted to fit the Klett-Summerson colorimeter, filled to capacity with supplemented Davis minimal medium and 25 mM $NaHCO_3$. Potassium nitrate (0.1%) was added where indicated. Maximum turbidity readings were recorded when growth of the cultures had ceased. Strain A428: aerobic (○), anaerobic (△), anaerobic + nitrate (□). Strain N_{144}: aerobic (●), anaerobic or anaerobic + nitrate (▲).*

adenosine triphosphatase activity of the parent was stimulated about threefold after solubilization with SDS. In contrast, even after SDS treatment, there was only slightly detectable adenosine triphosphatase activity in the mutant preparation. Mixing of membrane ghosts or solubilized preparations from N_{144} with corresponding preparations from A428 had no effect on the adenosine triphosphatase activity of the parent, suggesting that the defect is not due to the presence of a diffusible inhibitor. The mixing experiments do not rule out the possibility that the absence of activity in N_{144} is due to the presence of a tightly bound inhibitor.

The defect in N_{144} appeared to be due to a single-point mutation since the mutant reverted to growth on Krebs cycle intermediates with a frequency of 1 in 10^8. In addition, N_{144} could be transduced to growth on tricarboxylic acid cycle intermediates (10), and no differences in growth or adenosine triphosphatase activity could be observed between a transductant and A428. Butlin et al. (2) reported that *uncA* was cotransducible with *ilv* but not with *metE* and was located at 73.5 min on the *E. coli* chromosome. Similarly, the mutation in N_{144} was cotransducible with *ilv* at a frequency of 17%; no cotransduction was found with *metE*. The defect in N_{144} may thus be due to a mutation in the *uncA* gene or in a gene close to it.

We thank Eliora Z. Ron for the strain A428 and for her critical reading of the manuscript. We also thank Eugene Rosenberg and Joseph Neumann for their helpful suggestions and criticisms, and Tamar Tuito and Vanda Freudis for their expert technical assistance.

LITERATURE CITED

1. Bauchop, T., and S. R. Elsden. 1960. The growth of microorganisms in relation to their energy supply. J. Gen. Microbiol. 23:457-469.
2. Butlin, J. D., G. B. Cox, and F. Gibson. 1971. Oxidative phosphorylation in *Escherichia coli* K12: mutations affecting magnesium ion-or calcium ion-stimulated adenosine triphosphatase. Biochem. J. 124:75-81.
3. Cox, G. B., N. A. Newton, F. Gibson, A. M. Snowswell, and J. A. Hamilton. 1970. The function of ubiquinone in *Escherichia coli*. Biochem. J. 117:551-562.
4. Davis, B. D., and E. S. Mingioli. 1950. Mutants of *Escherichia coli* requiring methionine or vitamin B_{12}. J. Bacteriol. 60:17-28.
5. Evans, D. J., Jr. 1969. Membrane adenosine triphosphatase of *Escherichia coli*: activation by calcium ion and inhibition by monovalent cations. J. Bacteriol. 100:914-922.
6. Evans, D. J., Jr. 1970. Membrane Mg^{2+}-(Ca^{2+})-activated adenosine triphosphatase of *Escherichia coli*: characterization in the membrane-bound and solubi-lized states. J. Bacteriol. 104:1203-1212.
7. Fiske, C. H., and J. SubbaRow. 1925. The colorimetric determination of phosphorus. J. Biol. Chem. 66:375-400.
8. Kormančiková, V., L. Kováč, and M. Vidová. 1969. Oxidative phosphorylation in yeast. V. Phosphorylation efficiencies in growing cells determined from molar growth yields. Biochem. Biophys. Acta 180:9-17.
9. Lowry, O. H., N. J. Rosebrough, A. L. Farr, and R. J. Randall. 1951. Protein measurement with the Folin phenol reagent. J. Biol. Chem. 193:265-275.
10. Luria, S. E., J. N. Adams, and R. C. Ting. 1960. Transduction of lactose-utilising ability among strains of *E. coli* and *S. dysenteriae* and the properties of transducing phage particles. Virology 12:348-390.
11. Ota, A., T. Yamanaka, and K. Okunuki. 1964. Oxidative phosphorylation coupled with nitrate respiration. II. Phosphorylation coupled with anaerobic nitrate reduction in a cell-free extract of *Escherichia coli*. Biochem. J. 55:131-135.
12. Säsärman, A., K. E. Sanderson, M. Surdeanu, and S. Sonea. 1970. Hemin-deficient mutants of *Salmonella thyphimurium*. J. Bacteriol. 102:531-536.
13. Säsärman, A., M. Surdeanu, G. Szegli, T. Horodniceanu, V. Greceanu, and A. Dumitrescu. 1968. Hemin-deficient mutants of *Escherichia coli* K-12. J. Bacteriol. 96:570-572.

Part IV

ADAPTIVE RESPONSES

Editor's Comments
on Paper 29

29 MOSS
The Influence of Oxygen Tension on Respiration and Cytochrome a_2 *Formation of* Escherichia coli

ELECTRON TRANSPORT

The account of the work given by Frank Moss in Paper 29 is doubly interesting. He not only describes the effect of variation of dissolved oxygen concentration upon the cellular content of cytochrome a_2 (see Paper 10) but moreover provides, independently of Monod and of Novick and Szilard,[1,2] a derivation of expressions delineating the kinetics of growth in continuous culture. His results included the important observation that the cellular respiratory rate was independent of terminal oxidase content. The technique of varying the proportions of cytochromes o and a_2 (*d*) by altering the availability of dissolved oxygen has been recently employed to show that so-called "branched" electron transport chains conserve energy with an efficiency independent of the ratio of cytochrome *d* to cytochrome *o*,[3] a conclusion opposite to that reached by Jones (see Editor's Comments to Papers 12 and 13).

REFERENCES

1. Monod, J. *Ann. Inst. Pasteur,* **79**, 390–410, 1950. Paper 10 in P. S. S. Dawson, ed., *Microbial Growth.* Benchmark Papers in Microbiology, Dowden, Hutchinson & Ross, Inc. Stroudsburg, Pa., 1974.
2. Novick, A., and L. Szilard. *Science,* **112**, 715–716, 1950. Paper 11 in P. S. S. Dawson, ed. *Microbial Growth.* Benchmark Papers in Microbiology, Dowden, Hutchinson & Ross, Inc. Stroudsburg, Pa., 1974.
3. Rice, C. W., and W. P. Hempfling. *J. Bact.,* **134**, 115–124, 1978.

29

Reprinted from *Aust. J. Exp. Biol. Med. Sci.* **30**:531–540 (1952)

THE INFLUENCE OF OXYGEN TENSION ON RESPIRATION AND CYTOCHROME a_2 FORMATION OF *ESCHERICHIA COLI*

by F. MOSS[1]

(From the Institute of Medical Research, the Royal North Shore Hospital, Sydney).

(Accepted for publication 11th September, 1952.)

The experiments described in this paper arose as a result of information gained during attempts to prepare large quantities of *Escherichia coli* for the purpose of investigation of cytochrome a_2, and if possible to increase the cytochrome a_2 content of the bacteria. It is generally held that cytochrome a_2 has the function of a cytochrome oxidase. Carbon monoxide shifts the absorption band to 634 mμ, oxygen to 645 mμ, and aeration in the presence of cyanide causes the band to disappear.

Further evidence for the oxidase function of cytochrome a_2 of *Aerobacter aerogenes*, which has a similar cytochrome absorption spectrum to *E. coli*, was provided by Tissières (1951) who showed that on passing air into a cooled suspension of *A. aerogenes* cytochrome a_2 is oxidized before b_1, and on cessation of aeration cytochrome b_1 is reduced before a_2. However, Tissières has also shown that oxygen uptake is not directly related to the intensity of the a_2 absorption band in *A. aerogenes*, and suggested that cytochrome a_1 may also function as cytochrome oxidase. The same worker (1952) was able to prepare a cell-free suspension of particles, containing cytochrome a_1 and b_1 but no visible amount of cytochrome a_2. This suspension showed considerable respiratory activity.

The adaptive development of the cytochrome system of yeast has now been reported by a number of workers (Chin, 1950; Ephrussi, Slonimski and Perrodin, 1950; Ephrussi and Slonimski, 1950).

Schaeffer (1950) described an increase in the cytochromes of *Bacillus cereus* on aeration, and found that the medium from anaerobic culture contained much more free porphyrin than medium from aerobic culture. This suggested that porphyrins not used in the synthesis of cytochrome were excreted. In the case of *E. coli*, however, very little free porphyrin was found in the medium from anaerobic cultures, and none in aerobic culture.

Adaptive formation of the cytochromes of *E. coli*, and increase of respiration in the presence of oxygen was also found by the author, independently.

---

[1] This work has been carried out by the aid of a grant from the National Health and Medical Research Council of Australia.

MATERIALS.

The organism. The strain of *E. coli* used in this experiment was obtained from the diagnostic laboratory of the hospital. The organism showed the following properties: indole was 'not formed; M.R. positive; V.P. negative; citrate was not used as a sole source of carbon; H_2/CO_2 ratio, 1:1; acid and gas from glucose, lactose, maltose, mannitol; sucrose, dulcitol, and salicin were not fermented; gelatin was not liquified; catalase was present. This strain developed a particularly strong cytochrome spectrum on aeration.

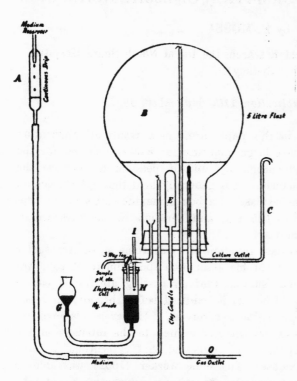

The medium consisted of: KH_2PO_4, 1·0 gm.; $(NH_4)_2HPO_4$, 4·0 gm.; s o d i u m citrate, 2·0 g.m.; $MgSO_4.7H_2O$, 0·7 gm.; NaCl, 1·0 gm.; $FeSO_4.7H_2O$, 0·125 gm.; tap water to one litre. Sterile glucose to make 0·5 p.c. and veal broth 5 p.c. were added after autoclaving the salt solution.

Apparatus.

The continuous culture apparatus is shown in the Figure. Medium from a 10-litre reservoir was admitted to the 5-litre flask B through the drip A. Rate of influx of medium was measured by counting drops of known volume. C is an overflow which maintained a constant volume of 1 litre. Various mixtures of 5 p.c. CO_2 in O_2 and 5 p.c. CO_2 in N_2, were admitted by a fine grade Berkefeld candle E, which, under 30-lb. pressure, produced a vigorous turbulence by very small bubbles. Unabsorbed gas escaped by the vent O. Samples of culture were admitted to the electrolysis cell of a polarograph H by lowering the mercury bulb G. This mercury served also as the anode. The volume of the sample was 10 ml. This was admitted in 10 seconds. 250 ml. of inoculum grown under N_2 were admitted anaerobically from a flask (not shown in Figure) by a positive pressure of nitrogen. Temperature was maintained at 37° C. by keeping the temperature of the incubator at 40° C., and that of the reservoir (which was the only part of the apparatus not in the incubator) at 39° C. by a pilot flame. The polarograph was of the simple manual type. The dropping mercury electrode (I) was constructed from a clinical thermometer. Sensitivity of the galvanometer was 1,100 mm. per microamp., with the scale at 1 metre. The period was 2 seconds. The calomel reference cell and salt bridges contained KCl saturated at 32° C. An E.M.F. of 0·5 V. was applied cathodically; this was the midpoint of the first wave of oxygen in the medium. Galvanometer deflections were measured for oxygen-saturated, and oxygen-free, solutions before each experiment. The difference was taken as proportional to the concentration of oxygen in solution. This was found to be a reliable measure of oxygen tension by the method of Lewis and McKenzie (1947): A saturated solution of oxygen in bacteria-free medium is mixed in various proportions with oxygen-free medium. The galvanometer deflection at 0·5 V. applied potential is found to be proportional to the amount of oxygen-saturated solution present.

EXPERIMENTAL PROCEDURES.

The problem of maintaining constant the rate of oxygen absorption during growth was overcome by a method of continuous dilution, while keeping the volume constant. The rate of dilution was such that bacterial density was kept constant.

This method of continuous culture was devised independently from and simultaneously to that by Monod (1950). Monod also described the mathematics and uses of the method.

Initially, oxygen tension and oxygen uptake rates were measured amperometrically as described by Skerman and Millis (1949) and Wise (1951).

However, it was found that Q_{O_2} measured by conventional manometry did not agree with that found amperometrically; consequently Q_{O_2} was measured by conventional manometry in this experiment (see polarographic measurement of Q_{O_2}).

5 p.c. CO_2 gas mixtures were used for aeration in all experiments. It was thought that the difference between amperometric and manometric results may be caused by the presence of CO_2 in the amperometric sample. Consequently manometry was also carried out in 5 p.c. CO_2 atmospheres by the use of CO_2 buffers. Oxygen tension during aeration was arrived at by a combination of manometric and amperometric methods.

The rate of solution of oxygen is equal to a (G—S), where G is the partial pressure of oxygen in the gas phase and S is the oxygen tension of oxygen in the solution. a is a constant dependent on the apparatus.

The rate of removal of oxygen by bacteria is qm, where m is the concentration of bacteria in mg. dry weight per ml. and q is the rate of oxygen uptake, here expressed in terms of decrease in oxygen tension per minute per mg. dry weight.

$$\frac{ds}{dt} = a(G-S) - qm \qquad \qquad 1$$

The solution of this equation is:

$$S = (G-mq/a)\,(1-e^{-at}) \qquad \qquad 2$$

The constant a was determined experimentally from an oxygen tension-time curve, obtained by measurement of oxygen tension amperometrically by passing oxygen into *sterile* oxygen-free medium. For the apparatus used here a had the value 1·75 min.$^{-1}$.

Oxygen tension during aeration of culture was then found as follows:

The expression $(1-e^{-at})$ was taken as 1, since equilibrium was established within a few minutes.

$$q = \frac{Q_{O_2}/60}{\text{solubility of } O_2 \text{ at } 37°\text{ C.}}$$

The solubility of oxygen in the medium at 37° C. was determined by the Van Slyke apparatus, and was found to be 23 cmm. per ml. Q_{O_2} is given its conventional meaning.

From equation 2 it follows that

$$S = G - \frac{Q_{O_2} \times m}{60 \times 23 \times 1·75}$$
$$= G - ·000414 \, Q_{O_2} \, m$$

The rate of influx of medium which was required to maintain constant bacterial density was found in the following manner:

The required condition is that

$$\frac{dm}{dv} = \frac{m}{v} \quad \cdot \quad \cdot \quad \cdot \quad \cdot \quad \cdot \quad \cdot \quad \cdot \quad \cdot \quad \cdot \qquad 3$$

where m is the required mass of bacteria present in volume v in the aeration flask.

Now

$$\frac{dm}{dt} = km \quad \cdot \quad \cdot \quad \cdot \quad \cdot \quad \cdot \quad \cdot \quad \cdot \quad \cdot \qquad 4$$

where k is the specific growth rate.

From equation 1:

$$\frac{dm}{dt} \cdot \frac{dt}{dv} = \frac{m}{v}$$

From this by substitution from equation 4:

$$\frac{dv}{dt} = kv \quad \cdot \quad \cdot \quad \cdot \quad \cdot \quad \cdot \quad \cdot \quad \cdot \qquad 5$$

The specific growth rate k was found from the formula

$$k = \frac{\ln m_2/m_1}{t_2 - t_1} \quad \cdot \quad \cdot \quad \cdot \quad \cdot \quad \cdot \quad \cdot \qquad 6$$

which is derived by solution of equation 4 between time t_1 and t_2 when density is m_1 and m_2 respectively. This growth rate of anaerobic culture increased on aeration until a constant value was reached, in a period which was dependent on the oxygen tension. Thus it was necessary to adjust the rate of influx of medium at frequent intervals until a steady state had been reached.

The initial rate of influx was estimated from equations 5 and 6 by measurement of the growth rate of an anaerobic culture in the aeration flask prior to commencement of aeration.

Manometry.

This was carried out in conventional Warburg manometers containing air, and simultaneously in manometers fitted with Dixon-Simer cups with 5 p.c. CO_2 buffered atmospheres as described by Krebs (1951).

It was assumed that growth commenced immediately when bacteria were transferred from the aeration flask to the manometer, and that the specific growth rate remained constant during the forty-minute period of measurement. Q_{O_2} was calculated as follows:

By solution of equation $4 : m = m_O e^{kt}$. By suitable choice of units, the oxygen uptake rate of culture in the manometer is equal to $Q_{O_2}.m_O e^{kt}$.

From this

$$Q_{O_2} = \frac{\triangle O_2 k}{m_0} \left(\frac{1}{e^{kt_2} - e^{kt_1}} \right)$$

$\triangle O_2$ is the observed oxygen uptake, t_1 is the period from commencement of equilibration to closing the manometer taps. t_2 is the period from the commencement of equilibration to the end of measurement.

Oxygen tension in the culture contained in the manometers was of the same order as that in corresponding culture in the aeration vessel. This was shown by increasing the bacterial density of culture in the manometer flask until the oxygen uptake became independent of further increase of bacterial density at a certain shaking rate which was used throughout. These flasks contained air. From this the constant *a* of equation (1) applied to the manometer flask was found to be $2 \cdot 2$ min.$^{-1}$.

Polarographic measurement of Q_{o_2}.

In general Q_{O_2} measured amperometrically was lower than that measured by manometry. This was most noticeable when p_{O_2} during culture was high, in which case values as low as 40 p.c. of manometric values were obtained at the commencement of aeration. After $4\frac{1}{2}$ hours, however, Q_{O_2} measured by both methods were usually similar.

Amperometric p_{O_2}–time curves for culture grown below 0·5 atm. were linear. However, when above 0·5 atm. the rate of oxygen uptake increased noticeably with falling p_{O_2}. Q_{O_2} in this case was calculated from the straight line of best fit.

It sometimes happened that points on the graph were so irregular that a smooth curve could not be constructed.

The difference between manometric and amperometric measurements may be due to the fact that invisible gas bubbles were withdrawn into the electrolysis cell, or that respiration was inhibited at high p_{O_2} from oxygen poisoning or from the formation of hydrogen peroxide. The first explanation is thought to be the more likely.

General procedure.

The amount of oxygen in the gas mixture necessary to give a certain oxygen tension was found amperometrically beforehand, by passing the gas mixture through *sterile* medium in the aeration flask and adjusting until the calculated galvanometer deflection was obtained. Gas was delivered from two cylinders containing 5 p.c. CO_2 in O_2 and 5 p.c. CO_2 in N_2. The main valves of the cylinders were opened fully and adjustments made by alteration of the fine adjustment valves. The main valve of the nitrogen cylinder was then shut off, and the galvanometer deflection for oxygen determined when the reading became steady again. The deflection corresponding to residual current was determined by shutting off the main valve of the oxygen cylinder and opening that of the nitrogen cylinder.

To 750 ml. of sterile oxygen-free medium contained in the aeration flask after adjusting the gas mixture, 250 ml. of anaerobic culture were added anaerobically. The added culture was prepared from a needle point inoculum grown at 37° C. for fourteen hours. This large inoculum ensured that sufficient essential metabolites were added, and that inhibitory substances were not present in amounts sufficient to limit growth.

Aeration and influx of medium were not commenced until the optical density of a sample indicated a bacterial content of 0·15 mg. per ml. Density was measured at 15 minute intervals during this period. The specific growth rate was calculated from these measurements by use of equation 6, when growth was established. The initial rate of influx was estimated from equation 5. This was usually about 6 ml. per minute, whereas 8 ml. per minute at this stage caused decrease of density. Increase of growth rate after aeration necessitated adjustment of influx at 15 minute intervals until it reached a maximum; the necessary dilution rate then reached was about 25 ml. of medium per minute when oxygen tension was low. Bacterial concentration was maintained between 0·15 mg. per ml. and 0·30 mg. per ml., which corresponded to that at the beginning of the logarithmic phase in culture not submitted to continuous dilution. pH remained between 6·6 and 6·9. 2 ml. samples were removed at intervals for manometry. The CO_2-buffered cups contained 3 ml. of 4 M diethanolamine previously equilibrated to 5 p.c. CO_2. These were gassed from a bye-pass from the gas used in aeration. The manometric measurements in air and 5 p.c. CO_2 were each in triplicate.

Anaerobic conditions were obtained for a control experiment during continuous dilution by aerating with oxygen-free nitrogen, prepared by passing nitrogen over a long column of yellow phosphorus pellets, followed by washing in water.

Examination of cytochrome a_2 during aeration.

In a separate experiment samples of paste were prepared from cultures grown at high and at low oxygen tension. Cytochrome a_2 was estimated by matching the intensity of the absorption band of *E. coli* at 640 mμ against the 630 mμ band of a standard solution of hem*i*globin contained in a wedge trough as described by Keilin and Hartree (1946).

Five litres of culture grown by the continuous culture method were aerated very vigorously by gas mixtures which produced oxygen tensions of approximately 0·75 atm. and 0·1 atm. respectively.

Two litres of culture were withdrawn at half-hourly intervals and centrifuged. The paste so obtained was placed under the microscope objective in a small wedge. The optimum depth of the paste for observation of the cytochrome a$_2$ band was 0·6 cm. This was maintained in all experiments, as was the optimal adjustment of the slit of the spectroscope, and the intensity of the light source. Adjustment of light through the standard matching solution was arranged so that background illumination was equal in standard and paste. Bacterial density of the paste was estimated from its protein content using the biuret method of Strickland (1951).

An attempt was made to estimate the amount of cytochrome b$_1$ present, by matching its band at 560 mμ against that of reduced cytochrome c at 550 mμ. However, optimal conditions for a$_2$ observations allowed poor distinction of the intensity of the b$_1$ band. The band of cytochrome a$_1$ at 590 mμ was too faint to attempt measurement.

RESULTS.

Respiration.

Table 1 shows the Q_{O_2} of *E. coli* grown for $4\frac{1}{2}$ hours in continuous culture at oxygen tensions between 0·09 and 0·95 atm. These results were taken from manometry in 5 p.c. CO_2. It was found that the Q_{O_2} of non-aerated cells at zero hours was slightly less in the 5 p.c. CO_2 buffered series when oxygen tension was high than in the CO_2-free air atmosphere of Warburg cups. The low Q_{O_2} of 540 and 520 at zero hours in two experiments may be due to the fact that in these experiments aeration was commenced somewhat earlier after adding the culture to the aerator than in the others. The highest values of Q_{O_2} reached between 3 and $4\frac{1}{2}$ hours were from 910 to 1,090.

The fact that increase of Q_{O_2} is not due to factors dependent on continuous culture is shown by the constant Q_{O_2} obtained in the anaerobic series.

TABLE 1.

Increase of Q_{O_2} during aeration.

P$_{O_2}$	Hours of aeration			
	0	$1\frac{1}{2}$	3	$4\frac{1}{2}$
0·90–0·95	670	960	1090	950
0·75–0·87	540	890	1000	940
0·42–0·45	640	—	970	980
0·1–0·3	520	830	910	1020
Anaerobic	650	650	680	—

Growth rate.

It was noticed during continuous culture that the rate of influx required for constant density was greatest when p_{O_2} was low. It was noticed during manometry also that the growth was higher when p_{O_2} was low. Table 2 shows the value of k in terms of specific growth rate per hour. These values were obtained during manometry. Growth of culture grown at oxygen tension 0·1 to 0·3 atm. was more rapid than that at 0·9–0·95 atm., and in the anaerobic culture. The Q_{O_2} of the latter was measured in 5 p.c. CO_2 and 95 p.c. O_2.

TABLE 2.

Specific growth rate per hour (k) during growth at different oxygen tension.

P_{O_2} of culture	P_{O_2} in Warburg flask	Hours of aeration			
		0	$1\frac{1}{2}$	3	$4\frac{1}{2}$
Anaerobic	0·95	0·53	0·55	0·37	0·4
0·1–0·3	0·1–0·3	0·80	0·84	1·44	1·56
0·90–0·95	0·90–0·95	0·35	0·82	0·86	1·17

Variation of cytochrome a_2 concentration with oxygen tension.

Table 3 shows the amount of cytochrome a_2 produced in two experiments during aeration for $4\frac{1}{2}$ hours, when oxygen tension was held at about 0·1 atm. and 0·75 atm. respectively.

TABLE 3.

Development of cytochrome a_2 during aeration.

P_{O_2}	Hours of aeration									
	0	$\frac{1}{2}$	1	$1\frac{1}{2}$	2	$2\frac{1}{2}$	3	$3\frac{1}{2}$	4	$4\frac{1}{2}$
0·1	0	0	0	10	—	20	—	22	32	32
0·75	0	8	8	16	16	16	16	16	16	16

The units of measurement used are mm. of a layer of haemiglobin solution being $4·85 \times 10^{-5}$ molar for haem, which matched the a_2 absorption band of a standard cell paste of 0·6 cm. thickness containing 100 mg. per ml. dry weight of bacteria. Each is the result of at least four readings.

It is seen that the a_2 band developed more rapidly at 0·75 atm. than at 0·1 atm. Absorption, equivalent to 8 mm., is reached in 30 minutes at 0·75 atm., whereas there is no a_2 detectable in the 0·1 atm. sample in 60 minutes. After 60 minutes, however, formation of a_2 became more rapid in the 0·1 atm. culture. At $4\frac{1}{2}$ hours the 0·1 atm. culture contained twice as much a_2 as the 0·75 atm. sample.

It was said earlier that the effluent from the continuous culture used for measurements of Q_{O_2} was examined for the presence of cytochromes. It was noticed repeatedly that the a_2 content was high when oxygen tension was low and that the band at 630 mμ could often not be seen when p_{O_2} approached saturation. Addition of broth to the medium appeared to increase a_2 formation.

The interval required for preparation of cell paste allowed ample time for reduction of cytochromes. It was found on many occasions that addition of dithionite or incubation with glucose failed to increase the strength of the a_2 band, when it was found to be poorly developed, after vigorous aeration. The a_2 band from cells produced at high oxygen tension was therefore produced by cytochrome a_2 in the fully reduced state. Cytochrome b_1 which was absent in anaerobic cells produced an intense band at 560 mμ, within 4 hours, on aeration.

DISCUSSION.

Table 4 shows the ratio of Q_{O_2}/a_2 during 4½ hours of aeration at low and high p_{O_2}. At low p_{O_2} the cytochrome a_2 content increased much more than Q_{O_2} between 1½ and 4½ hours, while at high p_{O_2} the Q_{O_2}/a_2 ratio remains steady. It is evident that the cytochrome a_2 content and the corresponding Q_{O_2} are not closely related, although both rise during aeration. It is possible that excess cytochrome a_2 may be formed at low p_{O_2}, and that this may be counterbalanced at high p_{O_2} by a destruction of cytochrome a_2.

TABLE 4.

Q_{O_2}/cytochrome a_2 units.

P_{O_2}	Hours		
	1½	3	4½
Low[1]	83	45·5	34
High[2]	60	68	59

[1] Q_{O_2} and cytochrome a_2 units at a p_{O_2} of about 0·1.

[2] Q_{O_2} at a p_{O_2} of about 0·9, cytochrome a_2 units at a p_{O_2} of about 0·75.

The higher growth rates of cells grown at low p_{O_2} shown in Table 3, which suggests at least superficially a relationship between a_2 content and growth rate, may also be explained by O_2 poisoning.

Another possibility is that cytochrome a_2 is concerned in directing aerobic energy towards cell synthesis and that cytochrome a_1 functions as the real oxidase.

SUMMARY.

A continuous culture apparatus is described which permits growth while maintaining bacterial concentration and oxygen tension within narrow limits.

The mathematical theory of the method is discussed.

A strain of *E. coli* was found to develop cytochromes a_2, a_1, and b_1 on aeration.

The Q_{O_2} of aerated *E. coli* was found to increase as the result of aeration. The Q_{O_2} reached was not closely related to the amount of cytochrome a_2 present.

Possibilities concerning the function of cytochrome a_2 are discussed.

Acknowledgments. The author wishes to thank Dr. R. Lemberg for his continued advice and interest in this work; also Mr. W. H. Lockwood and Dr. D. B. Morell for valuable discussion, Dr. J. Breyer for advice concerning the polarographic aspects of the experiments and Mr. P. Caiger for experimental assistance.

REFERENCES.

Chin, C. H. (1950): Nature, 165, p. 926.
Ephrussi, B., Slonimski, P. P. and Perrodin, G. (1950): Biochim. biophys. Acta, 6, p. 256.
Ephrussi, B. and Slonimski, P. P. (1950): Compt. rend. Acad. Sci. 230, p. 685.
Keilin, D. and Hartree, E. F. (1946): Nature, 157, p. 210.
Krebs, H. A. (1951): Biochem. J. 48, p. 349.
Lewis, V. M. and McKenzie, H. A. (1947): Indust. eng. Chem. Analytical Edition, 19, p. 643.
Monod, J. (1950): Ann. Inst. Pasteur, 79, p. 390.
Schaeffer, P. (1950): Compt. rend. Acad. Sci., 231, p. 381.
Skerman, V. B. D. and Millis, Nancy (1949): Austral. J. exp. Biol., 27, p. 183.
Strickland, L. H. (1951): J. gen. Microbiol., 5, p. 698.
Tissières, A. (1951): Biochem. J., 50, p. 279.
Tissières, A. (1952): Nature, 169, p. 880.
Wise, J. S. (1951): J. gen. Microbiol. 5, p. 167.

Editor's Comments
on Papers 30 and 31

30 BRAGG, DAVIES, and HOU
Function of Energy-Dependent Transhydrogenase in Escherichia coli

31 HEMPFLING and MAINZER
Effects of Varying the Carbon Source Limiting Growth on Yield and Maintenance Characteristics of Escherichia coli *in Continuous Culture*

ENERGY CONSERVATION

Like enzymatic components of respiration, it may be expected that associated energy-conserving reactions reflect environmental conditions. Here the ability to measure the efficiency of energy conservation becomes most important to the successful outcome of experiments testing for such phenomena. Papers 30 and 31 demonstrate that the nutritional circumstances of bacterial growth may change the activity of the energy-dependent transhydrogenase reaction or the efficiency of oxidative phosphorylation, but that the two reactions are under different controls.

P. D. Bragg, P. L. Davies, and C. Hou show, in Paper 30, that certain amino acids, alone or in combination, diminish the energy-dependent reduction of $NADP^+$ by NADH. Their attempt to assay oxidative phosphorylation by using subcellular preparations, however, does not show significant differences as the result of differences in growth conditions.

Kashket and Brodie[1] had remarked in 1963 that extracts of glucose-grown *Escherichia coli* exhibited poor phosphorylation efficiency. Consistent with that finding was the observation of Hempfling that intact, glucose-grown *E. coli* B exhibited less efficient oxidative phosphorylation than did organisms growing at the expense of amino acids.[2] In Paper 31 Hempfling and Mainzer apply the technique of substrate-limited continuous culture to the question of growth-yield[3] dependency upon the identity of the substrate. The notion of maintenance respiration, following Marr[4] and Pirt,[5] is introduced here. This was the first work to employ aerobic continuous culture in an attempt to estimate the effiency of oxidative phosphorylation, now a fashionable technique.[6]

REFERENCES

1. Kashket, E. R., and A. F. Brodie. *Biochim. Biophys. Acta,* **78**, 52–65, 1963.
2. Hempfling, W. P. *Biochem. Biophys. Res. Commun.,* **41**, 9–15, 1970.
3. Bauchop, T., and S. Elsden, *J. Gen. Microbiol.,* **23**, 457–467, 1960.
4. Marr, A. G., E. H. Nilson, and D. J. Clark. *Ann. N. Y. Acad. Sci.,* **102**, 536–548, 1963.
5. Pirt, S. J. *Proc. Roy. Soc. London,* ser. B, **163**, 224–231, 1965.
6. Hempfling, W. P., and C. W. Rice. Microbial bioenergetics in continuous culture. In P. Calcott, ed., *Continuous Cultures of Cells,* CRC Press, Inc., West Palm Beach, Fla., in press.

30

Reprinted from *Biochem. Biophys. Res. Commun.* **47**:1248–1255 (1972)

FUNCTION OF ENERGY-DEPENDENT TRANSHYDROGENASE IN ESCHERICHIA COLI

P.D. Bragg, P.L. Davies and C. Hou
Department of Biochemistry
University of British Columbia
Vancouver 8, B.C., Canada

Received May 8, 1972

SUMMARY

The activity of the energy-dependent transhydrogenase of membrane particles of E. coli varied markedly with growth conditions. The activity of the enzyme was not related to the efficiency of oxidative phosphorylation. The enzyme was not subject to catabolite repression but was repressed by mixtures of amino acids. It is suggested that the transhydrogenase has a role in generating NADPH for biosynthesis.

INTRODUCTION

The exact role of the energy-dependent transhydrogenase of

Escherichia coli (1-6) and other cells is unknown. Although it

could act in vivo as a source of NADPH, direct evidence in support

of this hypothesis is lacking, and a function as a proton pump has

been suggested (7).

There is a close relationship between the enzyme and oxidative

phosphorylation in mitochondria since both processes compete for

high energy intermediates (8). Thus, in E. coli also, a change in

one activity might be expected to affect the other. Now, Hempfling

(9) observed that the efficiency of oxidative phosphorylation in

E. coli varied with growth conditions. In log phase cells grown

on glucose it was low (P:O <0.4) but it was much higher in station-

ary phase cells (P:O >3). Cells grown on succinate showed maximal

P:O values of 1.9 during the log phase. These results indicated

301

that ATP formation by oxidative phosphorylation was subject to
catabolite repression. In line with this, the effect of glucose
was abolished by inclusion of 2.5mM cAMP in the growth medium (10).

We have investigated the effect of growth conditions on the
energy-dependent transhydrogenase of E. coli to see if variation
in the efficiency of oxidative phosphorylation affected this enzyme.
No clear relationship between the two processes was observed, and
the transhydrogenase was not subject to catabolite repression.
Moreover, it was repressed by growth in the presence of amino acids
suggesting that it had a role in providing NADPH for biosynthesis.

METHODS

E. coli NRC-482 was grown on a minimal salts medium with 0.4%
glucose as previously described (11) except that in some experiments 2% vitamin-free casein hydrolysate (Nutritional Biochemicals)
or L-amino acids (each at a final concentration of 0.1%) were
present. For growth on a minimal salts medium containing 0.8%
disodium succinate 0.1% ammonium sulfate was added also, and the
pH of the medium was maintained at pH 7.2-7.4 during growth by
additions of 5 N HCl. Except where noted, the above media contained 12μM ferric citrate. The complex glucose medium was 3%
trypticase-soy medium (BBL). The cells were grown at 37° with
vigorous aeration from a sparger except for growth on complex
media where a reciprocating water bath shaker was used. The cells
were harvested mid to late log or in the stationary phase of
growth and were washed once with 50mM Tris sulfate buffer, pH
7.8, containing 10mM $MgCl_2$ (TM buffer). The cells were suspended
in TM buffer (1 g wet weight per 10 ml buffer) and disrupted in a
French press (Aminco) at 20,000 psi. The suspension was centrifuged at 17,000 x g for 10 min to remove whole cells and large
cell fragments. The respiratory particles were obtained by cen-

trifuging the supernatant from the above step at 120,000 x g for
2 hours. The resultant pellet was suspended in TM buffer containing 1% bovine serum albumin at a concentration of 10-15 mg particle protein per ml.

Transhydrogenase activity was measured by a modification of
the procedure of Fisher and Sanadi (5). 1 ml TM buffer containing 0.1% bovine serum albumin, 0.1mM dithiothreitol and 0.7 M
sucrose was preincubated with 50 μl particle suspension in a
cuvette at 37° for 5 min. The cuvette was then transferred to a
Coleman 124 spectrophotometer equipped with recorder and the absorbance followed at 340 nm after addition of 5 μl ethanol, 50 μl
yeast alcohol dehydrogenase (4 mg per ml; Calbiochem) and 25 μl
3mM NAD. After 0.66 min 50 μl 16.3mM NADP was added and the reduction of NADP measured ("aerobic-driven transhydrogenase").
When the oxygen in the cuvette was exhausted the reduction of
NADP abruptly changed to a lower rate ("energy-independent transhydrogenase"). When this rate had been established 10 μl 60mM
ATP was added and the new rate of NADP reduction measured ("ATP-
driven transhydrogenase"). The rates of the two energy-driven
transhydrogenase activities were corrected for the contribution
made by the energy-independent transhydrogenase. NADH oxidase
activity was calculated from the time taken to deplete oxygen
in the cuvette. NADPH:O ratios were calculated from the amount
of NADPH formed during the aerobic phase.

ATPase activity was measured at 37° in the presence of 5mM
$CaCl_2$ as described before (12). P:O ratios given by respiratory
particles were determined at 30° by the method of Butlin *et al*.
(13) except that oxygen uptake was measured polarographically.
Cytochromes were quantitated using the extinction coefficients
given by Jones and Redfearn (14).

TABLE 1. Effect of growth conditions on energy-dependent transhydrogenase and other activities of respiratory particles

Medium	Additions	Harvested	ATPase	NADH oxidase	Cytochrome		Transhydrogenase		
					b_1	a_2	Aerobic	ATP	NADPH:O
Salts-succinate	No Iron	L	839	1160	0.23	0.08	21	33	0.07
	--	L	773	1230	0.49	0.16	33	55	0.04
Complex glucose	No Iron	L	397	1330	0.57	0.43	0	11	0
	No Iron	S	368	1030	0.85	0.56	0	17	0
Salts-glucose	No Iron	L	--	1730	0.27	0	84	60	0.15
	No Iron	S	--	1890	0.21	0.05	58	67	0.13
	--	L	406	1770	0.28	0.06	89	75	0.15
	--	S	476	1880	0.34	0.07	65	69	0.10
	2.5mM cAMP	L	783	1380	0.33	0.04	49	68	0.09
Salts-glucose (anaerobic)	--	L	686	--	--	--	61	80	0.14

L, logarithmic phase; S, stationary phase. Cytochrome concentration is expressed as nmoles/mg protein, ATPase and transhydrogenase activities as nmoles/min/mg protein, and NADH oxidase as nmoles/min/nmole cytochrome b_1.

RESULTS AND DISCUSSION

Table I shows the effect of growth conditions on the energy-dependent transhydrogenase activities of respiratory particles from E. coli. Cytochrome content, and NADH oxidase and ATPase activities are included since the aerobic-driven transhydrogenase derives its energy from oxidation of NADH via the cytochrome chain, and the ATPase has been implicated in the ATP-driven reaction (6). Both transhydrogenase levels (and cytochrome a_2) varied markedly with growth conditions and to a greater extent than did cytochrome b_1, ATPase and NADH oxidase. Highest transhydrogenase activities occurred during the log phase of growth on glucose and were somewhat lower when the cells had entered the stationary phase. Enrichment of the growth medium with 12μM ferric citrate did not significantly affect the transhydrogenase activities although it increased the cytochrome content. Addition of cAMP or growth on glucose under anaerobic conditions also did not greatly affect the transhydrogenase activities. When the cells were grown on succinate the energy-dependent transhydrogenase activities were lower.

Since these results suggested that there might be a reciprocal relationship between the aerobic-driven transhydrogenase and ATP-formation (P:O value) as predicted by Hempfling's results, we measured oxidative phosphorylation in our respiratory particle preparations (Table 2). The P:O values were low, probably due to lack of coupling factors (2), but could be measured reproducibly by the technique employed. No relationship was found between the aerobic-driven transhydrogenase activity and the P:O values. Thus, although the situation could be different in whole cells, the variation in the transhydrogenase activity with growth conditions does not seem to be due to variation in the ability of

305

TABLE 2. Effect of growth conditions on oxidative phosphorylation performed by respiratory particles

Medium	Harvested	P:O		
		NADH	D-Lactate	Succinate
Salts-glucose	L	0.082	0.082	0.076
	S	0.071	0.062	0.052
Salts-succinate	L	0.075	0.110	0.078
Complex glucose	L	0.091	0.067	0.044
	S	0.095	0.041	0.045

L, logarithmic phase; S, stationary phase

---

the various preparations to carry out oxidative phosphorylation,
or to differences in ATPase, NADH oxidase and cytochrome b_1 levels.

With respiratory particles prepared from cells grown on
trypticase-soy medium (Table 1) or on casein hydrolysate, with
or without glucose (Table 3), the aerobic-driven transhydrogenase
could not be detected and the ATP-driven reaction was much less
active. Growth on glucose in the presence of selected groups of
amino acids or single amino acids indicated that this effect could
not be attributed to any one amino acid. These data suggest that
the energy-dependent transhydrogenase has a role in supplying
NADPH for the biosynthesis of amino acids (and other intermediates),
and that formation of this enzyme is repressed when the preformed
end-product is supplied.

Further support for the function of the transhydrogenase in
anabolism was obtained using three catabolite derepressed mutants
(cat 5,6 and 11) derived from E. coli B. The energy-dependent
transhydroge:ase and ATPase activities of the mutants did not
differ significantly from those of the parent strain.

306

TABLE 3.   Effect of growth in the presence of amino
acids on the energy-dependent transhydrogenase
of respiratory particles

Medium	Additions	Transhydrogenase			ATPase
		Aerobic	ATP	NADPH:O	
Salts	Casein hydrolysate	0	18	0	668
Salts-glucose	--	89	75	0.15	406
	Casein hydrolysate	0	11	0	569
	His,ser,gly	16	33	0.05	670
	Tyr,phe	43	63	0.09	666
	Lys,met,pro,arg,glu	0	21	0	644
	Ileu,Val,leu,thr	0	16	0	625
	Ileu	23	25	0.05	633
	Val	19	21	0.05	539
	Leu	13	17	0.03	642
	Thr	23	25	0.06	622
	Met	23	43	0.06	

Enzyme activities are expressed as nmoles/min/mg protein

ACKNOWLEDGEMENTS

We wish to thank Dr. A. Kropinski for providing the catabolite derepressed mutants of E. coli B and the Medical Research Council of Canada for a research grant.

REFERENCES

1.   Murthy, P.S. and Brodie, A.F.   J. Biol. Chem. 239, 4292, 1964.
2.   Bragg, P.D. and Hou, C.   Can. J. Biochem. 46, 631, 1968.
3.   Fisher, R.J., Lam, K.W. and Sanadi, D.R.   Biochem. Biophys.
     Res. Commun. 39, 1021, 1970.
4.   Sweetman, A.J. and Griffiths, D.E.   Biochem. J. 121, 125,
     1971.
5.   Fisher, R.J. and Sanadi, D.R.   Biochim. Biophys. Acta, 245,
     34, 1971.
6.   Cox, G.B., Newton, N.A., Butlin, J.B. and Gibson, F.   Biochem.
     J. 125, 489, 1971.
7.   Skulachev, V.P.   FEBS Letters, 11, 301, 1970.

307

8. Lee, C.P. and Ernster, L. Eur. J. Biochem. $\underline{3}$, 385, 1968.
9. Hempfling, W.P. Biochem. Biophys. Res. Commun. $\underline{41}$, 9, 1970.
10. Hempfling, W.P. and Beeman, D.K. Biochem. Biophys. Res. Commun. $\underline{45}$, 924, 1971.
11. Bragg, P.D. Biochim. Biophys. Acta, $\underline{96}$, 263, 1965.
12. Davies, P.L. and Bragg, P.D. Biochim. Biophys. Acta, $\underline{266}$, 273, 1972.
13. Butlin, J.D., Cox, G.B. and Gibson, F. Biochem. J. $\underline{124}$, 75, 1971.
14. Jones, C.W. and Redfearn, E.R. Biochim. Biophys. Acta, $\underline{113}$, 467, 1966.

31

Reprinted from J. Bacteriol. **123**:1076–1087 (1975)

Effects of Varying the Carbon Source Limiting Growth on Yield and Maintenance Characteristics of *Escherichia coli* in Continuous Culture[1]

WALTER P. HEMPFLING* AND STANLEY E. MAINZER[2]

Department of Biology, University of Rochester, Rochester, New York 14627

Received for publication 27 May 1975

The magnitudes of Y_0 (grams [dry weight] formed per gram of atom O) and m_0, the maintenance respiration (milligram-atoms of O per gram [dry weight] per hour), of *Escherichia coli* B have been determined by growing the organism in aerobic continuous culture limited by a number of different substrates. The value found were as follows: glucose—$Y_0 = 12.5$, $m_0 = 0.9$; glucose plus 2.7 mM cyclic adenosine 3′,5′-monophosphate (cAMP)—$Y_0 = 31.2$, $m_0 = 9.3$; galactose—$Y_0 = 13.2$, $m_0 = 1.8$; mannitol—$Y_0 = 20.1$, $m_0 = 6.1$; L-glutamate—$Y_0 = 25.5$, $m_0 = 17.7$; glycerol—$Y_0 = 14.9$, $m_0 = 10.0$; succinate—$Y_0 = 11.2$, $m_0 = 12.1$; and acetate—$Y_0 = 14.7$, $m_0 = 25.4$. During growth in anaerobic continous culture with limiting glucose Y_{ATP} was found to be 10.3 g (dry weight)/mol of adenosine 5′-triphosphate (ATP) and m_{ATP} was 18.9 mmol of ATP/g (dry weight) per h. The aerobic growth yields of cells growing on glucose, glucose plus cAMP, mannitol, and glutamate were consistent with the hypothesis that carbohydrates partially repress oxidative phosphorylation, but the yields of cells growing on glycerol, succinate, acetate, and galactose were all lower than expected. We conclude that, like the efficiency of oxidative phosphorylation, both the maintenance respiration and the amount of ATP necessary to serve maintenance processes are determined by the identity of the growth substrates. Yields smaller than expected may be explained by the absence of respiratory control exerted by phosphate acceptors.

Several estimates of the efficiency of energy conservation during the aerobic growth of bacteria have appeared. The methods used to make such estimates have included the determination of the growth yield referred to oxygen consumption (8, 15, 21; A. M. Whittaker and S. Elsden, J. Gen. Microbiol. **31**:xxii), direct measurement of the P/2e⁻ value of oxidative phosphorylation in nondividing whole cell suspensions (1, 10, 31), and calculation of the stoichiometry of respiration-dependent proton extrusion of whole cells (19, 21). Each of these methods has yielded conflicting results when employed by different investigators, possibly as a result of the use of different growth conditions, different preparation procedures, different carbon sources, and different organisms. Especially important is the failure of many workers to take into account, during the estimation of growth yield referred to oxygen consumption,

the effect of a varying growth rate upon yield due to the diversion of energy to maintenance processes (13, 20, 26). The differential repressive effects of different carbon sources upon the efficiency of oxidative phosphorylation (9) have been ignored also.

We have undertaken an investigation of the effects of varying the composition of the growth medium, pH, and temperature of growth upon the growth yield and maintenance requirements of *Escherichia coli* B, an organism which in our hands exhibits dependency of oxidative phosphorylation efficiency on the nature of the substrate. To this end, we have employed the technique of substrate-limited continuous culture (14). This communication describes results obtained when the identity of the carbon source limiting growth is varied and when cyclic adenosine 3′5′-monophosphate (cAMP) is added to glucose-limited medium.

A preliminary report of some of these findings has appeared (S. E. Mainzer and W. P. Hempfling, Abstr. Annu. Meet. Am. Soc. Microbiol., G109, p. 38, 1974). (Some of the data reported

[1] Dedicated to the memory of our friend and teacher. Wolf Vladimir Vishniac (1922–1973).

[2] Present address: Department of Human Genetics. Yale University, School of Medicine, New Haven, Conn. 06511.

here are included in a dissertation submitted by
S.E.M. to the University of Rochester in partial
fulfillment of the requirements for the Ph.D.
degree.)

MATERIALS AND METHODS

Organism. *E. coli* B was maintained as previously
described (12).

Growth media. The minimal medium, described
elsewhere (9), was prepared in 15-liter batches and
sterilized at 121 C for 60 min. Potassium phosphate
buffer (1 M), pH 7.0, and 1 M solutions of the carbon
sources (neutralized when necessary with KOH) were
autoclaved separately. All solutions were added in the
proper proportions to the minimal medium contained
in a mixing reservoir and were thoroughly mixed by
means of a magnetic stirrer before addition to the
culture vessel. The final concentration of phosphate
was 15 mM. When cAMP was included in glucose-
containing medium it was added at a final concentration of 2.7 mM, and the entire medium was then
sterilized by passing it through a membrane filter
apparatus (Millipore Corp.) containing a filter of
$0.22-\mu m$ porosity.

The chemostat. The cylindrical Pyrex chemostat
vessels used were of 330- and 400-ml culture volume.
They were designed in this laboratory and were
fabricated by Blaessig Glass Specialties, Rochester,
N.Y.

The culture medium was pumped through an inlet
at the top of the vessel by means of a Harvard
apparatus peristaltic pump, using both channels to
minimize pulsation. Spent medium and organisms
were removed through an overflow tube protruding
from the side of the vessel at a point about halfway up
the side.

The culture medium in the chemostat vessel was
stirred by a Teflon-covered magnetic stirring bar
driven by a magnetic stirrer placed immediately
beneath the vessel.

The rate of air flow from the laboratory-compressed
air supply was controlled and measured by passage
through a low-pressure, single-stage gas regulator
(The Matheson Co., model 70) at about 2 lb/in^2 and a
Matheson flowmeter (no. 601 or 602). Air was sterilized by passage through two drying tubes (25 by 200
mm) linked in series and packed with sterile, nonab-
sorbent cotton.

Air was dispersed inside the vessel by means of a
centrally located glass tube terminating (about 1.5 cm
from the bottom) with a sintered glass sparger
("coarse" porosity) at rates of 1.0 to 1.6 liters/h.

Effluent gas was separated from the effluent liquid
by providing separate exits for the two components at
the end of the overflow tube. The lower aperture was
connected to a length of rubber tubing with a loop
placed in it so as to form a fluid lock. Once the loop
filled with effluent fluid, air passed out via the
second, upper outlet to either the atmosphere or the
gas analyzer. No restrictions were placed upon the
free exit of the gas from the vessel, thereby avoiding
significant pressure changes in the system.

When anaerobic culture conditions were required,
both chemostat vessel and mixing reservoir received a
continuous flow of N_2 which was first passed through
a gas-washing bottle containing a solution of 20%
(wt/vol) Na_2CO_3 and 20% (wt/vol) pyrogallol. The
flow rate of N_2 was between 1.5 and 3 liters/h.

The temperature of the chemostat vessel was maintained at 37 C ($\pm 0.1°$) by means of a heating tape
wrapped around the vessel. Current was supplied to
the tape by a Variac variable rheostat operated at
about 40% capacity and was regulated by a Yellow
Springs Instrument Co. temperature controller
(model 65 RC). The thermistor probe which served as
detector for the temperature controller was placed in a
water-filled glass well protruding deeply into the
culture fluid in the chemostat vessel.

The hydrogen ion concentration of the culture
medium was maintained at pH 6.8 (± 0.05) with the
aid of a Radiometer pH meter (model pHM 28 and
28b), combination pH electrode (model 5123c), im-
mersed in the growth medium and a titrator unit
(model TTT 11b) operating a magnetic valve (type
MNV 1c). When a valve opened in response to
deviation of the pH of the culture medium from pH
6.8, sterile 1 M KOH or HCl (depending upon the
direction of change) was admitted dropwise, thereby
restoring the hydrogen ion concentration to pH 6.8.
The concentration of alkali or acid used was sufficient
to prevent large volume changes as a consequence of
neutralization but not great enough to cause significant over- or undershoots of pH after addition.

The pH electrode was sterilized in air saturated
with ethylene oxide vapor for 12 to 18 h at 22 C or by
immersion in acidified ethanol (70% ethanol containing enough HCl to give a reaction of pH 2) for a period
of 8 to 12 h at 22 C. Either method gave satisfactory
results if the pH electrode was carefully washed free of
any organic matter that might have adhered to it
during the course of the previous experiment.

Growth in continuous culture. A complete discussion of the theory and operation of continuous culture
devices can be found elsewhere (14). Continuous
culture was initiated by inoculating the complete
medium contained in the chemostat vessel with 1 to 5
ml of suspension of *E. coli* B which had been grown
for 12 to 18 h in batch culture in glucose minimal
medium (9). When the population in the vessel
became visible, medium pumping began at the slowest dilution rate to be used in the experiment. A
minimum of 5 culture volumes was permitted to flow
through the vessel before sampling began; generally a
steady state was attained by the end of the third
culture volume replacement. After completion of
sampling at a given dilution rate, the pumping rate
was increased by a small amount, and the process
was repeated until the desired number of growth
rates had been examined. At this point the mixing
reservoir was drained and rinsed twice with 2 liters
of the minimal medium containing a different
carbon source. In no case was continuous culture
permitted to extend beyond 3 weeks.

Determination of oxygen consumption. The oxygen consumed in the chemostat vessel was measured
with either a Fisher-Hamilton gas partitioner or with
an IBC differential oxygen analyzer. When the gas

partitioner was used for the estimation of oxygen no conditioning of the effluent gas was necessary, but it proved imperative, when the IBC analyzer was employed, to pass the effluent gas through drying tubes containing, in sequence, silica gel, Ascarite, and indicator silica gel in order to remove moisture and CO_2. When these precautions were taken the results obtained with one instrument were indistinguishable from those obtained with the other.

Comparison of the amount of residual oxygen in the effluent gas with the amount of oxygen in the incoming air made it possible to determine the volume of oxygen consumed by the culture. The rate of air flow at the time of oxygen measurement was determined with a 10-ml "bubble meter" and was continuously monitored by means of the Matheson flowmeters. Individual rate measurements differed from the mean rate by ±5%. To calculate the number of moles consumed per unit time a volume of 22.4 liters/mol of O_2 was assumed. The measurements were done at room temperature, and each determination was accompanied by subsequent standardization using primary standard mixtures of O_2 in N_2 obtained from the Matheson Co. Using standards containing 16.6 and 20.4% O_2 (by volume) the typical resolution on a 10-inch (25.4-cm) chart recorder was 6% O_2 (i.e., between 15 and 21% O_2 by volume). The volume of oxygen in the effluent gas never sank below 15% by volume.

When it was desired to estimate the concentration of dissolved oxygen in the growth medium, a Clark electrode was sterilized in ethylene oxide vapor and then inserted in the vessel through a portal provided. The vessel was deoxygenated by flushing with sterile N_2 and then fully aerated by increasing the aeration rate to above 1 liter/min.

Determination of bacterial dry weight. To measure bacterial dry weight the rubber tubing attached to the overflow arm was disconnected and the effluent medium and cells were allowed to fall into a 50-ml polypropylene centrifuge tube surrounded with ice. Collection was continued until at least 15 ml of effluent medium accumulated in the tube, but for not longer than 30 min. Longer periods frequently resulted in significant loss of cell mass, probably through partial cell lysis. Duplicate portions of the effluent culture were collected in this way and then immediately centrifuged for 10 min at $12,000 \times g$ in a Sorvall RC2B refrigerated centrifuge held at 2 C. The volume of the resulting supernatant portion was determined by decantation, and the centrifuge tube containing the sedimented bacteria was allowed to drain. After the sides of the tube were freed of excess moisture, the pellet was suspended in 2.5 to 3.0 ml of 0.15 M NaCl, and duplicate aliquots were placed into dried, tared aluminum weighing pans (weighing approximately 400 mg) and dried to constant weight over a period of 12 to 18 h at 95 to 105 C. An equal volume of NaCl solution was placed on other pans and similarly dried. The weight of bacteria was calculated by subtracting the weight of the NaCl from the weight of the bacteria suspended in NaCl. No further moisture could be removed from the dried samples when

held in vacuo at 105 C for 24 h.

Early measurements of dry weight included saline to prevent possible lysis of cells during repeated washes. Although the weight of NaCl was great compared to the sample, reproducibility of sample weights after subtraction of saline blanks was acceptable. Later control experiments showed that no differences in weight occurred between unwashed samples and those washed once or twice with saline; therefore, washing of cell pellets was discontinued. The use of saline was continued so that the results of the two methods could be directly compared.

Estimation of the carbon content of dried bacteria. *E. coli* B, grown in batch culture on several different media, were harvested by centrifugation in the cold during the late log period of aerobic growth at 37 C in a New Brunswick Scientific Co. incubator-shaker. The bacterial pellets were resuspended to 20% of the original culture volume in distilled water and again centrifuged. The washed pellets were resuspended in a small volume of distilled water and then dried to constant weight. The carbon content of the dried bacterial masses was measured with a Hewlett-Packard CHN analyzer, model 185. Cyclohexa-none-2,4-diphenylhydrazone and L-arginine were used as standards.

Measurement of the concentrations of glucose, acetate, lactate, and ethanol. Glucose concentrations of samples of the medium contained in the mixing reservoir and of the effluent medium were determined by the Glucostat method, using reagents obtained from the Worthington Biochemical Corp.

Acetate in the supernatant fraction of the effluent medium was estimated using acetate kinase obtained from the Sigma Chemical Co. The reaction mixture employed was adapted from that described by Rose et al. (27); it contained, in a final volume of 1.0 ml: 0.5 to 2.5 µmol of tris(hydroxymethyl)aminomethane-chloride, pH 7.4; 10 µmol of $MgCl_2$, 10 µmol of adenosine 5'-triphosphate (ATP) (neutralized); 750 µmol of hydroxylamine (pH 7.4); 1.5 to 2.0 U of crystalline acetate kinase; and 20 µmol of 2-mercaptoethanol. After incubation of the mixture for 90 min at 37 C the reaction was terminated by the addition of 0.5 ml of 20% (wt/vol) trichloroacetic acid followed by 1.0 ml of 5% (wt/vol) $FeCl_3$ in 4 N HCl. The optical density of the solution at 510 nm was determined, and the value was compared with those given by carrying out the reaction with known amounts of sodium acetate.

Lactate and ethanol in the supernatant portion of the effluent medium were measured by enzymatic techniques as described by Hohorst (17) and Bonnichsen (3), respectively. Hydrazine hydrate replaced semicarbazide and hydrazine sulfate.

Spectrophotometric measurements were performed with a Hitachi-Coleman Perkin-Elmer model 124 dual wavelength spectrophotometer, using Pyrex cuvettes of 1.00-cm lightpath length.

Statistical treatment of data. The final graphical presentation of the data was chosen so as to provide an assessment of cumulative experimental error; to this end the linear regression coefficients are provided for each function. Graphical functions were obtained which best fitted the data by the means of the least-squares method. The linear regression coefficients were calculated (7) with the aid of a Hewlett-Packard calculator, model 9100A.

RESULTS

Estimation of Y_{ATP} through anaerobic continuous culture in glucose-limited minimal medium. Because different values of the growth "constant," Y_{ATP} (grams [bacterial dry weight] formed per mole of ATP synthesized), have been reported (6), it was necessary to establish the value of Y_{ATP} characteristic of *E. coli* B before proceeding to aerobic growth experiments. This was best accomplished in anaerobic continuous culture using limiting glucose, since the stoichiometry of ATP formation is known for the fermentative reactions carried out by that organism. Whereas the identity of the fermentation products varied with the growth rate, it was nevertheless possible to calculate ATP production simply by measuring the amount of glucose metabolized, the amount of glucose incorporated into cell material, and the amount of acetate formed (8). Only trace amounts of ethanol and lactate were formed; therefore, we have assumed the balance of carbon-containing fermentation products to be formate and CO_2. The following reactions were assumed to occur: (i) glucose + 2 adenosine 5′-diphosphate (ADP) + 2 P_i → 2 pyruvate + 2 ATP + 2 (2e⁻ + 2H⁺); (ii) pyruvate + ADP + P_i → acetate + formate + ATP.

A small correction for the assimilation of glucose into cell material was applied based on the finding that carbon comprises 45.6% (standard deviation = 2.6%) of the bacterial dry mass. This value was obtained from measurements of the carbon composition of *E. coli* B grown in batch culture in media containing eight different carbon sources over a range of specific growth rates of 0.4 to 1.2/h. It was assumed that cellular carbon was at the average reduction level of carbohydrate. Several measurements of the carbon composition of cells growing in anaerobic continuous culture have shown that the ratio of carbon to cell mass remains constant down to a specific growth rate of about 0.1/h.

The results of the experiment relating bacterial dry mass to ATP production in anaerobic continuous culture are given in Table 1. The amount of acetate formed per mole of glucose metabolized is strongly dependent upon the rate of growth. The yields referred to moles of glucose metabolized ($Y_{glucose}$) and to moles of ATP produced (Y_{ATP}) exhibit similarly strong dependencies upon growth rate. $Y_{glucose}$ and Y_{ATP}, when plotted versus the dilution rate on the abscissa, can be seen to vary hyperbolically with the specific growth rate, a phenomenon consistent with the view that part of the ATP produced is diverted to serve maintenance processes at a rate which is independent of the growth rate. An estimate of the amount of substrate required to serve maintenance processes can be obtained by means of the double reciprocal plot of $1/Y_{substrate}$ versus $1/D$ as suggested by Pirt (26). In Fig. 1 we show that such a plot ($1/Y_{ATP}$ versus $1/D$) yields a straight line. The intercept on the ordinate is $1/Y_{ATP}$ corrected for the diversion of ATP for maintenance purposes, and the slope of the function represents the rate of ATP utilization for purposes of maintenance (m_{ATP}). Using this linear transformation of the data, $Y_{ATP}(max)$ is 10.7 g (bacterial dry weight) per mol of ATP, and

TABLE 1. *Yield characteristics of E. coli B growing in glucose-limited anaerobic continuous culture*[a]

D (h⁻¹)	x (μg [dry wt]/ml)	Residual glucose (mM)	Glucose[b] metabolized (mM)	Acetate produced (mM)	ATP/glucose metabolized	$Y_{glucose}$[c]	Y_{ATP}[d]
0.087	107	ND[e]	12.7	9.5	2.75	8.40	3.05
0.153	135	ND	12.4	5.1	2.41	10.9	4.50
0.254	176	ND	12.2	4.3	2.35	14.4	6.13
0.364	188	0.015	12.1	4.7	2.39	15.6	6.53
0.570	129	4.67	7.8	1.7	2.22	16.5	7.43

[a] Conditions: 330-ml vessel; 13.5 mM glucose in medium.

[b] Glucose metabolized = glucose concentration in reservoir medium minus glucose concentration in effluent (residual glucose) minus glucose equivalent of incorporated carbon. Glucose incorporated (mM) = 0.456 x/(12) (6).

[c] x (micrograms/milliliter)/micromoles of glucose metabolized per milliliter.

[d] $Y_{glucose}$/moles of ATP per mole of glucose metabolized.

[e] ND, Not detectable.

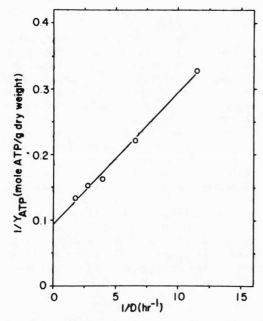

FIG. 1. *Relation of Y_{ATP} of E. coli B growing anaerobically with limiting glucose to dilution rate: double reciprocal linear transformation. Linear regression coefficient, 0.9968.*

m_{ATP} is 20.1 mmol of ATP/g (dry weight) per h.

To offset, in part, appreciable error introduced by the method used to plot the data we also have determined Y_{ATP}(max) and m_{ATP} by plotting Y_{ATP} versus Y_{ATP}/D according to the method recommended by Hofstee (16). A Hofstee plot gives Y_{ATP}(max) = 9.9 g (bacterial dry weight) per mol of ATP, and m_{ATP} = 17.7 mmol of ATP/g (dry weight) per h with a linear regression coefficient of −0.959. We will accept the means of the two plotting methods as the effective values; that is, Y_{ATP}(max) is 10.3 g (dry weight) per mol of ATP and m_{ATP} is 18.9

mmol of ATP/g (dry weight) per h.

Yield and maintenance in aerobic continuous culture limited by glucose and the effect of cAMP. The results of a representative experiment in which glucose served as the compound limiting growth are given in Table 2. It should be noted that the amount of oxygen consumed at each growth rate did not account for complete oxidation of glucose, even though only traces of glucose remained in the effluent medium. Assay of acetate in the effluent medium showed it to be a major end product, especially at higher growth rates, in addition to CO_2. Other oxidation products were not sought. From the double reciprocal plot of $1/Y_0$ versus $1/D$ of the data in Table 2 and data obtained from additional experiments (Fig. 2) we calculate that Y_0 corrected for maintenance respiration, that is, Y_0(max), is 12.5 g (dry weight)/g-atom of O and that the rate of maintenance respiration (m_0) is 0.9 mg-atom of O/g (dry weight) per h.

Addition of cAMP to the glucose-limited medium resulted in a marked increase in the rate of maintenance respiration and in Y_0(max). These results are also shown in Table 2 and Fig. 2. Y_0(max) reaches 31.2 g (dry weight)/g-atom of O (an increase of some 2.5-fold) and m_0 increases more than 10 times to 9.3 mg of O/g per h.

In these and in following experiments the amount of dissolved oxygen remaining in the growth medium was estimated by direct insertion of the Clark electrode into the chemostat vessel. At no time was the amount of oxygen found to be less than about 70% of air saturation. It should be pointed out that the respiratory rate in any dilution rate can be determined directly from the data provided according to the expression $D Y_0^{-1}/2$ = moles of O_2 per gram per hour.

Yield and maintenance in aerobic continu-

TABLE 2. *Estimation of Y_0 as a function of D in glucose-limited aerobic continuous culture in the presence and absence of 2.7 mM cAMP*

Condition	D (h^{-1})	x (μg [dry wt]/ml)	Output (mg [dry wt]/h)	Respiration (mmol of O_2/h)	Y_0 (g [dry wt]/g-atom of O)	Q_{O_2} (μmol of O_2/mg/h)
5.1 mM glucose,	0.090	234	7.30	0.33	10.9	4.34
330-ml vessel	0.190	310	19.5	0.82	11.9	8.02
	0.380	309	39.3	1.66	11.8	16.3
	0.510	306	51.7	2.12	12.0	21.0
	0.970	147	46.9	1.96	12.3	40.4
5.0 mM glucose +	0.095	111	3.48	0.23	7.75	6.01
2.7 mM cAMP	0.127	148	6.19	0.34	9.10	6.96
	0.162	177	9.46	0.43	11.0	7.36
	0.248	215	17.6	0.60	14.7	8.46

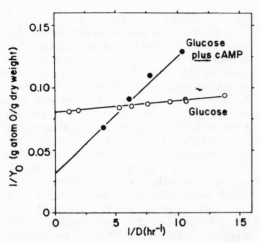

FIG. 2. *Relation of Y_0 of E. coli B growing aerobically with limiting glucose in the presence and absence of 2.7 mM cAMP to dilution rate:double reciprocal linear transformation.*

ous culture limited by carbon sources other than glucose. Experiments similar to those carried out with limiting glucose were performed with limiting galactose, mannitol, glycerol, L-glutamate, succinate, or acetate, and the results are given in Table 3. The data were then subjected to the two methods of linear transformation, and the values of m_0 and of $Y_0(max)$ thereby obtained are shown in Table 4.

Galactose and mannitol are compounds with the greatest similarity to glucose, and galactose-grown cells are characterized by values of Y_0 (max) and m_0 close to those of glucose-grown cells. Mannitol-grown cells differ significantly from hexose-grown cells: $Y_0(max)$ is nearly doubled and m_0 undergoes an even larger increase. The addition of cAMP to glucose-limited cultures elicits growth with the largest value of $Y_0(max)$.

Still larger values of the rate of maintenance respiration are observed when noncarbohydrate substrates are used to limit growth in aerobic continuous culture. Only when L-glutamate is employed as the substrate limiting growth, however, does the value of $Y_0(max)$ change substantially from that of glucose-grown cells. It is of interest that all of the m_0 values obtained with this set of substrates exceed even the rate of maintenance respiration observed in cultures growing with glucose and cAMP.

It can be seen that $Y_0(max)$ varies from 11.2 g(dry weight)/g-atom of O (succinate) to 31.9 g (dry weight)/g-atom of O (glucose plus cAMP), a difference of some 2.8-fold. Values of m_0 vary from 0.9 mg-atom of O/g per h (glucose)

to 25.4 mg-atom of O/g per h (acetate), a difference of some 28-fold.

Contribution of oxidative phosphorylation to $Y_0(max)$. We estimate the contribution of oxidative phosphorylation to $Y_0(max)$ values by correcting for the amount of ATP formed due to substrate-level phosphorylation and for the amount of ATP expended in the synthesis of monomers (6). These adjustments are made on the mean values of $Y_0(max)$ obtained by averaging the values derived from the double-reciprocal and Hofstee plots and result in a value called "$Y_0(max)$ corrected" in Table 4. After correction for the use of ATP for monomer biosynthesis and for the contribution of ATP from substrate-level phosphorylation, it is seen that the contribution of oxidative phosphorylation to $Y_0(max)$ varies from 9.2 g (dry weight)/g-atom of O (glucose) to 27.9 g (dry weight)/g-atom of O (glucose plus cAMP), a difference of threefold.

DISCUSSION

The results described here show that both the maintenance respiration rate and the growth yield referred to oxygen consumption of *E. coli* B are dependent upon the identity of the substrate used to limit growth in aerobic continuous culture. Among cells grown in carbohydrate-limiting medium there exists an apparent correlation between $Y_0(max)$ and m_0 in that cultures with higher yields also exhibit higher maintenance respiration. Such a correlation is not as strong in cultures grown on noncarbohydrate substrates.

Y_{ATP}. Fundamental to any attempt to derive the stoichiometry of ATP formation through substrate metabolism is the accurate and reliable estimation of Y_{ATP} during the metabolism of substrates through known pathways. The present findings indicate that $Y_{ATP}(max)$ is 10.3 g (dry weight)/mol of ATP formed during glucose fermentation. Such a value is typical of those reported by others, as given by Forrest and Walker (6). Lower values can in part be rationalized by the failure of the investigators to take into account expenditure of ATP for purposes of maintenance. The consequences of disregarding maintenance are seen in the low values for Y_{ATP} of the growth of *E. coli* calculated by Hernandez and Johnson (15).

Considerably higher values of Y_{ATP} can be found in the literature. Although some of these data arise from the failure to take into account the variation of fermentation products as a function of growth rate (see, for example, reference 23), such an explanation cannot be applied

TABLE 3. *Yield characteristics of E. coli B growing in aerobic continuous cultures limited by substrates other than glucose*

Substrate	Concn in reservoir (mM)	Culture vol (ml)	D (h⁻¹)	x (µg [dry wt]/ml)	Output (mg [dry wt]/h)	Respiration (mmol of O_2/h)	Y_0 (G [dry wt]/g-atom of O)
Mannitol	5.9	330	0.063	344	7.15	0.50	7.15
			0.087	355	10.2	0.62	8.27
			0.125	397	16.4	0.82	10.0
			0.254	409	34.3	1.30	13.2
	4.5		0.189	338	21.1	0.83	12.7
	2.9		0.573	233	44.0	1.28	17.2
Galactose	6.2	330	0.103	350	11.9	0.55	10.8
			0.135	357	15.9	0.69	11.5
	5.4		0.172	314	17.8	0.80	11.1
			0.232	342	26.2	1.11	11.8
			0.286	381	36.0	1.44	12.5
			0.476	326	51.3	2.02	12.7
Glycerol	3.9	330	0.100	92	3.03	0.24	6.31
			0.129	79	3.36	0.23	7.30
			0.171	91	5.16	0.32	8.07
			0.108	131	4.66	0.37	6.30
			0.136	161	7.24	0.51	7.10
			0.234	199	15.4	0.84	9.18
			0.467	215	33.1	1.44	11.5
	4.5	400	0.100	96	3.86	0.35	5.52
			0.236	139	13.1	0.73	9.00
			0.336	134	18.0	0.91	9.90
			0.474	162	30.7	1.30	11.8
	5.0		0.203	148	12.0	0.73	8.23
			0.322	164	21.1	1.07	9.86
Succinate	8.0	400	0.082	133	4.36	0.50	4.36
			0.125	120	6.00	0.56	5.36
			0.164	152	10.0	0.85	5.88
			0.227	158	14.4	1.04	6.92
			0.294	118	13.9	0.92	7.55
			0.378	116	17.5	0.97	9.02
L-Glutamate	3.0	400	0.080	70	2.24	0.28	3.90
			0.154	90	5.52	0.46	6.03
	5.0		0.173	107	7.39	0.56	6.60
			0.228	116	10.6	0.64	8.31
			0.238	118	11.2	0.64	8.60
			0.357	123	17.6	0.71	12.4
			0.475	107	20.3	0.80	12.7
	6.0	330	0.185	170	10.4	0.67	7.82
			0.244	192	15.5	0.84	9.20
			0.303	227	22.7	1.15	9.90
			0.435	240	34.5	1.24	13.9
Acetate	10	400	0.141	108	6.11	0.76	4.02
			0.172	116	7.96	0.86	4.63
			0.285	100	11.4	0.88	6.48
			0.367	75	11.0	0.77	7.14

to all experiments which lead to values of Y_{ATP} significantly in excess of 10 g (dry weight)/mol of ATP. For example, values of Y_{ATP} approaching the theoretical maximum of 25 to 30 g (dry weight)/mol of ATP (6) have been obtained during the anaerobic continuous culture with limiting glucose of *Lactobacillus casei* L3 (5) and during the anaerobic continuous culture with excess glucose and limiting tryptophan of *Aerobacter aerogenes* (30). In these experiments the growth rate was varied so that the maintenance expenditure of ATP could be determined, and fermentation products were assayed. Hadjipetrou et al. (8) had earlier reported a value of about 10.5 g/mol of ATP for the anaerobic yield of *A. aerogenes* growing in batch culture, but did not include a correction for maintenance in reaching that conclusion. An explanation for

Table 4. *Summary of yield and maintenance data and calculation of contribution of oxidative phosphorylation to $Y_0(max)$*

Substrate	m_0			$Y_0(max)$			r^c		ATP required[d] for monomer synthesis (mol of ATP/g)	ATP formed[e] at the substrate level (ATP/O)	$Y_0(max)$[f] corrected
	A^a	B^b	Mean	A	B	Mean	A	B			
Glucose	0.96	0.83	0.90	12.5	12.4	12.5	0.937	-0.930	0	0.33	9.2
Succinate	13.1	11.0	12.1	12.0	10.4	11.2	0.985	-0.991	0.012	0.14	10.0[g]
Galactose	1.75	1.90	1.82	13.1	13.3	13.2	0.874	-0.824	0	0.17	11.5
Glycerol	10.2	9.70	10.0	15.0	14.7	14.9	0.972	-0.964	0.012	0.29	12.2
Acetate	25.9	24.9	25.4	15.1	14.2	14.7	0.998	-0.966	0.038	0	15.2
Mannitol	5.73	6.50	6.12	19.3	21.0	20.1	0.995	-0.984	0	0.31	17.0
Glutamate	17.1	18.2	17.7	24.0	27.0	25.5	0.986	-0.887	0.012	0.33	22.5
Glucose plus cAMP	9.31	9.40	9.35	31.2	31.3	31.2	0.990	-0.947	0	0.33	27.9

[a] $1/Y_0$ versus $1/D$.

[b] Y_0 versus Y_0/D.

[c] Linear regression coefficient.

[d] ATP required for the net synthesis of 2.5 mmol of glucose from the starting substrate (equivalent of the carbon content of 1 g [dry weight] of bacteria).

[e] Assuming complete oxidation of the substrate through the Embden-Meyerhof-Parnas pathway (where applicable) and the Krebs tricarboxylic acid cycle (substrate level phosphorylation equivalent to cases where acetate is a major end product of oxidation).

[f] Calculated by adding to $Y_0(max)$ an amount of dry weight equivalent to the ATP requirement for monomer synthesis and then subtracting an amount of dry weight equivalent to the ATP formed at the substrate level.

[g] Additional correction of 0.01 mol of ATP/g (dry weight) applied to offset redox imbalance of $2e^-$/succinate.

the large difference between the "average" value of Y_{ATP} and those reported by Stouthamer's group (5, 30) is not available.

In the present anaerobic experiment and in those of others with *L. casei* (5) and *A. aerogenes* (30), appreciable corrections in the growth rate-dependent values of Y_{ATP} were made because of relatively large demands of substrate purposes of maintenance. This does not mean, however, that all earlier estimates of Y_{ATP} are rendered invalid because of failure to correct for m_{ATP}, because similarly large maintenance requirements are not exhibited by all microorganisms. Bauchop and Elsden used *Streptococcus faecalis* to obtain some of the earliest estimates of Y_{ATP} (2). We have observed that the Y_{ATP} value of *S. faecalis* 10C1 is invariant down to a specific growth rate of 0.1/h, a good indication that m_{ATP} is small enough to have little effect upon Y_{ATP} (W. P. Hempfling, S. E. Mainzer, and P. J. VanDemark, Bacterial. Proc., p. 143, 1969).

Substrate dependency of $Y_0(max)$. We have suggested that the efficiency of oxidative phosphorylation in *E. coli* B is determined by the identity of the energy source used for growth through a mechanism similar to catabolite repression (9). This hypothesis was based upon the observations that glucose-grown cells showed $P/2e^-$ values of 1.7, and cells grown at

the expense of Casamino Acids plus succinate, glycerol, or acetate showed $P/2e^-$ values of about 3. The addition of 3 mM cAMP to cultures growing in glucose-containing media (in the presence or absence of Casamino Acids) overcame the repressive effect of glucose and brought about the growth of cells with a $P/2e^-$ value of about 3 (11).

Current experiments indicate that the level of oxidative phosphorylation efficiency of glucose-grown cells which we reported previously was, in fact, an underestimate. Using a procedure which allows the direct measurement of total oxygen consumption and total inorganic phosphate esterification in the first 3 s after oxygenation of anaerobic cells, we now find that the maximum P/O value of glucose-grown cells is 1.0 (W. P. Hempfling and T. A. Kurtz, manuscript in preparation).

In Table 5 we present the P/O values predicted for each continous culture, assuming complete oxidation of substrate and based upon the hypothesis that glucose-grown cells carry out oxidative phosphorylation with a P/O value of 1.0, galactose- or mannitol-grown cells with P/O values of 2.0, and the remaining cells with values of 3.0. Predictions have been made with assumptions which give the largest possible quantities; that is, glucose-grown cells have a single site of phosphorylation associated with

TABLE 5. *Comparison of observed and predicted P/O values*

Substrate	Predicted P/O[a]	Observed P/O[b]	Observed/ predicted
Glucose	1.0	0.89	0.89
Galactose	2.0	1.12	0.56
Mannitol	2.0	1.65	0.83
Glycerol	2.7	1.18	0.44
Succinate	2.7	0.97	0.36
Acetate	2.8	1.48	0.53
Glutamate	2.8	2.18	0.80
Glucose plus cAMP	2.9	2.70	0.93

[a] Calculated by assuming complete oxidation of substrate and one "site" of phosphorylation associated with cytochrome b_1 oxidation in glucose-grown cells, two "sites" of phosphorylation associated with flavoprotein oxidation in mannitol- and galactose-grown cells, and three "sites" of phosphorylation associated with pyridine nucleotide oxidation in the remaining cultures (9–11). In some cases the values are not integral because of flavoprotein-linked oxidation of intermediate succinate or α-glycerophosphate.

[b] Observed P/O = "Y_0(max) corrected"/Y_{ATP} (see Table 4).

the oxidation of cytochrome b_1 or cytochrome o, and galactose- or mannitol-grown cells have an additional site associated with the oxidation of flavin. The predicted efficiencies of oxidative phosphorylation are compared with observed efficiencies taken from the data in Table 3.

Reasonable agreement between the predicted and observed P/O values was obtained for cells grown at the expense of glucose, glucose plus cAMP, mannitol, and glutamate. The observed P/O values of the remainder of the cultures fall short of the predicted values. The poorest agreement is found between the observed and predicted P/O values of succinate-grown cells. In addition, the discrepancy between predicted and observed results with galactose-grown cells is particularly difficult to explain, since energy-consuming reactions in biosynthesis of monomers are thought to be less important during growth on carbohydrates than during growth on simpler compounds; hence, unanticipated corrections are less likely to be necessary.

In spite of the obvious discrepancies with some substrates, it does not seem justified to discard the hypothesis which led to the predicted values of P/O. In no case did the observed value exceed the predicted value, and glucose-grown cells exhibited the lowest efficiency as predicted by the hypothesis. The agreement found during growth on glucose, glucose plus cAMP, mannitol, and glutamate prompts us to consider reasons why the capacity

for oxidative phosphorylation is not used fully by cells growing on acetate, glycerol, succinate, or galactose. Even though washed suspensions of *E. coli* are no longer growing at significant rates, they are still capable of rapid respiration when mixed with their growth substrate (6, 9). ATP is synthesized, but at low efficiency (12). These observations suggest that no obligatory coupling exists between phosphorylation and respiration in the sense that it exists in mitochondria with high "respiratory control ratios." Those cultures which fall short of the predicted P/O ratio by a significant margin are also those in which respiration is fastest at a given specific growth rate, but this may be a cause or a consequence of low P/O values. Rottenberg et al. (28) have pointed out that the conditions of an experiment designed to measure the efficiency of oxidative phosphorylation—temperature, concentrations of reactants, and respiratory rate—may well diminish the observed P/O values significantly below the predicted ones. It is probably unreasonable to predict all the features of the behavior of bacterial oxidative phosphorylation systems from results of experiments with mitochondria.

Maintenance respiration. We have measured that fraction of respiration which satisfies those energy-requiring processes of maintenance operating at rates independent of the rate of growth and have shown that the magnitude of that maintenance respiration rate is a function of the identity of the substrate limiting growth. Only a few reports describing estimation of the maintenance respiration are extant. Schulze and Lipe (29) cultivated *E. coli* continuously with limiting glucose and in the presence of oxygen and found that a plot of Q_{O_2} versus growth rate yielded a straight line with positive slope which intersected the ordinate above the origin at a value of about 1 mg-atom of O/g (dry weight) per h at 37 C. Their value compares nicely with our own of 0.9 mg-atom of O/g (dry weight) per h. Meyer and Jones (21) cultivated several bacteria in media containing excess glycerol or succinate and set the growth rate by varying the rate at which oxygen was made available to the cell population. When *E. coli* was grown in succinate-containing medium, a value of about 10.4 mg-atom of O/g (dry weight) per h (30 C) was obtained at specific growth rates below 0.3/h. At faster growth rates, however, the apparent maintenance respiration rate increased markedly, so much so that extrapolation of Y_0^{-1} to the ordinate of the double reciprocal plot resulted in a negative value, making application of the Pirt expression meaningless. The reasons for this deviation are not apparent. Nevertheless, Meyer and Jones obtained a value at slow growth rates which compares well with our own estimate of 12.1 mg-atom of O/g (dry weight) per h for the maintenance respiration rate of succinate-grown cells.

Since m_0 varies with the growth substrate, either the amount of energy necessary for maintenance changes with the substrate or the efficiency of energy conservation associated with respiration changes with the substrate, or both phenomena occur. Let us first assume that the amount of energy required for maintenance is independent of the substrate used for growth. If that be true, then changes in m_0 are a consequence of the changes of P/O with growth substrate. To test this hypothesis we calculate the amount of ATP expended for maintenance on the basis of an estimate of P/O derived from $Y_0(max)$ (assuming that Y_{ATP} equals 10 g [dry weight]/mol of ATP) and find that m_{ATP} is not constant but varies from 1.1 mmol of ATP/g per h (aerobic glucose) to 41.1 mmol of ATP/g (acetate) per h. The assumption that P/O varies with substrate and is equal to 1, 2, or 3 (9) likewise leads to the conclusion that m_{ATP} is not constant. Therefore, since $Y_0(max)$ varies according to the substrate used for growth, and since Y_0 (max) is generally taken to reflect P/O, we conclude that both m_{ATP} and P/O are determined by the substrate used for growth and by the presence or absence of oxygen. As a consequence of this dual variation, m_0 also varies with the growth of substrate.

To calculate a value of P/2e$^-$ for nitrate respiration Stouthamer and Bettenhaussen assumed that m_{ATP} of *A. aerogenes* was the same during anaerobic growth in the presence or absence of nitrate (30). The present results suggest that attempts ought to be made to verify that assumption.

It is of interest to consider possible explanations for the variation of m_0 (and m_{ATP}) with the growth substrate. Such a consideration must recognize that the maintenance processes served are independent of the rate of growth, a conclusion made necessary by the linearity of all double reciprocal plots of $1/Y_0$ versus $1/D$ which have been presented here. Since growth rates approaching μ_{max} were not examined (with the exception of aerobic glucose medium), however, the results reported here do not exclude the possibility that small but significant amounts of energy might be diverted to support growth rate-dependent maintenance functions.

Two kinds of reactions are likely to require energy in a manner which fulfills the kinetic restrictions: turnover of macromolecular constituents and membrane-associated transport

processes which are "active" in nature. Protein is known to comprise about one-half of the cell's dry mass and undergoes destruction and resynthesis (turnover) during growth, but it is unlikely that increased maintenance respiration is caused by increased protein turnover. Pine showed that, in *E. coli* B growing in a balanced manner in glucose-containing medium ($\mu = 0.84/h$) or in acetate-containing medium ($\mu = 0.25/h$), protein turnover was 2.5%/h and 3.0%/h, respectively (25). This increase of only 20% contrasts strongly with an increase in maintenance respiration rate of about 28-fold. Marr et al. found an increase in the rate of protein turnover at low growth rates (20), but such a process as the one described by them does not fulfill the necessary kinetic requirements to be the reaction we seek. Nevertheless, calculations show that protein turnover comprises a major fraction of the maintenance requirement of cells growing aerobically on glucose: assuming a requirement for protein synthesis of 27 moles of ATP/g (dry weight) (6), a turnover rate of 2.5%/h gives m_{ATP} of 0.6 mmol/g per h, or about one-half of the total m_{ATP} of 1.12 mmol of ATP/g per h. The ATP requirement for protein synthesis was calculated by Forrest and Walker assuming 3 mol of ATP per amino acid and a constant requirement of about 2 mol of ATP per amino acid for purposes of messenger ribonucleic acid (mRNA) turnover. Nierlich (24) has pointed out that no obligately stoichiometric coupling appears to exist between protein synthesis and messenger ribonucleic acid synthesis; hence the assumption of Forrest and Walker may well be invalid for all culture conditions, especially if it is found that the noncarbohydrate carbon sources enrich the population of messenger ribonucleic acid molecules with species of very short half-lives. An accurate assessment of the possibility of differential contributions of messenger ribonucleic acid turnover to maintenance requirements during growth at the expense of different energy sources must await further experiments.

"Active" transport of solutes into and out of the cell is another process which may require significant amounts of energy. Such transport processes must, however, satisfy the kinetic criterion of independence of the rate of growth. Unfortunately, little information is available about the rate of, say, acetate uptake and extrusion as a function of growth rate, nor are data extant which relate respiration and the rate of uptake of growth substrate under our conditions of growth. It is of interest that those substrates thought to be transported by the phosphoenolpyruvate phosphotransferase system (18) yield cells with the lowest aerobic values of m_{ATP}.

The active nature of transport of ions such as K$^+$ has recently been questioned by Minkoff and Damadian (22). Should their arguments be substantiated, ion transport could then be ignored as a major energy-requiring maintenance process. At high external ion concentrations (e.g., 60 mg-ions of K$^+$/liter, as in the present experiments) it is not likely that differences in the efficiency of ion transport might explain the differences of m_{ATP}, since DiGiacomo (Ph.D. dissertation, University of Rochester, Rochester, N.Y., 1973) observed a constant ratio of K$^+$ taken up to oxygen consumed after the addition of glucose, mannitol, or glycerol to washed suspensions of nondividing *E. coli* B which had been grown at the expense of the substrate added. However, at low K$^+$ concentrations (e.g., less than 100 μg-ions of K$^+$/liter), some variation of m_0 but not of Y_0(max) becomes apparent (S.E. Mainzer and W.P. Hempfling, manuscript in preparation), suggesting that m_{ATP} is changed.

Finally, as there appears to be no obligatory coupling between respiration and phosphorylation, so there may exist a similar relationship between respiration and energy-requiring maintenance processes. This interpretation of the change of m_0 with substrate is consistent with the observation that those cultures respiring most rapidly at a given specific growth rate exhibit the highest values of m_0 as well as the largest deviations of observed from predicted P/O values.

ACKNOWLEDGMENTS

We are grateful to Diane K. Beeman, Judith N. Conners, and Theresa A. Kurtz for their patience and their excellent technical assistance.

This work was supported by a grant from the National Science Foundation (GB-25582).

LITERATURE CITED

1. Baak, J. M., and P. W. Postma. 1971. Oxidative phosphorylation in intact *Azotobacter vinelandii*. FEBS Lett. **19**:189-192.
2. Bauchop, T., and S. Elsden. 1960. The growth of micro-organisms in relation to their energy supply. J. Gen. Microbiol. **23**:457-467.
3. Bonnichsen, R. 1965. Ethanol. Determination with alcohol dehydrogenase and DPN, p. 285-287. *In* H. U. Bergmeyer (ed.), Methods of enzymatic analysis. Academic Press Inc., New York.
4. Chance, B., L. Smith, and L. Castor. 1953. New methods for the study of the carbon monoxide compounds of respiratory enzymes. Biochim. Biophys. Acta **12**:289-298.
5. deVries, W., W. M. C. Kapteijn, E. G. van der Beek, and A. H. Stouthamer. 1970. Molar growth yields and fermentation balances of *Lactobacillus casei* L3 in batch cultures and in continuous cultures. J. Gen. Microbiol. **63**:333-345.
6. Forrest, W. W., and D. J. Walker. 1971. The generation and utilization of energy during growth, p. 213-274. *In* A. H. Rose and J. F. Wilkinson (ed.), Advances in microbial physiology, vol. 5. Academic Press Inc., New York.
7. Freund, J. E. 1971. Mathematical statistics, p. 361-367. Prentice-Hall, Englewood Cliffs, N. J.
8. Hadjipetrou, L. P., J. P. Gerrits, F. A. G. Teulings, and A. H. Stouthamer. 1964. Relation between energy production and growth of *Aerobacter aerogenes*. J. Gen. Microbiol. **36**:139-150.
9. Hempfling, W. P. 1970. Repression of oxidative phosphorylation in *Escherichia coli* B by growth in glucose and other carbohydrates. Biochem. Biophys. Res. Commun. **41**:9-15.
10. Hempfling, W. P. 1970. Studies of the efficiency of oxidative phosphorylation in intact *Escherichia coli* B. Biochim. Biophys. Acta **205**:169-182.
11. Hempfling, W. P., and D. K. Beeman. 1971. Release of glucose repression of oxidative phosphorylation in *Escherichia coli* B by cyclic adenosine 3',5'-monophosphate. Biochem. Biophys. Res. Commun. **45**:924-929.
12. Hempfling, W. P., M. Hofer, E. Harris, and B. Pressman. 1967. Correlation between changes in metabolite concentrations and rate of ion transport following glucose addition to *Escherichia coli* B. Biochim. Biophys. Acta **141**:391-400.
13. Hempfling, W. P., and W. Vishniac. 1967. Yield coefficients of *Thiobacillus neapolitanus* in continuous culture. J. Bacteriol. **93**:874-878.
14. Herbert, D., R. Ellsworth, and R. C. Telling. 1956. The continuous culture of bacteria: a theoretical and experimental study. J. Gen. Microbiol. **14**:601-622.
15. Hernandez, E., and M. J. Johnson. 1967. Energy supply and cell yield in aerobically grown microorganisms. J. Bacteriol. **94**:996-1001.
16. Hofstee, B. H. J. 1959. Non-inverted *versus* inverted plots in enzyme kinetics. Nature (London) **184**:1296-1298.
17. Hohorst, H.-J. 1965. L-(+)-lactate. Determination with lactic dehydrogenase and DPN, p. 266-270. *In* H. U. Bergmeyer (ed.), Methods of enzymatic analysis. Academic Press Inc., New York.
18. Kundig, W., S. Ghosh, and S. Roseman. 1964. Phosphate bound to histidine in a protein as intermediate in a novel phosphotransferase system. Proc. Natl. Acad. Sci. U.S.A. **52**:1067-1074.
19. Lawford, H. G., and B. A. Haddock. 1973. Respiration-driven proton translocation in *Escherichia coli*. Biochem. J. **136**:217-220.
20. Marr, A. G., E. H. Nilson, and D. J. Clark. 1963. The maintenance requirement of *Escherichia coli*. Ann. N.Y. Acad. Sci. **102**:536-548.
21. Meyer, D. J., and C. W. Jones. 1973. Oxidative phosphorylation in bacteria which contain different cytochrome oxidase. Eur. J. Biochem. **36**:144-151.
22. Minkoff, L., and R. Damadian. 1973. Caloric catastrophe. Biophys. J. **13**:167-178.
23. Moustafa, H. H., and E. B. Collins. 1968. Molar growth yields of certain lactic acid bacteria as influenced by autolysis. J. Bacteriol. **96**:117-125.
24. Nierlich, D. P. 1972. Regulation of ribonucleic acid synthesis in growing bacterial cells. II. Control over the composition of the newly made RNA. J. Mol. Biol. **72**:765-777.
25. Pine, M. J. 1970. Steady-state measurement of the turnover of amino acid in the cellular proteins of growing *Escherichia coli*: existence of two kinetically distinct reactions. J. Bacteriol. **103**:207-215.
26. Pirt, S. J. 1965. The maintenance energy of bacteria in growing cultures. Proc. R. Soc. London Ser. B **163**:224-231.
27. Rose, I. A., M. Grunberg-Manago, S. R. Korey, and S.

Ochva. 1954. Enzymatic phosphorylation of acetate. J. Biol. Chem. **211**:737-756.

28. Rottenberg, H., S. R. Caplan, and A. Essig. 1967. Stoichiometry and coupling: theories of oxidative phosphorylation. Nature (London) **216**:610-611.

29. Schulze, K. L., and R. S. Lipe. 1964. Relationship between substrate concentration, growth rate and respiration rate of *Escherichia coli* in continous culture.

Arch. Mikrobiol. **48**:1-20.

30. Stouthamer, A. H., and C. Bettenhaussen. 1973. Utilization of energy for growth and maintenance in continuous and batch cultures of microorganisms. Biochim. Biophys. Acta **301**:53-70.

31. van der Beek, E. G., and A. H. Stouthamer. 1973. Oxidative phosphorylation in intact bacteria. Arch. Mikrobiol. **89**:327-339.

AUTHOR CITATION INDEX

SUBJECT INDEX

About the Editor

WALTER P. HEMPFLING is an Associate Professor of Biology at The University of Rochester, where he teaches courses in biochemistry, microbial physiology, and general biology. His research interests include the regulation of growth and continuous culture of pro- and eucaryotes, the biochemistry and physiology of respiratory energy conservation in procaryotes, and the general microbiology of highly stressed environments, especially cold deserts.

After receiving a B.S. degree with High Honors in Bacteriology from the University of Cincinnati, Hempfling completed the Ph.D. degree in Microbiology as a Predoctoral Fellow of the National Science Foundation at Yale University and The University of Rochester. The late Wolf V. Vishniac was his major professor. The period 1963–1966 was spent as NIH Postdoctoral Trainee, Pennsylvania Plan Scholar and Research Associate in Physical Biochemistry at the Eldridge Reeves Johnson Foundation for Medical Physics, University of Pennsylvania. During the academic year 1978–1979 Hempfling was a Visiting Investigator in Cellular Biology at the Scripps Clinic and Research Foundation, La Jolla, California.